The

Dr Roy Macgregor has worked for twelve years as a G.P. in a busy inner-city health centre. He has presented ITV's health series *The Full Treatment* for five years, as well as presenting the 'Doc Spots' on TVam and making numerous successful health videos. He writes on health for a number of popular magazines.

The Treatment Handbook for 300 Common Ailments

Dr Roy Macgregor

Cedar

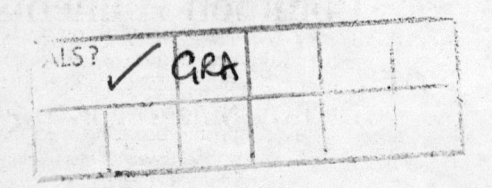

A Mandarin Paperback
THE TREATMENT HANDBOOK

First published in Great Britain 1988
by Methuen London Ltd
in association with Thames Television International
This Cedar edition published 1993
by Mandarin Paperbacks
an imprint of Reed Consumer Books Ltd
Michelin House, 81 Fulham Road, London SW3 6RB
and Auckland, Melbourne, Singapore and Toronto

Copyright © 1988 Roy Macgregor

A CIP catalogue record for this title
is available at the British Library

ISBN 0 7493 1340 4

Printed and bound in Great Britain
by Cox and Wyman Ltd., Reading, Berks

This book is sold subject to the condition
that it shall not, by way of trade or otherwise,
be lent, resold, hired out, or otherwise circulated
without the publisher's prior consent in any form
of binding or cover other than that in which
it is published and without a similar condition
including this condition being imposed
on the subsequent purchaser.

Preface

This book which emanates from the television series *The Treatment*, attempts to improve our understanding of common complaints and the effects they have on us. In my work as a family doctor I am continually struck by the extent to which a lack of simple information can make minor problems assume a worrying importance. This book attempts to set down much of what I would say in a consultation and to explain all aspects of illnesses and their treatment.

Deciding what to include has been very much a matter of personal choice. It is more a reflection of the problems that are brought to me than an attempt to include only those items that occur most commonly.

Some topics may not be considered strictly ailments, but are problems or questions that are often raised with me. Some items listed cover several ailments, so it will usually be easier to use the index to find a particular problem, despite the alphabetical listing of major items. Wherever appropriate I have used 'he' rather than 'he or she' when referring to either doctor, child or sufferer.

While I don't believe a doctor's consultation can ever be fully replaced, I do hope that using this book will enable many people to manage their illnesses or difficulties with greater ease.

Roy Macgregor

Acne

This is a term used to describe spots, usually on the face, commonly occurring in adolescence. It may persist into the early twenties and be troublesome in pregnancy. There are many myths surrounding acne, which has nothing to do with being dirty and little to do with what you eat. More than half of all teenagers will be affected, and there is often some family history of acne. It is the commonest skin problem; the best thing to be said for it is that it always improves.

Symptoms

* Found on face particularly, also back, chest and upper arms.
* Whiteheads.
* Blackheads.
* Red pimples.
* Pustules.
* Boils.
* Scarring.

Causes

- The exact cause is unknown.
- The skin is covered with tiny hairs, barely visible in places. Grease is secreted by the skin on to the surface around these hairs. In acne the grease-producing gland on the skin is blocked, but grease is still produced leading to a build-up. This produces spots, known as acne.
- Hormonal changes in puberty make the skin produce more grease.
- Certain foods such as chocolate are found by some people to make the acne worse. Unfortunately, most people find it makes little difference what they eat.

Treatment

There is no real cure, but certain measures can help.

- Washing:
  - ordinary soap usually adequate
  - twice a day at least, or more often if the skin is abnormally oily
  - a good routine for washing is to use very hot water, make a good soapy lather, rub well in, rinse with hot water, then cold; dab dry without rubbing.
- Hair care – regular shampooing helps to clear the skin. (See **Hair problems**.)
- Sunshine is well recognised as helpful.
- Acne creams sold at chemists can help.
- Don't squeeze spots, particularly the larger red pustules or boils.
- Medicated anti-acne soaps are sold but often, if condition is severe, a visit to the doctor may be necessary.

The Doctor

- May prescribe stronger, slightly abrasive creams but these are sometimes a problem in themselves (e.g. benzoyl peroxide), causing red angry patches of skin.
- May prescribe antibiotics, e.g. tetracycline and erythromycin, which act by stopping infection in the gland that secretes the oil, and can prevent blocked glands becoming pustules. Improvement will be slow with antibiotics. They should be taken for at least three months before any judgement as to how they are working is made. Doses of antibiotics can be reduced when acne has improved,

a low dose often keeping the skin relatively clear. Tetracycline tablets are absorbed less well if taken with milk. All antibiotics can interfere with the absorption of the contraceptive Pill.
- The Pill consists of hormones. In some people taking the Pill can improve acne, but this is not always the case.

Adenoids

The adenoids are fleshy lymph glands which are found at the back of the nose in children. Their exact function is not clear, but they are thought to be part of our defence mechanism against germs entering the body via the nose. They are not usually troublesome but in some children enlarge abnormally and cause a variety of problems from the age of around five years. If chronic adenoid infection is not treated adequately ear troubles may occur. By early adolescence the adenoids have normally shrunk by themselves.

Symptoms

* Snoring is usual if the adenoids are enlarged.
* Breathing through the mouth is common in children with enlarged adenoids, though people do not normally breathe in this way.
* The nose appears to be permanently runny.
* There is a persistent cough as the normal drainage of secretions does not occur and drips from the back of the nose enter the throat. This may be more noticeable at night.
* Ear infections are more common if the adenoids are enlarged. Stagnant secretions become infected and infection reaches the ear via a tube called the Eustachian tube which connects the ear and nose.
* The child who used to be described as 'adenoidal' is less common since the widespread treatment of infections with antibiotics. A typical 'adenoidal child' has nasal speech, runny nose and mouth hanging open.

Causes

☐ The overgrowth of adenoids in some children occurs without any obvious explanation.
☐ The obstruction of nasal secretions in the nose and air passages makes infection more likely. The main problem occurring as a result of this is the increased tendency to ear infections. If these are inadequately dealt with glue ear and decreased hearing may result. (See **Ear problems**.)

Treatment

- Frequent blowing of the nose helps to clear nasal secretions and cannot but help to clear away germs, making ear infections less likely.
- Steam inhalations (see **Cough**) can help loosen nasal secretions, allowing them to be cleared more easily, and diminish cough.
- If your child appears persistently to have symptoms suggestive of enlarged adenoids, or has repeated ear infections, see your doctor.

The Doctor

- As well as treating each episode of infection with antibiotics, the doctor may arrange for you to see an ear, nose and throat specialist to have the adenoids checked.
- The adenoids can be seen by looking in a mirror held at the back of the throat. This may be difficult to do in some children and often a specialist can tell from the symptoms that the adenoids are causing problems, but this is only confirmed when the adenoids are checked during an opera-

tion for the insertion of grommets, for example. (See **Ear problems**.)
- Removal of the adenoids is less common than it used to be. This is for the same reasons as explain the less frequent removal of the tonsils. As the adenoids shrink down of their own accord by puberty it is usually not necessary to remove them.
- If there are persistent infections, hearing or speech problems the adenoids can be removed by operation under general anaesthetic. This normally requires a hospital stay of two or three days. It is often combined with an operation on the ear or removal of the tonsils. (See **Tonsillitis**.)

AIDS

AIDS is a viral infection which has reached epidemic proportions in America. It is likely to reach similar proportions here. There is no cure for AIDS. It is not just a disease of homosexuals and is increasingly found amongst heterosexuals. In AIDS the body's defence system is attacked, leading to a variety of illnesses. This explains the word AIDS, which is made up as follows:

- A – Acquired: caught from someone or something, as opposed to inherited.
- ID – Immune Deficiency: the body's defence system is not able to work to protect you against illness.
- S – Syndrome: the particular pattern of illnesses you can get as a result of becoming infected with the virus.

Symptoms

* You can catch the AIDS virus and develop no symptoms. Current thinking suggests that about 30 per cent of those infected with the AIDS virus will develop symptoms within five years. It may be that all those infected with AIDS will die of the disease. Only time will give us the answer as to how many people infected by the AIDS virus will die as a result. This is a new disease, only recognised around 1980.
* The most common early symptoms of AIDS illnesses are:
  - recurrent thrush in the mouth and certain skin troubles
  - sweats and marked weight loss usually with fever
  - swollen glands and profound exhaustion lasting for several weeks

Many of these symptoms may occur as a result of other illnesses and do not necessarily mean you have AIDS.

* Two particular illnesses which are more specific to AIDS patients are:
  - Kaposi's sarcoma – a rare form of cancer, mainly of the skin but also affecting other parts of the body. Hard pink/purply skin blotches appear
  - *Pneumocystis carnii* pneumonia – a serious lung infection with prolonged shortness of breath and cough; lasts much longer than a simple infection

Causes

- HIV I is the name of the most common virus causing AIDS. This is the cause of AIDS in Europe and America. See below.
- HIV II is the virus causing AIDS in West Africa and is the cause of some cases in France and Sweden. Different tests are required for this virus and these are only available at clinics for sexually transmitted diseases.
- It may be that generally decreased immunity and the presence of other sexually transmitted diseases, such as syphilis with open sores, increases the likelihood of catching AIDS. This

may explain the very high incidence of AIDS infection in some parts of Africa.

How do you catch AIDS?

☐ It is most frequently caught by having sexual intercourse. This may be anal, vaginal or oral intercourse. The virus is present in semen and vaginal fluid.

☐ Another important way the virus is spread is by sharing infected equipment when taking drugs, including syringes, needles and mixing bowls.

☐ Babies of mothers who are carrying the AIDS virus can catch the virus through the placenta during pregnancy, at birth, or through their mother's breast milk.

☐ In the past some people have become infected with the AIDS virus from infected blood or blood products. Some haemophiliacs have caught the virus in this way. Now all donated blood products are tested and treated before being used, to reduce the risk of infection.

☐ Travel abroad may put you at risk, not only if you have intercourse but if you require medical treatment involving injections or blood transfusions. Not all countries have facilities to provide new or sterilised equipment or checks on blood and blood products.

The AIDS virus is not caught from:
– normal social contact
– kissing and cuddling
– sharing cups and cutlery
– toilets and baths
– giving blood

Prevention

- The more partners you have the more you are at risk.
- In both homosexual and heterosexual intercourse you should use a condom (sheath or rubber). This will reduce the risk of catching the virus. It is also advisable to use a water-based lubricating gel with the condom. Oil-based gels can weaken the rubber. No other contraception provides protection.
- If you are misusing drugs never inject. If you do, never share equipment.
- If you are a woman carrying the AIDS virus you are advised not to become pregnant. If you do, you should inform the doctors and health workers looking after you.
- Do not share a toothbrush or razor with someone who is infected.
- Ear-piercing or tattooing can put you at risk unless the equipment has been properly sterilised or has not been used before.

Testing for the AIDS virus

- It is now possible to test for the presence of the HIV I virus in the bloodstream. This can be done by your own doctor or at a clinic for sexually transmitted diseases. The test is not normally positive (showing infection with the virus) until about three months after contact with an infected person. A false negative result, suggesting you have not got the infection when you have, is extremely unlikely. A false positive result is, however, possible. If you have a positive test this needs to be confirmed by a special test done at your local clinic for sexually transmitted diseases.
- A positive test shows that you have been in contact with the HIV I virus but cannot predict whether you will go on to develop the AIDS illnesses.

Treatment

- Minor symptoms of AIDS may be treated in the normal way – treatment for thrush or skin infections, for example.

- Infected children can be given an injection of a substance called gamma globulin to try and help them fight off infections.
- Severe weakening of the body's defence system can be treated using a new drug called AZT. This has unpleasant side-effects but may control the disease for a time.

☎ Terence Higgins Trust, BM/AIDS. London WC1N 3XX. Tel: 071 242 1010. (Phone between 3–10 p.m.)

☎ SCODA, Standing Conference on Drug Abuse, 1–4 Hatton Place, Hatton Garden, London EC1N 8ND. Tel: 071 430 2341. (This is a national organisation providing information of services for drug-users thoughout the country.)

☎ Sexually Transmitted Disease Clinics. (Listed in phone book under Venereal Disease or under Sexually Transmitted Disease, or phone your local main hospital or London Lesbian and Gay Switchboard.)

☎ National AIDS Helpline. Tel: 0800 567123. (24 hour service offering advice and counselling on AIDS and HIV infection. Can also provide numbers for local helplines.)

☎ Scottish AIDS Monitor. Tel: 031 555 4850 (Edinburgh), 041 353 3133 (Glasgow).

☎ MASTA (Medical Advisory Services for Travellers Abroad), London School of Hygiene and Tropical Medicine, London WC1E 7HT. Tel: 071 631 4408. (Phone for details of AIDS travel pack.)

Alcoholism

At what stage does having a drink 'now and then' become alcoholism? This is one of the questions people most frequently ask doctors. A small amount of alcohol is perfectly all right for your health, and can even have good effects. There is no doubt that too much alcohol is harmful. One in five of all men in hospital have an alcohol-related problem. The commonest age at which problems caused by alcohol occur is between thirty-five and fifty-five years old. Contrary to popular belief, alcohol is a depressant drug. Despite 'feeling better' for a drink, largely because you relax, the alcohol has had a deppressant effect. In the long term not only will this increase your chances of having an accident but it will affect your health and self-esteem.

How much is too much? This varies enormously from individual to individual and between men and women. Alcohol can be considered in units. If you exceed either 21 units spread over a week, for men, or 14 units spread over a week, for women, your chance of running into problems increases dramatically. 1 unit of alcohol is equal to:
- half a pint of beer
- one (pub) measure of spirits
- one glass of wine
- small glass of sherry
- one measure of vermouth or aperitif

The rate at which the body consumes alcohol, and at which the level in the blood diminishes, is about 1 unit per hour. Someone drinking six pints of beer on a night out, and driving to work the next morning, may very easily be over the legal limit. For some people 3 units of alcohol, or less, may, render their driving illegal. Any alcohol interferes with your driving.

Symptoms
* Decreased concentration.
* Personal and social difficulties.
* Sexual difficulties.
* Need to have a drink to feel 'normal'.
* Irritability.
* Aggression.
* Repeated assertions that you have

stopped drinking (when in fact you have not!).
* Feeling jealous and paranoid.
* Depression and other psychiatric conditions.

Physical consequences
* Flushed and/or veiny face.
* Pot belly.
* Bruises on body and limbs from falls.
* Husky voice.
* Trembling hands.
* Liver inflammation (hepatitis) or permanent liver-scarring (cirrhosis).
* Stomach disorders, repeated vomiting or indigestion symptoms, gastritis, bleeding and ulcers. (These items are covered elsewhere in detail.)
* Cancer of the mouth, throat and oesophagus.
* Brain damage.
* High blood pressure.
* Muscle disease.
* Nerve problems, pains in legs and arms.
* Vitamin deficiency.

Causes

☐ Alcoholism usually starts when having a drink has provided temporary relief from everyday stress in your personal, business or social life. The alcohol then provides relief every time the tension occurs. As the frequency of drinking increases, so your ability to cope with tension decreases. This leads to further drinking. At this stage addiction occurs, which may often be either denied or not acknowledged.

☐ At the stage when alcohol has led to a deterioration in your work performance or personal life you need urgent help. The physical consequences for your body will also be significant at this stage.

☐ The physical effects of alcohol are a result of its action on various parts of the body, including the liver, stomach and brain. The chemicals in the liver which are used to process alcohol are present in increased quantities if you are drinking excessive amounts. One such chemical is called glutamyl transferase and can be easily measured by a blood test (see below).

Treatment

- This can only start when the person drinking can admit there is a problem. Sadly, it often takes the loss of a job or the breakdown of a relationship for someone to realise they need help. Despite the efforts of family and friends, no help can be given to alcoholics unless they really want to help themselves.

- Start by keeping your 'score'. Using the unit system described above, keep a diary over one week of how much you drink. (Home measures are often double pub measures.) If you are honest you will almost certainly be astonished at how easily your drinking exceeds 21 units, or 14 for women. If it exceeds 36(22) health damage is likely, without your necessarily being aware of it.

- Reducing the amount of alcohol you drink can often be done without any adverse effects. The more you have been drinking, however, the more likely you are to find it difficult. Withdrawal symptoms include 'the shakes' and anxiety symptoms. In severe alcohol addiction complete withdrawal may lead to hallucinations or fits (delirium tremens, 'the DTs').

- Noting where and when you drink may often suggest an area of your life which you could alter in order to decrease your drinking. Try rearranging your schedule or taking up other activities.

- Noting who you drink with can be very helpful in indicating a particular relationship or friendship that is in-

creasing your intake. A change can often lead to a large decrease in your overall consumption of alcohol.
- Avoid buying drinks in rounds, opt out, or drink more slowly so your glass stays fuller and you can say, 'I'm OK for now.'
- Pace your drinking throughout the evening, only allowing yourself three pints in one and a half hours instead of your usual four or five, for example. Setting total limits is often helpful.
- When you succeed in cutting down your drinking use the money for a special event, better food, a cinema trip or new clothes, for example.

The Doctor
- It is never too late, nor too early, to ask your doctor for advice on decreasing or stopping your drinking.
- Tranquillisers are sometimes necessary, but should only be taken as prescribed, and for a short period. (See **Tranquilliser addiction**.)
- Your doctor may prescribe a drug which will make you ill if you take alcohol. This is sometimes a useful deterrent. One such drug is disulfiram, which should only be taken if you are determined not to drink and must be taken every day. Even very small amounts of alcohol can cause extremely unpleasant symptoms.
- Counselling is helpful in planning your withdrawal and maintaining your improvement afterwards. This can be arranged by your doctor, or the agencies listed below may be helpful. If at first you do not find support keep trying: the variety of agencies available usually means it is possible to find an organisation or individual that suits you. Often significant changes in the work or social pressures that have created your drinking habits must be made.

- Blood tests can be done before and after a period of altered drinking to watch the changes in the liver that occur due to excess alcohol in the body. Over a period of six to eight weeks there may be significant changes for the better if you stop drinking alcohol completely.

Hangovers
Not only do alcoholic drinks lead to dehydration, thus contributing to a hangover, but they also contain many other ingredients. Any of these ingredients may contribute significantly to hangovers.

There is no one remedy that suits everyone, as individual reactions to alcoholic drinks vary enormously. Everyone knows that the only way to be sure of avoiding a hangover is to drink less. (See **Headaches**.)

- ☎ Alcohol Concern, 275 Grays Inn Road, London WC1X 8QF. Tel: 071 833 3471.
- ☎ Al Anon Family Groups, 61 Great Dover Street, London SE1 4YF. Tel: 071 403 0888.
- ☎ ACCEPT, 724 Fulham Road, London SW6 5SE. Tel: 071 371 7477.

Allergies

Allergies are an exaggerated reaction by the body to a substance which would normally be tolerated without any ill-effects. This over-reaction, or hypersensitivity, to substances may occur when they are inhaled, eaten or touch the skin. For some unknown reason the body responds inappropriately to the substance, as if it was defending you against a germ or harmful substance.

Infants may develop allergies which may either remain all their lives or disappear as they reach adolescence. Older people may also develop allergies. Sometimes an allergy may develop to a substance which has previously caused no reaction despite repeated contact.

There is very often a history of others in the family who have had some form of allergic reaction. Usually allergic reactions are minor or can be controlled with treatment. Rarely, a very severe allergic reaction called anaphylactic shock may occur. This leads to collapse and death if treatment is not given immediately. (See **Shock**, **Bites** and **Stings**.)

Symptoms

* Symptoms depend on the area affected.
  - inhaling substances like pollen may lead to symptoms of asthma or hayfever
  - certain foods can cause allergic reactions (shellfish and seafoods are particularly troublesome)
  - contact with the skin may lead to eczema or dermatitis
* Specific symptoms of allergy vary enormously. They include: sneezing, runny noses, sore throat, catarrh, conjunctivitis, colitis, mouth ulcers, skin rashes, itching, headaches, migraine, joint problems, indigestion, breathing and skin problems.

Causes

☐ When an allergic reaction takes place the body's defence cells release chemicals, including histamine. It is these substances that cause the symptoms of allergy.

Treatment

● If you can avoid contact with the substance concerned, the allergic reaction will be avoided. Unfortunately, this is not always possible, and treatment of the resultant symptoms must be attempted.
● Most people adapt their lives to avoid contact with substances provoking allergic reactions as much as possible, e.g. wearing pure metal jewellery instead of nickel or avoiding certain foods.

The Doctor

● Some medicines may be helpful in interfering with the allergic reaction, e.g. sodium cromoglycate or antihistamines.
● Your doctor may be able to arrange for you to be tested for allergies if you feel that one substance may be causing your problems. However, the situation is usually more complex and several factors are involved.
● Desensitising injections are sometimes used. They have to be aimed at a specific allergic reaction. One of the reasons why they are not always helpful is because it is not possible correctly to identify the main cause of the allergic reaction. The injections usually have to be continued over three years and are by no means a complete cure. There is a small risk of dangerous shock reactions with these injections and they should only be carried out where there is adequate medical supervision at the time of injection and for a short time after it.
● For details of specific treatment for allergic reactions see the sections on **Asthma**, **Eczema**, **Hayfever**, **Hives**, **Gastroenteritis**.
● ☎ Food and Chemical Allergy Association, 27 Ferringham Lane, Ferring by Sea, BN12 5NB.

Anaemia

Anaemia may occur at any time in life. It is not usually serious and can almost always be corrected. It develops either slowly over many months or may occur quite suddenly. More uncommonly it may be present throughout life as part of an inherited family problem giving no significant problems.

Symptoms
* Pallor of the skin and the red part of the inside of the eyelid.
* Tiredness.
* Weakness.
* Fainting.
* Breathlessness, initially only on exertion.
* Palpitations.
* The mouth and tongue may be uncomfortable.
* Rarely, in deficiency of vitamin B12, there may be symptoms of loss of weight, decreased appetite, tingling of hands and feet, difficulty in walking and even mental confusion.

Causes
☐ Anaemia is caused by a problem in the production of blood, which is a continuous process taking place in the bone marrow. Production problems can occur either on the supply side – insufficient ingredients, e.g. from diet, to make haemoglobin – or in the production process itself – with the formation of abnormal blood cells, for example.

☐ Anything which leads to an imperfect production of blood will diminish the oxygen-carrying capacity of the blood. It is this inability of the blood to supply adequate oxygen that gives rise to the majority of the symptoms of anaemia.

Difficulty in haemoglobin production
☐ This may be caused by lack of iron supplies or increased use of the iron available. This occurs if there is:
– inadequate iron in the diet
– increased blood loss, as occurs after injury or persistently heavy periods (see **Periods**)
– internal blood loss from a bleeding ulcer or cancer (see **Ulcers, stomach and duodenal**)
– chronic disease such as rheumatoid arthritis (see **Arthritis**)
– pregnancy, when more iron is required for the baby's growth (see **Pregnancy problems**)

☐ Defects in haemoglobin production may be present from birth, such as in sickle-cell disease and thalassaemia. Both these illnesses in their mild form produce few, if any, symptoms. The severe forms are associated with repeated difficulties and medical treatment throughout life.

Difficulty in red cell production
☐ Red cell production may be faulty from birth, as in a rare condition called hereditary spherocytosis.

☐ The difficulty may be caused by a lack of essential ingredients such as folic acid deficiency – usually due to an inadequate diet. There are no large reserves of folic acid in the body. Eating plenty of green vegetables prevents the problem. Elderly people not uncommonly have a folic acid deficient diet. In pregnancy there is an increased need for folic acid for the developing baby.

☐ Vitamin B12 deficiency is a possible cause of problems though dietary lack of vitamin B12 is very rare indeed. Normally the liver contains nearly three years' supply. To help absorb vitamin B12 the stomach secretes a chemical called intrinsic factor. Pernicious anaemia is the name given to the anaemia that develops when the stomach fails to produce adequate intrinsic factor to enable vitamin B12 absorption to take place. Removal of part of the stomach may also interfere with vitamin B12 absorption (see **Ulcer, stomach**) and hence anaemia may develop.

Other causes of anaemia
- ☐ Certain drugs may damage red cells and lead to an increased turnover of blood cells, causing an anaemia.
- ☐ Illnesses may affect the production centre of blood cells in the bone marrow, e.g. leukaemia.
- ☐ Certain treatments such as radiotherapy or chemotherapy may also produce anaemia.

Prevention
- If you eat a normal diet it is unlikely that anaemia will develop, unless one of the above causes is present. Foods that are rich in iron include red meats, particularly beef and liver, dark-leafed vegetables, dried fruit and wholemeal bread.
- If you suspect you may be anaemic it is unwise to take iron medicines or tonics without seeking your doctor's advice.
- Self-administered iron can significantly interfere with the necessary tests that must be done to establish why you are anaemic.

The Doctor
- Will do a blood test to establish whether you are anaemic and how bad the condition is.
- Blood tests also help to indicate what type of anaemia is present, and the levels of iron stored in the body.
- Examining the blood may also indicate whether the fault producing anaemia rests with the haemoglobin production or the red cell production (see above).
- Less commonly it is necessary to examine the site of blood production in the bone marrow. This is done by a small needle being inserted, under local anaesthetic, into the marrow and some marrow being withdrawn for examination.
- The doctor may arrange tests, such as those described under **Ulcer, stomach** and **duodenal**, to ensure that internal bleeding is not causing anaemia.
- Usually treatment of the cause corrects the anaemia.
- If iron is given it will usually be in tablet form. Iron by mouth may cause indigestion; this can be helped by taking it after food. It may also cause constipation, and a high-fibre diet is advisable while you are on iron treatment. (see **Constipation**.)
- Rarely, it is necessary to give iron by injection. This is painful and unpleasant. Persist with the oral tablets if possible.
- In pregnancy both iron and folic acid will be given in a combined form. This is because both are required by the developing baby.
- If anaemia is caused by inadequate vitamin B12 absorption, the vitamin will be given by injection every few months. This must be continued for life as the ability to absorb vitamin B12 from the stomach does not return.
- If large amounts of blood are lost due to injury, or during an operation, a blood transfusion may be given to correct anaemia.

Angina

Angina is a heart pain in the chest felt at times of exercise or emotion. The heart is complaining because not enough blood is coming into its muscles to let it do the work required. It is caused by furring-up of the arteries supplying blood to the heart. Just as scale in a central heating system makes it less efficient, so the heart works less well when its pipes are furred up by heart disease. Deposits of material, including fat, build up in the heart's arteries to such an extent that the blood supply to its muscles is limited.

Symptoms
* Pain in central chest, which can be crushing, tight and severe.
* Pain on exercising, after heavy meals, at emotional times.
* This can be accompanied by:
  - difficulty in breathing
  - palpitations
  - tiredness
  - 'having to stop', and when you do pain usually goes in around five minutes

Treatment
- Stop smoking. This is essential. Smoking causes the already narrowed heart arteries to constrict and be narrowed further. Narrowing causes angina.
- Change your lifestyle, avoiding events or activities which provoke the pain. It may be necessary to:
  - stop driving (particularly for HGV drivers)
  - lose weight (See **Obesity**)
  - avoid stress (See **Stress**)

The Doctor
- See the doctor immediately.
- He will ask you to describe the pain. This is often so typical of angina that it may clearly suggest the diagnosis to the doctor.
- He may give you a drug called glyceryl trinitrate which, if you take it when you have the pain, and the pain then disappears, confirms the diagnosis.
- He may arrange other tests:
  - chest X-ray to see if the heart is bigger than normal as it has been working extra hard
  - heart tracing (ECG) – normal in half of those with angina but may tell the doctor a lot about how well the heart is working
  - blood pressure – if higher than normal can put you at increased risk of heart disease and angina (see **Blood pressure, high**)
  - blood tests – to check on your level of cholesterol, which is known to contribute to your arteries being furred up
  - other blood tests to check other organs of the body to see if they are affected by heart disease
- The doctor may prescribe glyceryl trinitrate, to be taken at the onset of an attack. This can be taken in tablet form dissolved under the tongue (it only lasts six weeks after the bottle is opened), or as a spray under the tongue (increasingly popular and easy to use; the dispenser lasts months, not weeks). It can also be taken from a sticking plaster which is applied to bare skin, usually on the chest. The drug is slowly absorbed from the plaster over twenty-four hours.
- Delayed-action nitrates may be prescribed,(e.g. isosorbide mononitrate,) usually taken twice daily. Tablets slowly release the drug, decreasing the number of attacks and the need to use under-the-tongue tablets.
- There are drugs which make the heart work less hard. This category includes a large number of different families of drugs. Many are also used for lowering blood pressure. All may help angina.
- Don't stop taking angina drugs suddenly; first consult your doctor. Angina drugs should always be stopped slowly.
- In some cases X-rays of the heart's arteries show the narrowing to be in places where it is possible to remove the narrowed artery and replace it with a fresh piece of pipework. Your doctor can tell you if you are a suitable person for this treatment, or refer you to a specialist.

Ankle-swelling

Many people suffer from swollen ankles. If the swelling is persistent and unexplained it is always advisable to see your doctor. The swelling may be a sign of a problem with the ankle, but can also indicate a much more general problem with health. Most of the reasons for ankle-swelling improve significantly with treatment.

Symptoms
* One or both ankles may be affected.
* Swelling may be with, or without, pain.
* Swelling may extend up the leg or into the foot.
* There may be redness or bruising.
* Associated symptoms of illness such as fever may also be noted.

Causes
- Injury, sprain or fracture. For up to six months or more after an injury recurrent swelling may be a problem.
- Fluid retention in pregnancy or before periods may cause ankle-swelling. In pregnancy it may be a sign of raised blood pressure. Hormone changes on the Pill may also cause fluid retention. (See **Pregnancy problems**.)
- Thrombosis may cause swelling of the ankle and leg. (See **Thrombosis**.)
- Varicose veins may exacerbate ankle-swelling due to poor circulation. (See **Varicose veins**.)
- Ankle-swelling may occur in heart failure. Breathlessness may also be noted.
- Arthritis may also cause swelling. (See **Arthritis**.)
- Kidney problems may lead to fluid retention and ankle-swelling.

Treatment
- This is aimed at the underlying cause. If it is not apparent and swelling persists, see the doctor.

The Doctor
- Will check for the various causes. For example, a blood test is often required to check the balance of minerals and chemicals in the body. These greatly affect fluid retention.
- May prescribe a water tablet (diuretic) if it is felt that the swelling could be safely treated in this way.
- Elevation of the leg often helps to decrease swelling. The foot needs to be higher than your bottom to have a significant effect.
- Further management will depend on the cause.

Anorexia nervosa

This is a complaint which has three main features: a fear of being fat, excessive dieting, and weight loss. The weight falls well below the average for height. Anorexia usually begins between the ages of fourteen and nineteen years old. Girls are more commonly affected than boys, although boys may also develop it. The outcome for about one-third of people with anorexia nervosa is full recovery; another third may continue to be obsessed with dieting and have personality problems. The other third never fully recover, having occasional lapses of severe illness and sometimes dying.

Symptoms
* Steady weight loss.
* Excessive exercising.
* Skin becomes pale and sallow, fine downy hair may appear.
* Periods cease and constipation may occur.
* Elaborate measures may be taken to achieve the desired weight loss:
  - food may be hidden or thrown away
  - laxatives may be taken

- vomiting may be induced
* Baggy clothes are frequently worn to conceal the shape of the body.
* Food may be cut up into tiny pieces and sufferers may take an excessively long time eating a meal.
* Family arguments and friction over food are common.
* Despite enormous weight loss, a person with anorexia nervosa still sees themselves as being considerably overweight. One part of the body, such as thighs or breasts, may cause more concern than others.
* Severe illness may develop owing to the lack of nourishment. The body chemistry is upset and infections may occur more easily. Death sometimes occurs.

Causes
- Why anorexia nervosa should occur is not fully understood. A number of factors may play a part in causing the condition.
- Frequently people with anorexia have a fear of their body changing shape, forcing them to become an adult. There may be an early sexual experience which has created feelings of fear or guilt. This may lead to a desire to keep the body shape that of a child or adolescent.
- Someone may develop anorexia after overhearing a chance remark about their being overweight. One person in a group of friends dieting may lose weight considerably faster than the others, and consequently develop anorexia nervosa.
- Genetic factors may be involved; it is known sometimes to run in families. The brothers or sisters of someone with anorexia have a higher chance of developing anorexia than other individuals. It occurs more commonly in middle-class families, particularly if there is a strong 'moral' atmosphere at home with the emphasis on working hard. This is not always the case, however, and anorexia may develop in other circumstances.
- Sufferers are often quiet, studious and interested in sport.
- There may be chemical factors in the brain which affect the tendency to develop anorexia nervosa.

Treatment
● Many adolescents diet and exercise with great enthusiasm; this is usually quite harmless. It is only when the preoccupation with weight loss starts to dominate a person's life that treatment is needed. If the fear of weight gain becomes effectively a phobia, anorexia nervosa may develop.
● If you feel someone in your family or a friend is developing anorexia, seek help early. Not only is early treatment more likely to help but an early response to treatment is associated with a better long-term outlook.

The Doctor
● By discussing the situation with the family, and by examination, will be able to establish if anorexia nervosa has developed.
● If anorexia nervosa is present, early referral to hospital for out-patient or in-patient treatment is likely.
● The treatment will involve all the family, usually over a considerable period of time. A target weight will be established. Special dietary assistance may be needed, but in general a normal attractive diet agreed amongst everyone is used. A few dislikes can be accepted. Weight is measured about twice weekly and the person with anorexia nervosa will need to be reassured that they will not become overweight.
● It is unwise to comment on the

improved appearance of someone with anorexia as this may precipitate a relapse. Psychotherapy can often be used during treatment and benefits are likely to be greater when there is some improvement in weight. The whole family will be asked to participate in some of the sessions. Often a number of previously unexpressed tensions and anxieties are aired with considerable benefit.

- Follow-up over a period of months, or even years, after the target weight is reached is usually advised.

Bulimia nervosa

This is a related condition which is characterised by over-eating excessive quantities of food and then making oneself vomit. People with bulimia may consume extraordinary quantities of food, going to several different shops to conceal their habit. At other times normal quantities of food may be eaten, followed by self-induced vomiting. It is rare in children and young adolescents.

Vomiting is usually induced by sticking fingers down the throat. In severe cases the teeth may be damaged by acid from the stomach and there may be marks on the back of the fingers caused by the teeth.

☎ Eating Disorders Association, 11 Priory Road, High Wycombe, Bucks. Tel: 0494 421431. Also at Sadville Place, 44–48 Magdalen Street, Norwich NR3 1JU. Tel: 0603 621414.

☎ Overeaters Anonymous and Women's Therapy Centre, 6–9 Manor Gardens, Holloway Road, London N7. Tel: 071 275 8008. For meetings outside London write to P.O. Box 19, Stretford, Manchester M32 9EB.

Anxiety

Anxiety is a normal reaction to difficult situations. If a lion jumps out of the jungle at you the body uses a hormone called adrenalin to get you ready to run like mad, or fight back, depending on your situation. The adrenalin causes many of the symptoms of anxiety. Anxiety only becomes a problem when it starts to interfere with normal daily living. For most situations treatment is not required, but nearly everyone, at some stage in their lives, needs help in order to cope with the symptoms of anxiety. It is not dangerous to suffer from prolonged anxiety, but if left untreated depression or other mental illness may develop.

Symptoms

* Feelings of apprehension and worry. Tension.
* Poor concentration.
* Disturbed sleep, including nightmares. (See **Sleep problems**.)
* Palpitations.
* Sweating and shaking.
* Difficulty swallowing or breathing.
* Nausea, aches and pains.
* Panic attacks, which occur when anxiety and fear reach a peak. Hyperventilation may occur. (See **Hyperventilation**.)
* Psychosomatic symptoms may develop; this means that the mind affects the body. For example, children may experience a rapid heart beat and go to the toilet more often when they are frightened. Almost any physical symptom can be brought on by anxiety. Stomach-aches and headaches are amongst the most common psychosomatic symptoms, particularly common in children. (See **School refusal**.)
* Phobias are an example of an anxiety symptom which has become irrational. Such anxiety as produces a

phobia may prevent you from going out (agoraphobia) or going in lifts or confined spaces (claustrophobia). Children may have fears of specific situations such as being in the dark or going to the doctor. Phobias in children under ten years old may come and go rapidly without the need for treatment. In adults, treating phobias may take many years of concentrated effort from psychiatrists, psychologists, friends and relatives.

Causes

- Individuals' responses to situations vary enormously. What may produce severe anxiety symptoms in one person may have little or no effect on another. In many instances the reason for this is never clear.
- Anxiety can be communicated from others. This is certainly true of infants. If a baby is held by an anxious mother the baby may often appear tense and feed poorly, thus creating more tension and anxiety in the situation.
- Anxiety is sometimes caused by your past experiences. Familiar situations are less likely to cause anxiety than new ones.

Treatment

- Ideally, the stressful situation should be removed. (If someone shot the lion mentioned above you would be very relieved.) Often it is not easy to remove the cause of anxiety, and a compromise has to be reached whereby it is possible for you to cope with the situation and lead a normal life.
- It is often possible, by carefully analysing a job or family situation, to discover not only the source of stress but a means of avoiding or decreasing it. For example, taking an earlier train or different route to work can decrease anxiety built up over years about missing a regular connection. At times when there may be other anxiety-provoking factors, such as threatened job loss, such a minor adjustment can often provide the necessary decrease in tension to allow you to continue working.
- Making a careful diary of events, over a period of days or weeks, can sometimes reveal areas of your life that are causing anxiety which you were not aware of.
- Relaxation through exercising, deep breathing or meditation may help. Other methods and suggestions are listed under **Sleep problems**.
- If anxiety symptoms are preventing you from leading a normal life it is important to see your doctor before they worsen. It is a very common and justifiable reason for people to see their doctor.

The Doctor

- May suggest you return on several occasions for further discussions, and will examine you to exclude any other causes of anxiety symptoms (see **Thyroid problems**, for example).
- Often discussing the situation with the doctor can provide sufficient reassurance for you to make adjustments on your own that decrease anxiety.
- The doctor can put you in touch with information on relaxation techniques.
- It may be helpful to discuss your anxiety further with a social worker, psychotherapist or psychologist. Your doctor is well placed to arrange for you to see the appropriate person.
- Drugs may be used but, except in cases of very acute short-term anxiety symptoms, are unlikely to be of great benefit. Drugs may temporarily relieve the symptoms but they will not affect or remove the source of

anxiety. With long-term use tranquillisers can be addictive and difficult to discontinue. Their beneficial effect may also decrease considerably after several weeks' use. In short-term situations, such as before travelling by air, the use of a mild tranquilliser may be justified for some people.
- In situations where you are required to perform well, such as during a driving test, tranquillisers cannot be used. In fact a normal level of anxiety in such a situation may improve your performance.
- The beta-blocking drugs have been used by sportsmen and women to improve their performance. For example, they help prevent a hand shaking through anxiety. They are banned for use in pistol-shooting and archery competitions, for example, and certain types are also banned for snooker players. These drugs can make you feel less anxious, by decreasing symptoms without having a strong tranquillising effect on the brain. They should only be used under a doctor's supervision. The same group of drugs is widely used for lowering blood pressure. Side effects include:
  - exacerbating asthma and heart failure
  - cold fingers and toes
  - stomach upsets, skin rashes
  - if taken in combination with other drugs, various side-effects

Consult your doctor before discontinuing a beta-blocking drug. If your anxiety symptoms include palpitations, tremor and a fast heartbeat one of this group of drugs may be helpful (propranolol is an example of a beta-blocking drug.)

☎ The Phobics Society, 4 Cheltenham Road, Chorlton-cum-Hardy, Manchester M21 1QN. Tel: 061 881 1937.

☎ Phobic Action, Claybury Grounds, Manor Road, Woodford Green, Essex IG8 8PR. Tel: 081 559 2459/0452 856021.

Appendicitis

The appendix is a small pouch area around three inches long which is attached to the intenstine. It is thin and rather worm-like in shape. Appendicitis is caused when this pouch becomes inflamed and causes pain; it then has to be removed. It can affect all ages but is rare under two years old. There is little risk involved in appendicitis, provided that diagnosis is made early. If the appendix bursts it leads to peritonitis, which is a more severe infection throughout the abdomen. The appendix in rabbits is much larger and helps in digesting grass, but in humans it is of no use at all – we are no worse off without it.

Symptoms
* Pain in the lower right-hand corner of the tummy, often severe, may start off all over abdomen and then become more noticeable in the corner over the appendix.
* Often rapid onset over twenty-four hours.
* Nausea.
* Vomiting.
* Fever.
* More pain when you press on the tummy, particularly over the appendix.
* Constipation or sometimes diarrhoea.
* Pain worse on movement.
* Symptoms are variable. Doctors can often, quite reasonably, have great difficulty in making the diagnosis because of the many different ways it can develop.

Causes
- A number of suggestions have been made as to why the normally quiet, useless, untroublesome appendix becomes angry and inflamed.
- One suggestion is that the entrance to the pouch may be blocked by a lump of digesting food from the intestine. The contents of the pouch then become stagnant, swell up and cause the problem.
- The real reason why appendicitis actually happens is never clear.

The Doctor
- A doctor should be seen if you have lower-right tummy pain and other symptoms mentioned above. Do not take a laxative as this could make the appendix burst.
- The treatment is to remove the appendix.
- This is done through a surgical operation under general anaesthetic. It is a simple operation with little risk of complications.
- You will normally be eating and drinking again within twenty-four hours and home within five days.
- Normal life can be fully resumed within two to three weeks.

What is a grumbling appendix?
The short answer is that it is probably not anything to do with the appendix. Although the appendix is occasionally removed because of recurrent lower-right tummy pain it is rarely inflamed. A more likely explanation of the repeated pains that are described as grumbling appendix is a more general disturbance of the intestine. (See **Irritable colon**.)

Arthritis

There are two main types of arthritis which can affect any of our joints. It is important when talking about arthritis to be clear whether you have a wear-and-tear arthritis called osteo-arthritis or a more serious and progressive disease called rheumatoid arthritis.

Osteo-arthritis

This arthritis is often called wear-and-tear as it is a natural part of the process of growing older. Almost all elderly people are affected. The extent to which you are troubled is affected by how much you use certain joints. For example, ballet dancers get it more in their feet, rugby players in their knees. Whatever age it starts, it will not go away and its future course is unpredictable. A rusty hinge may give intermittent trouble – in the same way a joint affected by osteo-arthritis may give variable amounts of trouble. This kind of arthritis is by far the commonest joint problem, but is seldom so severe that it interferes significantly with a normal way of life.

Symptoms
* Pain, which is generally worse with exercise.
* Restricted movements – osteo-arthritis may only become apparent when it is increasingly difficult to tie shoe laces, get dressed, climb stairs or get in and out of the car.
* The pain and arthritis is generally limited to the large joints which carry the body's weight, such as hips and knees. The spine is also affected.
* Pain from the hip can be transmitted to the knee.

Causes
- The smooth shiny white surface seen over the ends of a chicken leg joint when it is broken open is the joint lining. Humans have similar joint linings.
- In osteo-arthritis the joint lining is flakey, cracked and uneven.

- ☐ This becomes worn down by use of the joint and eventually the adjacent bone is thickened and distorted.
- ☐ The symptoms of osteo-arthritis are all a result of the damage that has occurred to the joint in this way.

Treatment

Once the osteo-arthritis has taken hold the bone will not return to normal, but symptoms can be greatly helped by:

- Simple painkillers.
- Local remedies of lints and creams – often felt to help, though it is not really understood why they should.
- Heat in the form of hot-water bottles, infra-red lamps, keeping warm.
- Rest when a joint is particularly troublesome, but not so much rest that stiffness sets in.
- Losing weight – any joint that is worn and torn should be given as light a load to bear as possible if it is to go on working.
- Exercises and physiotherapy help.
- Unstable joints need to be supported by a stick, stick with a tripod base or a U-shaped frame called a Zimmer.

The Doctor

- Can help confirm that the arthritis is a wear-and-tear type and not rheumatoid arthritis. X-rays and blood tests can help in this.
- Stronger painkillers may help on prescription.
- Anti-inflammatory drugs do work, but exactly why is not clear as this is a wear-and-tear joint problem rather than an inflammatory one. (Gout, for example, is an inflammatory joint disease, as is rheumatoid arthritis.)
- Advice can be given on the use of gadgets around the home, from special tin-openers to rails in the bathroom.
- Dietary advice is important.
- Physiotherapy can be of enormous benefit to help settle a particularly troublesome joint.
- Hip-joint replacement is possible for those severely affected by osteo-arthritis. It can transform you from a person unable to be active and go out to someone able (in theory!) to climb mountains. Other joints can be replaced, but this is less common and less successful.

Rheumatoid arthritis

This is the second main type of arthritis. Whereas osteo-arthritis is a normal, 'growing older' arthritis, rheumatoid arthritis is an inflammatory joint disease. It is a long-term disease and the diagnosis is important as there is a lot that doctors can do about it. It affects people at any age and there is a varying degree of severity and disability. Only one in ten of those with rheumatoid arthritis develop such bad joint deformity that it makes it difficult to lead a normal life.

Symptoms

* Typically, an early symptom is that the small joints of both hands are affected.
* You may feel generally unwell, with loss of appetite and loss of weight, and only notice difficulty with your hands and other joints in the morning.
* Stiffness and joint swelling tend to improve as the joints are used during the day.
* More rarely, a single joint can suddenly swell, and become red and tender.
* The disease may either gradually progress, damaging the joints and leading to deformity, or the more fortunate may have one attack and no more.

Causes
☐ What causes rheumatoid arthritis is not fully understood.

Treatment
- Rest the joints where possible.
- Swimming in heated pools can help.
- Physiotherapists can help, particularly during bad spells.
- Using a firm mattress with light bed covers is helpful.
- Aids are available, both gadgets for household tasks and fitments for the home.

The Doctor
- A rheumatologist who specialises in the management of joint diseases will usually try to prevent the arthritis progressing or damaging the joints too severely.
- He may splint affected joints.
- Diagnosis is made by a combination of blood tests and X-rays. These are not necessarily certain to confirm the diagnosis, so it is often made as the picture of the illness becomes clear over a period of several months or even years.
- Drugs used include:

Drugs for pain-relief
- aspirin
- non-steroid, anti-inflammatory drugs (see *Gout*)
- stronger painkillers

Drugs used to try and control the progress of the disease
- Gold
- penicillamine
- chloroquine
- salazopyrine

All drugs in this category need to be closely supervised as they can have side-effects on the blood.

☎ Arthritis and Rheumatism Council, Copeman House, St Mary's Court, St Mary's Gate, Chesterfield S41 7PD. Tel: 0246 558033.

☎ Arthritis Care, 18 Stephenson Way, Euston, London NW1 2HD. Tel: 071 916 1500.

Asthma

This is a long-term illness which affects the breathing. Asthma occurs when there is narrowing of the breathing passages in the lungs. Each passage or airway is surrounded by muscles, and in asthma these muscles contract, narrowing the passage so that less air can pass through. Asthma tends to cause intermittent problems, and a sufferer may go for long periods without any difficulty.

Asthma is usually first seen in childhood, and many children outgrow it before puberty. Adults may also develop asthma in middle age or later. A small proportion of those with asthma as a child, who outgrow it, may develop it again as adults. Very often there is a family history of asthma, hayfever or eczema. You are more likely to develop asthma if you have hayfever, or eczema or an allergic tendency.

Symptoms
* Signs of possible asthma include:
    - repeated cough at night
    - repeated attacks of wheezy bronchitis
    - cough and shortness of breath following exercise
* Asthma may also occur suddenly as a wheezy attack when no previous breathing difficulties have been noted.
* Symptoms during an asthma attack include:
    - shortness of breath
    - painless tightness in the chest
    - wheezing, although sometimes this may only be heard with a stethoscope
    - breathing may require a lot of effort, muscles in the neck and

tummy can be seen to be working hard; speech may become broken up as gasps for air are taken
- in severe asthma there is sweating and the pulse rate increases; dangerous signs are if you become bluish, pale and clammy (go to hospital or call help immediately if these symptoms occur)
- cough is not always a prominent feature but is often brought on by exercise or effort
- when asthma is severe the chest may be relatively silent but the affected person may be working very hard to breathe and become exhausted; this can often lead to the severity of the asthma being underestimated

Causes
☐ Asthma is a complex illness, and the cause of bad attacks is very likely to be a combination of many different factors rather than one specific cause. There may be no obvious cause for asthma symptoms.
☐ It is understood that certain factors do exacerbate asthma, though why some people should have muscles in their airways which respond to certain situations by contracting, while others remain unaffected, is not clear.
☐ Allergies to many substances may provoke asthma, e.g. pollens, animal fur and feathers. The house-dust mite has also been implicated in causing asthma (see below).
☐ Infections such as common colds, or more serious chest infections, may precipitate asthma attacks.
☐ Certain drugs may make asthma worse (some beta-blockers, e.g. propranolol, for example).
☐ If asthma is not adequately controlled by treatment, exercise can provoke symptoms.

☐ Emotional factors do play a part in asthma, but usually combine with other causes of asthma when they affect breathing. It is important never to dismiss asthma symptoms as an emotional reaction. Not only is this incorrect and misleading, but it may be very dangerous. Children and adults still die of inadequately treated asthma.

Prevention
- Avoid exacerbating factors such as substances causing allergic reactions. A change of bedding, including the mattress, to synthetic materials can help. Keeping down the quantity of house-dust mite, which is found in dust in most houses, can help some people. This can be achieved through:
  - regular vacuuming, of bedrooms particularly
  - wet-dusting to remove dust rather than shifting it from place to place
  - using plastic covers around mattresses and pillows and avoiding feather quilts
- Keeping a careful diary of events surrounding each attack may reveal an unexpected link between something you do, eat or drink, or are exposed to.
- The role of breast-feeding in the prevention of allergy and asthma is not clear. It has been suggested that prolonged breast-feeding and the late introduction of solids may reduce the incidence of asthma and allergies in some infants. The evidence for this is not as strong as was once thought.

Treatment
- With regular treatment many of the effects of asthma can be prevented. If you have severe or prolonged symptoms not responding to treatment seek help immediately.

The Doctor

- When a first attack of wheezing occurs in a child in the presence of infection the doctor may prescribe antibiotics. This may help, but if the wheezing is due to asthma and there is no infection, the antibiotics will have no effect. Antibiotics only have a very limited role to play in asthma and are not part of the specific treatment of asthma. If infection develops in the airways beyond the area of narrowing caused by asthma, antibiotics may, however, be used.
- More than one attack of wheezy bronchitis makes the diagnosis of asthma more likely. If the doctor considers asthma a possible diagnosis the height and weight of the affected person will be noted and a chest X-ray may be taken.
- The amount of breathing capacity, or puff, someone with asthma has can be measured by blowing into a simple meter. This is called a peak-flow meter and is an indicator of how much air the lungs can expel in one puff. Comparison of the meter reading and height and weight can be used not only as an indicator of whether asthma is present, but also to monitor how well treatment is working.
- In severe asthma steroids may be given as a course of tablets or by injection in order to gain control of symptoms. When given as a short course, if this is not repeated too frequently, steroids do not have the side-effects, such as growth problems, associated with their prolonged use.
- Rarely, if symptoms are not controlled, breathing has to be assisted by using a mechanical ventilator.

Asthma is treated in two main ways:
Treatment of symptoms
- The most commonly used drug is salbutamol. This works rapidly to relieve the muscle spasm which causes the airway to narrow. Salbutamol and terbutaline are both examples of drugs called sympathomimetics. (This group can be inhaled.)
- Another group of drugs called xanthines includes aminophylline and theophylline. These also work rapidly and may have a preventative effect. (This group cannot be inhaled.)

Prevention of symptoms
- The most commonly used drug is beclomethasone by inhalation. This is a steroid drug but, because it is taken by inhalation into the lungs, does not tend to cause the side-effects of steroids taken by mouth. This drug will be difficult to take when the airways are in spasm.

  Because there is no dramatic relief of symptoms using inhaled steroids many people abandon their use too quickly. Rather as cleaning your teeth can prevent you from developing tooth decay, so use of an inhaled steroid can prevent you from developing airway-narrowing. Regular use of such a drug can often greatly diminish the need for frequent use of salbutamol.
- Sodium cromoglycate is another drug which is used for the prevention of symptoms.
- Medicines in asthma may be given by: inhalation, tablets and capsules, nebuliser or injection.

If someone has a severe asthma attack

- If no relief is obtained from inhalers which you have to hand, call help immediately.
- Dial 999 and arrange hospital admission, particularly if there is blueness or pallor and clamminess.
- In all cases of severe asthma, even if the sufferer seems to cope by leaning

forward and sitting upright resting on their arms, seek medical help. Don't allow others to crowd anyone suffering an asthma attack and allow plenty of fresh air. One person should stay with the patient until help can be obtained.

Athlete's foot

An infection caused by fungi leading to an itchy, peeling condition found between the toes. Wet toes confined in shoes grow fungi in much the same way as rotten tree-stumps sprout fungi due to the damp and poorly ventilated atmosphere found there. It can be spread from person to person and to other damp, poorly aired parts of the body.

Symptoms
* Itchy skin.
* Scaling or peeling.
* White colour.
* Often starts and is worst between the smaller toes.
* May bleed on scratching.
* Can become infected by other germs, leading to more pain and needing more treatment.

Causes
☐ Infection with a fungus, a kind of ringworm called *tinea pedis*.

Prevention
- Don't leave inside-out socks on top of pants to be worn later. This can lead to groin itching (dhobie itch) as the fungus spreads to grow there and between the legs.
- It can similarly spread to armpits.
- Avoid barefoot activities in public areas, especially swimming baths, bathrooms and changing rooms.

Treatment
- Mild irritation can clear by scrupulous attention to:
  - drying between the toes
  - wearing clean cotton or wool socks
  - wearing well-ventilated clean shoes or sandals (that smelly old pair of trainers is a haven for fungi)
- Anti-fungal powders and creams are available from chemists to apply regularly and often. These must be continued after the skin has cleared for at least two weeks to ensure that the fungus doesn't return – from traces left in the skin.
- Try another preparation if the first one correctly applied doesn't work.

The Doctor
- Can prescribe anti-fungal creams combined with anti-itch creams, which may be more effective.
- In severe cases other germs may be making it worse, and an antibiotic cream or tablet needs to be given as well as anti-fungal cream.

Baby blues and post-natal depression

Baby blues

Half or more of all mothers go through a patch of mild depression soon after their baby is born, usually within the first week.

Symptoms
* You are unable to be cheerful.
* You are easily upset and tearful. Small things which would not normally matter upset you a great deal.
* You may feel very anxious and tense, often over small things.
* Sleeping may be difficult.

* General feeling of being unwell and tired.

Causes
- It may be caused or exacerbated by hormone changes.
- Often the sheer exhaustion and excitement of the birth leaves you feeling very drained. This, combined with the early problems and weariness of child care, are more than enough to make you feel down.

Treatment
- Baby blues can almost be considered normal, but can certainly be helped by support and practical help from family or friends.
- Normally the baby blues only last for a few days and then quickly improve. They sometimes persist for longer, but symptoms usually remain very mild.
- More severe symptoms of depression, including deep despondency and persistent tearfulness, may indicate post-natal depression (see also **Depression**).

Post-natal depression

This is a very distressing condition affecting as many as one in ten mothers. It is important to seek treatment to prevent symptoms becoming more severe. It does get better with treatment and the bad days gradually become fewer and fewer.

Symptoms
* Repeated tearfulness.
* Difficulty being cheerful, sometimes persistent deep despondency.
* Difficulty judging how you are coping or the baby is progressing.
* Poor appetite and weight loss.
* Loss of interest in sex.
* Irritability and continual exhaustion.
* Difficulty coping, which may extend to having aggressive feelings towards the baby. You may become detached and uninterested in the baby and the home.
* Symptoms last longer than a couple of weeks and generally persist. Depression becomes more severe and more difficult to treat.

Causes
- Why post-natal depression should affect some mothers and not others is not clear. Hormonal factors are important but it seems likely that your circumstances and general state of health prior to having the baby may affect whether or not post-natal depression develops.

Treatment
- It is very important to seek the advice of your health visitor, midwife and/or doctor at an early stage. There is no point in suffering distressing symptoms in the hope that they will go on their own.

The Doctor
- Anti-depressant drugs can significantly improve post-natal depression, though they may take a week or more before the maximum benefit is obtained. Adjustments in dosage may also have to be made.
- Talking to family, friends and your health visitor can often help. You may be able to meet other mothers who have had similar difficulties.
- (See **Depression**.)

☎ National Childbirth Trust, Alexandra House, Oldham Terrace, London W3 6NH. Tel: 081 992 8637. (For post-natal support only, not depression.)

☎ Association for Post-Natal Illness, 25 Jerdan Place, London SW6. Tel: 071 386 0868. (Open 10.00 am to 2.00 pm; answerphone at other times.)

Backache

Backache is one of the commonest complaints, affecting nearly everyone at some stage in their lives. It is also one of the commonest reasons for people to have to stay off work. When the complex nature of the spine is considered it is not surprising that difficulties and pain arise from time to time. There are more than thirty separate bones in the spine, called vertebrae. Each vertebra is separated from the next by a disc which acts like a washer between the bones. Between and around the bones there is a network of muscles, ligaments and nerves. Any excessive or awkward movement of the vertebrae can have effects on these surrounding structures. The spinal cord passes through a channel in the vertebrae. Injury or displacement of the back bones can therefore have important effects elsewhere. Backache can be prevented, and when it does occur, a number of treatments may be effective in giving relief.

Symptoms

* Backache may slowly develop over a period of weeks or months. What starts as a niggle may develop into severe pain passing right down the leg. (See **Sciatica** below.)
* It may come on very suddenly after lifting or stretching. Further movement may be impossible until the pain and muscle spasms wear off. This can be very frightening when it first occurs.
* The pain varies, not only in intensity, but also in position. It may be localised to one spot in the back, or to a larger area, or may be felt in the arms or legs.
* Movement usually exacerbates pain.
* Coughing or sneezing may exacerbate pain.
* Danger signs indicating pressure on nerves or spinal column include weakness, tingling and numbness. Bowel and bladder control may be affected. If these signs occur contact the doctor as soon as possible.

Causes

□ Long-term poor posture is one of the commonest reasons for backache developing. The spine will react badly if it is constantly held in an awkward or unnatural position. (See '**Prevention**' below.)
□ Strain injuries may arise from lifting incorrectly, pushing or pulling an object awkwardly, or movement in an unusual direction. Injuries may have minor effects on the muscles, which heal quickly, or more serious injury may occur to the ligaments which strap the bones and muscles together. Severe injuries can occur to the discs between the vertebrae causing pressure effects on the nerves or spinal cord. (See **Prolapsed disc**, **Sciatica** below.)
□ Stress and tension can lead to muscle spasm which may exacerbate or cause back problems, particularly if the back was already weakened by previous injury or long-term poor posture.
□ Wear-and-tear changes in the bones of the spine such as occur in osteoarthritis may cause backache to occur. Other types of arthritis may also affect the spine. (See **Arthritis**.)

Prevention

● Both before backache occurs and when you've had back problems, prevention is of the utmost importance.
● Kitchen work surfaces should be at the correct level for your height. There should be space for your feet to pass below the surface, in order to avoid stooping over. If possible keep one foot bent on a stool or foot rest

below the surface, e.g. when you are ironing.
- Seats are very important. Adequate back support and correct posture, rather than slouching, can go a long way towards avoiding back problems. Visual display unit (VDU) operators and typists are particularly vulnerable if their seating is inadequate.
- Lifting should always be done from the crouching position; lift by straightening the legs up rather than leaning over and pulling up an object with your back bent. A good rule is to try and keep your back upright and straight while lifting. Always test the weight of an object before lifting and carry it close to you.
- Rest your back correctly at night. You may be able to do more for your backache by changing your bed than by any other single measure. The back must be firmly supported throughout its length on a firm surface. Use a rigid board under your mattress or, preferably, use an 'orthopaedic' mattress. (For the best position to adopt to rest your back see 'Treatment' below.)
- Watching your weight can have enormous benefits in both preventing and treating backache. Any excess weight makes you more liable to develop back problems.

Treatment
- As seen under 'prevention', there is a considerable amount you can do yourself for backache.
- Resting in bed should be your first priority. Lie on a firm surface, with the mattress on the floor or a solid surface (see above):
  - if on your back: lie with one pillow only below your head; it can be helpful to put a pillow behind your knees, which allows the back muscles to relax
  - if on your side: bend the uppermost knee up towards you, resting it on one or two pillows; it may help to place a pillow in front of your chest, wrapping your arm round it; supporting the upper leg and arm in this way helps to keep the back in the best posture to allow the muscles to relax
- Resting is essential to relieve pressure on injured structures. By relaxing, muscle spasms which were previously forcing injured surfaces together will wear off. As the muscles relax the injured surfaces can separate, which allows healing to take place more easily. Resting should be complete; getting up for meals or to watch a favourite TV programme renders it useless.
- Regular painkillers should be taken. Start with aspirin or paracetamol. It is important to take these by the clock, rather than waiting to see if you can manage. If you do wait you may well require stronger painkillers, or larger doses, in order to get the pain under control. It may be necessary to take them alternately every three hours, i.e. two aspirin, followed three hours later by two paracetamol, then two aspirin and so on. Do not exceed the doses stated on the packet for a twenty-four-hour period.
- Use ice packs or hot packs to relieve pain and muscle spasm.
  - icepacks: frozen peas are useful, but do not eat after refreezing
  - hotpacks: a hot-water bottle wrapped in a towel or cloth can give relief
- After three or four days, if you are not improving, seek medical help. If at any stage you have weakness, tingling or numbness, or bowel or bladder difficulty, seek medical help at once.

The Doctor
- May prescribe stronger painkillers which, as mentioned above, are best taken regularly.
- Muscle relaxants may be prescribed. These can give great benefit by relieving muscle spasms which otherwise maintain pressure on a nerve or injured structure.
- Physiotherapy may be helpful. Ultrasound may be used to treat injured muscles. Exercises and correct posture may be taught to strengthen and relax the back. Massage may be helpful. Traction is sometimes used.
- X-rays are often taken to reveal any underlying problem, but often the results are not helpful. (See **Neck, problems**.)
- Use of a corset can sometimes be beneficial.
- Referral to an orthopaedic surgeon or neurosurgeon who has special interest in back problems may be arranged if symptoms do not improve. Very rarely, special X-ray tests, injecting die around the spinal column, can reveal any pressure on nerves and help to pinpoint the problem. In some rare cases surgery is performed to relieve pressure. This should not be undertaken lightly. Not only is it a major operation, but the results are not always very satisfactory.
- Conventional medicine may not be successful in treating backache. A number of other treatments can give considerable benefit, particularly osteopathy. The Alexander technique, which concentrates on your posture and the correct physical positioning of muscles, can be enormously helpful.

Prolapsed disc (slipped disc)

This refers to what happens when part of the washer-like structure separating the vertebrae protrudes on to surrounding structures. The effects may be severe if the disc presses on nerves or on the spinal cord. If bowel or bladder function is affected, for example, the pressure on the nerves must be urgently relieved.

'Slipped disc' is used as a common term to describe backache when it may not be possible to determine to what extent the disc is actually damaged.

True prolapse of the disc is more likely to occur if the disc becomes hardened and less supple with the changes of osteoarthritis. The soft cushion in the middle of the disc may then be pushed out into surrounding structures. Treatment is similar to that described above for backache. Traction may be used to separate the vertebrae and take pressure off the affected disc.

Sciatica

This is a nerve pain also called neuralgia. People often experience sciatica as part of backache problems. The sciatic nerve is quite large, almost as thick as a biro in places. As it leaves the spinal cord it may be subjected to pressure, thus causing the symptoms of sciatica.

Pain is felt as a severe burning sensation which may shoot down the leg. Normally felt through the buttock, down the back of the thigh towards the ankle. Treatment is as described for backache, and is aimed at relieving pressure on the nerve.

☎ National Back Pain Association, 31–33 Park Road, Teddington, Middx. Tel: 081 977 5474.

Bad breath

It is usually very upsetting when someone tells you that you have bad breath. Fortunately, most causes of bad breath are easily put right. Everyone has bad breath at some stage, from the garlic-eating gourmet to the tipsy tramp.

Symptoms
* Foul-smelling breath, which may only be noticed by others.

Causes
- One of the commonest and least recognised is the build-up of plaque (see **Toothache**). This creamy white paste stuck to teeth is made up of saliva and food. It can harbour lots of germs which give off unpleasant smells as they damage the teeth.
- Food particles stuck between teeth.
- Poorly cleaned dentures.
- Tooth decay or abscesses.
- Gum diseases.
- Infection or ulceration in the mouth.
- Smoking, food, alcohol.
- Fever often leads to bad breath. This is frequently noted in children.

Treatment
- This is aimed at the underlying causes listed above.
- Keeping your teeth clean and free of plaque is the most important way to avoid bad breath.
- If you cannot find any cause for your bad breath before seeing your doctor try using 'disclosing tablets'. These tablets contain a dye which shows up plaque on the teeth, often with surprising results even for those who think they have clean teeth.
- Infections in the mouth or elsewhere should be treated. (See **Mouth ulcers**, **Tonsillitis**, **Toothache**.)

Bedwetting

There are few common problems in childhood as distressing as persistent bedwetting. The important thing to remember is that it always improves. The label 'bedwetter' is often applied far too early. It is quite acceptable still to have some wet nights at five years old. If the child is having fewer wet nights, then there is less need for action than if the child appears to be making no progress at all. Sometimes there are others in the family who have been affected. Boys appear to be slower to stop bedwetting than girls. It is a myth that bedwetting children sleep more deeply. The importance of restricting fluids has also been exaggerated in the past; usually this has little effect. (In adults, see **Incontinence**.)

Symptoms
* By two years old most children have occasional dry nights.
* During the third and fourth years more and more nights are dry.
* Three-quarters of children are dry by three and a half years old.
* If bedwetting returns after a period of dryness seek help earlier than if it is slow to improve.
* If bedwetting still occurs when the child is five years old, this is the time for discussing the problem. Although many of the one in ten children still wetting between five and seven years old improve without help, a doctor's advice may be helpful.
* Bedwetting at seven years old needs professional advice from a doctor or special bedwetting clinic (also called an enuresis clinic).

Causes
- The bladder has to learn to hold the urine and the child has to learn to wake up when it is full.
- The mechanism by which bedwetting improves has to come naturally, as with so much else involved in growing up.
- Rarely, diabetes or infections in the urine, may produce bedwetting.
- Bedwetting that starts again after a period of dryness is almost always due to a nervous upset. The commonest reason is the arrival of a new

baby at home; others are separation from a parent or starting school.

Treatment
- Most importantly, do not scold or show your upset when the bed is wet. Avoid showing your frustration indirectly by making remarks such as, 'I know you can do it if you try', which suggests a lack of effort on the child's part and irritation on yours.
- Encouragement when there are dry nights helps.
- Lifting the child to pass urine when you go to bed can sometimes help, but if it makes no difference after a time abandon this.
- Using a calendar, allow the child to stick gold stars or favourite cartoon stickers on it for each dry night.

The Doctor
If the problem starts after dryness, or is still present and not improving between five and seven years old a doctor should be consulted.

- He will take a urine sample to check for infection and may advise a visit to a special enuresis clinic.
- An alarm may be recommended. This is a buzzer that is set off by the wet sheets and wakes the child, who has to get out of bed to turn off the buzzer. The child may quickly learn to wake up when the bladder is full, rather than staying asleep and bed-wetting. Uncomplaining family and neighbours, and the cooperation of the child can make this method very effective.
- Drugs are sometimes used, e.g. imipramine, but when the course ends there is often little improvement. The drugs are dangerous in overdose.
- Neither alarms nor drugs are advised in children younger than seven years old. Both require enthusiasm and patience in large measure.

Bereavement

The months following the death of someone close to you are always difficult. Because people die in such different ways, perhaps suddenly or very slowly after a long illness, reactions vary enormously. However, there are various stages of grief which are common to everyone. Nothing can alter the reality of a death, but an understanding of what it is perfectly acceptable to feel helps towards the eventual rebuilding of your life.

Symptoms
After a sudden death, symptoms may include:

* A sense of shock, numbness and feeling empty.
* Intense grief.
* Feeling of guilt that 'you could have done more' or anger towards others.
* You might often look for the deceased and behave as if he or she were alive.
* At around six weeks depression and apathy are common.
* At around six months feelings tend to be less intense but are still often overwhelming.
* At around one year you can begin to see the future without the deceased and plan, albeit slowly, a life for yourself.

After death following a long illness, symptoms may include:

* Relief that the moment has come.
* During the time that relatives are around and helping with affairs you may feel calm and relaxed.
* Strong feelings of anger and frustration are often felt, e.g. 'you could have done more' or 'the doctor could have come sooner'.

* From around three months there is usually a period of remembering and trying to relive the good moments and happy times together.
* At around one year some desire to live for yourself and make a future emerges more strongly.

Other symptoms, which can be very upsetting but are very common, include:

* Severe sleep difficulty.
* Vivid dreams.
* Feeling that you hear and see the deceased person very clearly. More than half of those who have lost someone close to them feel this.
* You may have worries that you have the same illness as the deceased and develop similar symptoms.

Symptoms are variable and may appear at any time after the death.

Causes

Your reactions and grief are greatly affected by:

- The time you had to prepare for the deceased person's death.
- Your sense of usefulness to the deceased.
- The support you have around you from family and friends.
- Your previous personality.
- The type of relationship you had with the deceased.

Treatment

- Above all, it is family and friends who can help.
- Talking is important. Too often feelings are not expressed and worse grief feelings occur later and hinder a return to normal life. However, you should recognise that other people may find it hard to talk about bereavement, and it is often up to you to show you are willing to talk about it.
- After the first few weeks the times when friends are most needed is at, say, six weeks, three months and six months. Bereavement is a long process and relatives who are often wonderfully supportive intially often forget the need to help, even if only briefly, at these intervals.

The Doctor

- Can help to reassure you that the frightening feelings, voices or visions you experience are in fact normal.
- Can put you in touch with special agencies who can be of great help if you are isolated and without support (see below).
- Does not generally give drugs, as nothing can remove the pain of your sense of loss. However, if you are in great difficulty over sleeping, may be able to help. It is so easy to become dependent on medicines, particularly at this time, it is best to avoid repeat prescriptions.

The child and bereavement

It is often wise to talk to your doctor about how you should react or behave when you are with a child who has lost a relative or friend. Some simple rules are:

- allow the child to grieve in his own way
- show your emotions in front of the child or he will feel excluded
- discuss things with the child as he will often feel, however wrongly, that in some way it is his fault
- if possible avoid any further changes for the child in the following six months

☎ Cruse-Bereavement Care, Cruse House, 126 Sheen Road, Richmond, Surrey TW9 1UR. Tel: 081 940 4818.

☎ The Compassionate Friends, 6 Denmark Street, Bristol BS1 5DQ. Tel: 0272 292778.

Birthmarks

This is a general term referring to a skin blemish appearing either at birth or during the following months. Birthmarks may persist permanently or may fade over a period of months or years. Forceps used to assist the birth often cause bruising, which can easily be mistaken for birthmarks; bruising will clear quickly over a period of days. Birthmarks are of no sinister medical significance; their main problem always lies in their appearance, which may be distressing but is usually easily masked. The majority of marks fade with time; others can be well camouflaged with modern cosmetics. The temptation to have a birthmark removed by a surgeon should be resisted until you are sure it will not go on its own. All surgery causes scars, but not all birthmarks cause scars.

There are six main types of birthmark:

brown (simple) mole
café au lait spot
Mongolian blue spots
port wine stain
stork mark (salmon patch)
strawberry naevus (cavernous haemangioma)

Brown (simple) mole

Symptoms
* Usually circular and small.
* Often appear several months after delivery.
* May have hairs growing out of them.
* Permanent.

Causes
□ Unknown.

Treatment
- None.
- Unless in adult life there is a change in a mole – particularly itching, increase in size or bleeding – these should be left alone.

Café au lait spot

The name derives from the similarity of appearance to a coffee stain. Indeed, the mark may be so mild that people ask, 'What is that on your skin?'

Symptoms
* One or two flattened areas of skin with a diffuse brown coloration.
* Very variable size.
* Occasionally there are a group of marks together.
* Can cover a large area of skin.
* Hair can sometimes be seen in the pigmented area and may be much thicker or longer than on surrounding skin.

Causes
□ Unknown.

Treatment
- These marks are generally permanent.
- Occasionally, for larger areas or where the appearance is distressing, a plastic surgeon may be able to help with a variety of techniques including laser treatment, tattooing, and skin grafting.

Mongolian blue spots

These are a group of spots which can easily be mistaken for bruising. Many people are alarmed when they first see these on a young child, and may even infer that the child has been injured. They have nothing to do with bruising. They are found in Asian and black people.

Symptoms
* Usually on lower back or buttocks.
* Can be grouped as patches of bluish flat skin, 4–6 cm across or smaller.
* The colour in all the patches is even (unlike bruising which would vary).

Causes
- Unknown.

Treatment
- None.
- Fade with time.

Port wine stain

Perhaps the most distressing of all birthmarks. The distress is only made worse by the lack of any treatment.

Symptoms
* Purply red discoloration of skin, flat on surface of skin.
* Present at birth.
* Permanent.
* Size varying from tiny to whole of one side of face.
* Rarely, blood vessel malformations are found in association with this stain.

Causes
- Unclear.

Treatment
- Cannot be removed.
- Cosmetic camouflage techniques are now highly developed. Your doctor can arrange for you to see a skin department and have specialist advice. Some camouflage cosmetics are available on prescription.

Stork mark (salmon patch)

These are extremely common, their name referring to the bite of the stork that delivered the baby to hospital! As true of a bite, these marks generally fade with time.

Symptoms
* Common on bridge of nose, eyelids.
* If on nape of neck may be more persistent.

Causes
- Not caused by storks.
- Actual cause unknown.

Treatment
- Leave alone.
- Usually fade with time.

Strawberry naevus (*cavernous haemangioma*)

This is one of the most distressing birthmarks for parents, and consequently one which is often unnecessarily interfered with in order to remove it. As these marks disappear with time, leaving at worst a slight puckering or pallor of the skin, they should be left alone.

Symptoms
* Raised red squashy area.
* Varies in size from small pea to 50p. piece.
* Usually appears in first or second month.
* Has three recognised phases:
  - rapid growth phase, when it may increase over a matter of weeks from a minor blemish to become an unsightly reddish lump
  - no change phase, which may last variable amounts of time
  - disappearing stage, the redness of the lump is gradually replaced by more white parts until the lump and discoloration resolves.

* The lump sometimes appears to sit on top of a fatty lump which gives it a peculiar appearance. The red/purplish surface may protrude half an inch above the skin surface.
* It can occur anywhere on the skin.

Causes
- These birthmarks are made up of dilated blood vessels.
- Why they should appear is unknown.

Treatment
- Without treatment about half of strawberry marks will appear flat on the skin by around five years old, and usually go completely by puberty.
- If bleeding occurs it should be stopped as for any cuts with sustained pressure from a clean piece of material. Bleeding will stop due to the blood's normal clotting mechanism. It is a myth that bleeding is unstoppable. (See Cuts.)
- Rarely, a mark can interfere with the eyes or air passages, in which case surgery is required.

Bites and stings

Everyone has the experience of being bitten at some stage by anything ranging from a mosquito to a horse. This is very rarely serious, but simple measures can make the difference between discomfort lasting for hours and much more serious infection needing urgent medical attention.

Symptoms
* Reddening.
* Swelling around the bite.
* Itching.
* Tingling and burning (from jelly fish particularly).
* They may appear in crops where skin is exposed, e.g. from fleas and bedbugs.
* Rarely, a sting can give rise to a severe local (allergic) reaction with very pronounced swelling. More rarely, a type of shock can occur. Medical help should be summoned immediately.

Causes
- Whatever causes the injury introduces poison into the body. The resulting reaction is due to the body defending us and trying to limit the spread of infection.

Treatment
- This should be aimed at limiting the spread of poison and preventing infection.
- Remove any stings left in the skin, e.g.:
  - bees and wasps: look for and remove sting with tweezers
  - jellyfish: scrape skin with wood or sand
- Apply ice or cold compresses with icy water and any clean cloth you have to hand.
- Calamine lotion can be cooling and soothing.
- Don't squeeze the spots – this spreads the poison.
- Try not to scratch as this may introduce infection or even cause scabbing and scarring.
- If it is an animal bite it is important to ensure that you are up to date on tetanus immunisation. Animal bites in this country will not result in rabies but often cause infection, and antibiotics may be necessary.
- Antihistamine ointments are widely available from chemists. While these may prevent itching they very often cause a skin reaction, particularly if used a lot, which may lead to more itching. Dermatologists advise against

antihistamine ointments, preferring giving antihistamine in tablet form to preventing itching; a side effect is drowsiness.
- The few people who suffer very severe reactions that endanger their lives can carry with them a small kit containing a drug to be injected into them if they have a reaction to a particular sting (called anaphylactic shock). This is available on prescription.

Blisters

Blisters form as a result of skin injury. The body releases fluid into a small bubble of skin which is pushed above the normal skin surface. A new layer of skin forms at the base of the blister. The fluid released to some extent cushions the new layer of skin as it forms. The size of blisters varies according to the cause.

Symptoms
* Simple blisters on the hands or feet on wearing new shoes are common to everyone.
* Blisters which develop over a large area can weep and interfere with clothing and activity.
* If red swollen skin develops around the blister, or it becomes pus-filled, this is a sign of infection.

Causes
□ Friction.
□ Burns (including sunburn).
□ Bites.
□ Allergic reactions.

Treatment
- Protect if possible with a soft dressing. Many varieties are available from chemists.
- Keep clean and dry.
- Avoid further friction over the same area.
- If the blister is broken there is a risk of infection.
- Normal healing leads to the fluid being absorbed, and the old skin drying and peeling off to reveal new skin.

The Doctor
- May, if the blister is very large, drain the blister using a sterile needle. The skin is left in place to protect the new skin forming underneath.
- Can provide suitable dressings, some of which are available on prescription.
- Will prescribe antibiotics if there are signs of infection.

Blood pressure, high (hypertension)

Having raised blood pressure (or hypertension) is extremely common. In Scotland as many as 15 per cent of the population may have raised blood pressure. Men are more at risk than women of having raised blood pressure. The heart pumps blood through the arteries under pressure in order for the body's circulation to work. Just as pumping air into a tyre under too much pressure causes damage so, if the heart pumps the blood around the circulation under too much pressure, damage may occur.

There are two numbers used to describe a blood pressure reading: 110 over 75, for example. The first number refers to the blood pressure as the heart pumps blood out, the second refers to the pressure as the heart relaxes and fills up with blood again. These are referred to as the systolic and diastolic blood pressures. Both numbers are important in indicating possible risk if they are raised.

Blood pressure is very variable between individuals and in different situations. Being anxious or nervous may raise your blood pressure temporarily. Brief periods of raised blood pressure are harmless, but in some people the pressure remains high and this can put you at risk of having a stroke, for example. High blood pressure is what is called a risk factor, making you more prone to illness in the same way as smoking increases the risk of your having certain illnesses.

What is raised blood pressure?

- Many factors influence the blood pressure level in an individual. Raised blood pressure that may be 'normal' or acceptable in the elderly may be very unacceptable in the young. Your doctor knows what your particular pressure should be and can explain how much it can go up before treatment should be started.
- In general, in a young healthy adult, 110/75 is normal. A blood pressure of 150/100 would be a cause for concern. (See 'treatment' below.)

What are the dangers of high blood pressure?

- The most important danger of having raised blood pressure is that you are very much more at risk of having a stroke.
- Raised blood pressure is thought to have an exacerbating effect on any blood vessel disease or heart disease. Heart failure may be made worse by raised blood pressure. Exact links between blood pressure and heart attacks have not been fully established.
- Raised blood pressure may also cause problems in the eyes and kidneys and elsewhere in the body. Damage to the kidneys may also in itself lead to further raised blood pressure.
- (Also see **Pregnancy problems**.)

Symptoms

* Usually there are none. Raised blood pressure is almost always discovered while having your blood pressure checked for some other condition.
* Very rarely, symptoms of headache and palpitations occur, but usually only if the pressure is dangerously high.

Causes

□ Blood pressure tends to rise slowly as you grow older.
□ There is sometimes a tendency for high blood pressure to run in the family.
□ Nearly all high blood pressure, about 95 per cent, is due to an unknown cause. This is called essential hypertension.
□ In a few people high blood pressure may be due to other problems such as kidney disease, hormonal problems, pregnancy or use of the contraceptive Pill. This is called secondary hypertension. (See **Pregnancy problems**.)
□ Other factors which may influence blood pressure and cause it to be higher than normal include:
  – excessive alcohol
  – depression
  – obesity
□ If you smoke, as well as having raised blood pressure, you are putting yourself at double the health risk of someone who doesn't smoke and has normal blood pressure. An exact link between smoking and blood pressure has not been made, but they are both considered important risk factors.

Prevention

• Everyone, particularly those over thirty years of age, should have regular checks of their blood pressure, about every three years. Checks should be done much more often if

your blood pressure is raised or slightly raised. If you are on treatment for hypertension, having checks every three months is not unreasonable.
- Ask the doctor or nurse to tell you what the reading is and make a note of the numbers so you can compare them with a future reading.

Treatment
- One reading of blood pressure is not enough to make a diagnosis of hypertension. Usually three to five readings are taken on separate occasions. If the average of these readings suggests a persistently raised pressure, not only will a cause be sought but active steps to lower the pressure will be considered.
- Investigations to discover the cause may include a variety of tests. These will vary according to your age and any other illnesses you may have had. Blood tests, urine tests, chest X-rays, and heart recordings may all be done. The eyes will also be examined.
- Treatment of the cause may help, but in most cases no cause is found (see 'causes' above). Initially, a look at your lifestyle may help to plan a way of lowering your blood pressure. Loss of weight and taking exercise may contribute to your being able to reduce your blood pressure. It is important, however, to have regular check-ups because after an initial improvement the pressure may rise again.
- Often treatment with drugs designed to lower the blood pressure is required. If treatment is started it is necessary to continue it for life.
- Various families of drugs are available, including:
  - beta blockers
  - diuretics
  - calcium antagonists
  - vasodilators
- Many drugs have side-effects, or some may not be suitable for you because of another illness – for example, asthma, which makes beta blocker treatment unsuitable. It may take some time to discover the best drug for you as an individual. Often troublesome symptoms such as ankle-swelling, cold hands and feet, dizziness or even depression may occur.
- It is, however, usually possible to find a drug which can be safely continued for life without undue side-effects.
- Regular check-ups will enable any further increase in blood pressure to be noted, and sometimes a dose adjustment of your drug or the addition of another drug is required.
- ☎ British Heart Foundation, 14 Fitzhardinge Street, London W1H 4DH. (Send s.a.e. for publications list.)

Boils

Boils are formed as a result of skin infection. They are not serious but can be very painful, particularly if continually subjected to friction – on your bottom or below a shirt collar, for example. A carbuncle is merely a large boil or several boils which have merged into one. Boils contain bacteria which are infectious to other people. They are infected skin and so are different from the spots found in acne (see **Acne**). Boils may occur either singly, in crops or recurrently.

Symptoms
* Red sore skin, gradually swelling over a few days.
* A large, tender, red lump forms, which may throb.
* A white or yellow head forms, which may burst over the next two to three days. It may not burst but slowly disappear on its own over

about ten days.
* More boils may appear on surrounding skin or elsewhere on the body.

Causes
☐ Boils are made up of germs (usually a particular bacteria called *staphylococcus*) and the body's own defensive cells, which combined are what forms pus.
☐ The build-up of the bacteria inside the boil causes pressure and consequently pain.
☐ It is usually the hair follicles that are infected.

Treatment
- Most boils will go on their own over a few days without treatment.
- Keep the boil and the area around it clean, particularly after it bursts.
- Avoid friction or rubbing over the boil.
- Do not squeeze boils as this will only spread the infection beyond the limited area of the boil.
- Hot compresses, as well as relieving discomfort, may help the boil to burst.
- Wash hands before cooking, as the germs of a boil can cause food poisoning.

The Doctor
- If a boil is particularly painful or not improving the doctor may:
  - lance it with a small scalpel blade
  - and/or prescribe antibiotics to fight the infection
- Swab tests may be taken from the boil to ensure that the correct antibiotic is given.
- If the boils are recurrent the doctor may:
  - take a nose swab (as germs are sometimes carried in the nose) to test if you are what is called 'a carrier' of the particular germ causing the boils
  - test the blood and urine for sugar, because you are more prone to boils if suffering from diabetes
- The prescribed treatment for boils consists of:
  - antibiotics
  - nasal cream to use in each nostril several times a day until you are clear of the infection; this will only usually be given if boils are recurrent and/or nose swabs reveal germs that cause boils
- Dressings will be applied to the boil to keep the area clean and absorb any discharge.
- If the boil is large a sterile gauze strand, called a wick, up to 20 cm long, may be packed into the boil. This ensures that the boil heals from the inside towards the surface and avoids the opening on to the skin healing while the boil re-forms on the inside.

Bowlegs

These are very common in infancy. The legs curve outwards and there is a gap between the knees. Infants may have a pad of fat on the outer leg below the knees which makes the bowing more pronounced. Most infants will grow out of this, but there are some pointers to bone disease which should make you take your baby to the doctor.

Symptoms
* The legs appear to sag under the weight of the infant.
* On lying down the gap between the knees becomes less.
* This gap should be less than two inches.
* There may be associated pigeon toes.
* The legs are usually equally curved.
* You should see your doctor if:

- one leg is more curved than the other
- the curvature is great
- the child is very short
- there is pain or difficulty with walking

Causes
- Most commonly normal, occurring in late infancy.
- May be present at birth owing to the baby being cramped in the womb.
- Rickets may also cause bowlegs because thin bones are bent into a bow.

Treatment
- A mild degree of bowing does not need treatment.

The Doctor
- If there is severe bowing your doctor will look for bone disease.
- X-rays will be taken of the legs and wrists.
- Blood tests will be taken to look for rickets.
- Wedged supportive shoes may rarely be needed.
- Very rarely, an operation is needed.
- Rickets is treated by a special form of vitamin D.

Does my child have rickets?

Rickets is very rare in healthy, well-nourished children, and may present as either knock knees or bowlegs. It is caused by a diet poor in vitamin D, which is needed to absorb calcium. Vitamin D is found in fish, eggs and butter. Baby milks have added vitamin D.

- Rickets is most common amongst Asian children, because dark skins cannot form vitamin D very well, and chapatti flour blocks the absorption of calcium.
- Premature babies have low vitamin stores.
- Some drugs taken to stop fits may cause rickets.
- Chronic digestion problems may cause rickets.
- Rickets has become less common since vitamin D has been added to baby milks.
- Vitamin D drops can be given to those at special risk.
- Some people recommend them for breast-fed babies up to one year old.

Breast problems

In this section we will consider:

Breast infection
Breast lumps
Breast-feeding problems
Breasts and adolescence

Breast infection

This is also called mastitis and generally refers to the development of an abcess in the breast tissue. It usually responds well to treatment. Although commonly occurring in breast-feeding mothers, those not breast-feeding may also develop an abscess.

Symptoms
* A tender area of the breast develops.
* This may appear red and inflamed. The redness may fan out in a wedge shape from the point of infection. There may be red lines spreading from the abscess across the breast surface.
* There is usually some swelling of the affected breast.
* The lymph glands under the arm become tender, swollen and start to ache.
* Fever may occur, with general feelings of being unwell.
* Affected area may feel hot.
* Pain can be severe.

* (See also **Breast lumps**, below.)

Causes
- Germs (bacteria) enter the breast tissue from the outside. Once in the milk ducts and glands they multiply until the symptoms of infection occur.
- A variety of different bacteria cause the infection, which if left unchecked may lead to the collection of a large amount of pus.
- A break in the skin surface such as a cracked nipple may make the breast infection more likely. All too often there is no obvious reason why germs should have either entered or developed to such an extent that an abscess forms. Many people have cracked nipples without breast infections.

Prevention
- There is no sure way to guard against development of a breast infection.
- Nipple care to prevent cracking during breast-feeding may be helpful, but some of the cleanest, best kept nipples may still permit a breast infection.

Treatment
- If signs of a breast infection do develop it is important to seek help early. In this way treatment is more likely to be effective and to work more quickly.
- Wearing a good supportive bra, although initially uncomfortable, may help overall.
- Massaging the breast during breast-feeding can help to clear the milk and ease the discomfort of infection.
- You can continue breast-feeding when you have a breast infection. Indeed, it may be better to do so to prevent engorgement while you have an infection. The baby is not usually affected.

The doctor
- Will prescribe an antibiotic to take by mouth. Only small amounts appear in breast milk and it is recommended to continue breast-feeding unless your doctor advises against it.
- Painkillers such as aspirin and paracetamol will help with the pain and reduce fever.
- Rarely, if the infection does not clear with antibiotics, surgical drainage may be required through a small incision on the breast. Seek help early to try and avoid a large abscess developing.

Breast lumps

Any woman finding a breast lump may naturally fear that she has cancer. This fear often deters people from either looking for or reporting a breast lump to their doctor. Although there is a very much greater chance that a lump will be benign than malignant, all breast lumps must immediately be checked by a doctor. Some people have naturally lumpy breasts. The breast is a complicated structure which can be visualised like a tree with its base at the nipple. Ducts fan out from the nipple like branches from a tree; blockages or changes along these ducts cause one or many lumps throughout the breast.

Symptoms
* There may be no symptoms whatsoever from a breast lump.
* Slight pain or tenderness.
* Discomfort, worse around period time.
* Skin changes, crinkling or puckering.
* Nipple changes.
* Nipple discharges.

Any of these last three symptoms, even

in the absence of a lump, should be reported to your doctor immediately.

Causes
The main causes of breast lump are:
- [ ] Cysts. If one of the ducts leading to the nipple is blocked, fluid builds up to form a bulging sac or cyst, which may be felt as a lump.
- [ ] Lumpy breasts or fibro-adenosis. If the ducts are generally thickened the overall texture of the breast may be lumpy. Individual lumps may be difficult to feel.
- [ ] Another cause of breast lumps is infection; usually easy to distinguish from other causes of breast lump by the associated symptoms of pain, redness, swelling and fever. Usually only occurs while breast feeding. (See **Breast infection**, above.)
- [ ] Some benign breast lumps occur which may be impossible to distinguish from malignant ones until removed and examined under a microscope.
- [ ] If the lump is cancerous there is much more than people realise that can be done about it. It is important and helpful that the lump has been found and treatment should begin straight away.

Treatment
- Self-examination is very important because of the frequent absence of symptoms. Lumps are often discovered through self-examination. Unfortunately, they are also often missed because it is not done, and a cancer is not discovered until it is too late to give adequate treatment.
- Regular examination should be carried out after each period or, after the menopause, choose a fixed day each month.
- Any lump must be immediately reported to your doctor.
- Any changes in a lump or in the breast should be reported.

The Doctor
- Will examine the breasts to try and discover what kind of lump is causing the problem.
- Will prescribe antibiotics for infection. It is usually best to continue breast-feeding, if possible.
- Is likely to refer you to a breast clinic for further examinations and tests.
- The tests include ultrasound examination, mammography, needle examination and removal of the lump (biopsy) for microscopic examination.
- Ultrasound and mammography are techniques which provide doctors with an image of the internal structure of the breast. This can provide important clues as to the nature of the lump.
- A needle examination may be done immediately. If the lump is a cyst the needle may withdraw fluid from inside the cyst, making the 'lump' disappear. The fluid will then be sent for microscopic examination.
- Removal of the lump by no means indicates that you have cancer. Because the examination and tests cannot give a definite answer, lumps are routinely removed for examination, many turning out to be benign.
- Regular check-ups will be arranged after attendance at a breast clinic, whatever the result of the tests.

☎ Dept of Health, Health Publications Unit, No. 2 Site Heyward Stores, Manchester Road, Heyward, Lancs OL10 2PZ. (Send s.a.e. for free leaflet 'Be Breast Aware'.)

Breast-feeding problems

Some people appear to breast-feed with ease and have few problems. Others find it a long, difficult period, eventually abandoning breast-feeding full of disillusionment. There is no doubt that breast-feeding has considerable advantages, including providing the baby with important antibodies which help to fight infection. Many people do not, however, realise that the numbers of people still breast-feeding some weeks or months after leaving hospital is very much less than might be expected. If you have to cease breast-feeding for one reason or another you should not feel guilty because 'everyone else manages' – this is not the case.

Simple management of some of the problems associated with breast-feeding can go a long way to helping you continue to breast-feed and enjoy doing so. It is wise to ask unashamedly for help early, rather than get into difficulties which will increase the likelihood of your giving up.

Symptoms

* Blocked duct – a swollen, tender segment of the breast. Pain may increase between feeds as milk builds up behind the blockage. There should be no redness on the skin, nor fever-signs of infection.
* Breast engorgement: one whole breast or both may become overfilled with milk. This can occur quite suddenly. Veins on the surface may be prominent. Pain can be intense.
* Cracked nipples, when a break in the skin of the nipple occurs. This may be a very small slit or a larger fissure. It is painful to feed the baby. Bleeding may occur.
* Breast infection. (See **Breast infection**, above.)

Causes

- Blocked duct: it is not fully understood why this should happen. Some people appear to be more prone to this than others. Often very brief in duration, but can be persistent.
- Breast engorgement: the release of milk and its build-up in the breast is under delicate hormonal control. Anything upsetting this control can produce engorgement. It may occur when attempting to stop breast-feeding. It may also occur unexpectedly on one side when breast-feeding has been previously problem-free.
- Cracked nipples: it is partly true to say that some nipples crack while others don't. Nipple care and the position of the baby during feeding are important. However, cracks often appear unexpectedly. Try to keep the nipples dry between feeds.
- Breast infection. (See **Breast infection**, above.)

Treatment

- Seek help early, particularly if there is fever, redness or signs which make you suspect infection (see **Breast infection**, above). Your midwife or health visitor can often give useful advice on coping with the discomfort of all these conditions.
- Blocked duct: massage the affected area while breast-feeding. Continue breast-feeding. Seek help if symptoms do not improve.
- Engorged breasts: continue wearing a bra if possible. Some degree of engorgement is common when you start breast-feeding. The baby may have difficulty fixing on the nipple because of engorgement. It may be necessary to express milk from the breast using a pump (available on prescription) or by hand. As the feeding becomes established the supply of milk to the breast and its withdrawal during feeding is correctly balanced. Engorgement is then less likely to occur. Painkillers are often

necessary; start with aspirin or paracetamol. Ask your doctor to prescribe stronger painkillers if you do not get relief. All painkillers should be taken regularly until the problem is controlled; in this way they are more likely to give relief. This is preferable to waiting to see if you can manage and then requiring even larger doses. If you wish to stop breast-feeding or if the engorgement is severe your doctor can prescribe a drug called bromocriptine. This stops milk production by affecting the hormonal control.

- Cracked nipples: thankfully, this problem often heals quickly. Continue breast-feeding, although a short rest or shorter feeds on the affected side may be helpful for twenty-four to thirty-six hours. Various creams and ointments are available. A cold antiseptic spray is available which can ease the discomfort of a cracked nipple. Your doctor can prescribe these products, which are also available from chemists. The doctor may prescribe an anti-fungal cream if thrush is suspected. See your doctor if there is bleeding or if blood appears in the baby's vomit or stool. These symptoms are common and not usually serious; breast-feeding can usually be continued.
- Breast infection (see **Breast infection**, above): antibiotics will normally be given. Breast-feeding can be continued.

☎ Association of Breast-feeding Mothers, 26 Homeshaw Close, London SE26 4TH. Tel: 081 778 4769.

Breasts and adolescence

Problems with breasts may occur in boys or girls at puberty. Any difficulties have to be considered in the context of other changes that may or may not be occurring in an individual. These other sexual changes may lead to greater anxiety over breast development than expected.

Symptoms
* Breasts may develop unequally. This is not at all uncommon. It does not necessarily mean they will remain unequal, although many people do have some difference in size between right and left. It is normal for one breast to 'bud' before the other.
* In both sexes small lumps may appear, particularly below the brown 'aureola' which surrounds the nipple. These lumps are formed as a consequence of uneven breast gland development.
* Pubertal mastitis is a descriptive term for a short-lived tenderness of breasts that may occur in boys or girls in adolescence. It does not indicate infection, and usually settles quickly without treatment.

Causes
☐ The hormonal changes of adolescence lead to the breast changes described.
☐ The average age at which first signs of breast development are noted is around ten to eleven years old. Noticeable changes have usually ceased by fifteen years old.

Treatment
- It is usually possible to reassure any young person if their breast changes are worrying them. A good understanding of what is happening and

what is likely to happen can greatly help to dispel fears and anxieties.

The doctor
- May be able to confirm the parent's reassurance and check for signs of normal adolescent development.
- Consult your doctor if puberty appears to be delayed, particularly if there are no signs of breast changes by fifteen years of age.

Broken bones

Everyone is likely to break a bone at some stage in their life. The risk of doing so increases as we grow older. If you break a branch of a tree various things can happen: it can break cleanly with a snap, or splinter only on one side, the other side holding it in place. Human bones are similarly variable in the way they break. A child's bone is bendy and often just cracks on one side, called a greenstick fracture. An elderly person's bones are brittle and weak and tend to break completely. When the broken ends are moved away from each other more damage is done to other body tissues and more treatment is generally required. A doctor is always needed to advise on a broken bone and treatment is important to minimise the damage done.

Symptoms
* Pain is usually severe, but occasionally in a small undisplaced break of a wrist bone may not be severe and only revealed on X-ray.
* Swelling occurs rapidly after a break and is nearly always a pronounced feature.
* The area is tender to touch and especially to move.
* Deformity of the bone or joint may indicate that the bone ends have been moved away from each other.
* Bruising, which often appears worst a day or two after the injury, is evident.

Causes
- Usually an accident or injury.
- Also, particularly in the elderly, thinning and weakening of the bones makes a break quite possible with very little or no additional force. This is called a 'pathological fracture', often seen in the hips of older people owing to aging making the bones weaker, disuse, and sometimes disease in the bone itself.

Treatment
- Always avoid any movement of the broken bones.
- Go to the nearest hospital casualty department, where an X-ray will be taken.
- If the broken ends are in an incorrect position they will need to be re-aligned into a good position for healing (usually done under general anaesthetic).
- If the bone is in several pieces, or broken severely, pins may be put in during an operation to stabilise the pieces.
- It is important that no food or drink is taken after a possible break occurs as this could delay your having a general anaesthetic.
- Plaster casts or synthetic splints will be applied to immobilise the broken bones. Pain usually decreases after this. If pain is increasingly severe during or after twenty-four hours have the plaster checked; swelling may have made it too tight or the bones become displaced again.
- When the plaster comes off is just the start of getting back to normal. Do not overuse muscles which have been out of action for so long or there is risk of further injury. Listen carefully to advice on strengthening exercises

and timing of return to normal work or school activities.

Specific breaks

Wrists
- One of the commonest.
- Often displaced, needing anaesthetic to re-align properly.
- At least six weeks' healing time.

Fingers
- Often strapping to neighbouring ones is sufficient treatment.

Thumbs
- Injuries are common when the thumb is pulled back too far in a fall. A particularly difficult break to see on X-ray – called a scaphoid fracture – may be suspected and the arm and hand put in plaster to ensure good healing without an obvious break being seen.

Collarbone
- May be treated only by putting arm in a sling.
- Four to six weeks' healing time.

Arms
- Generally a full plaster is needed, including the elbow, as elbow movements can pull broken bones out of place. Sling also used.
- Six weeks' healing time.

Legs
- Plaster required.
- Traction, where straps and weights are attached to the legs to pull the broken bones into place, is often necessary – in hospital.
- May be twelve to twenty weeks' healing time.

Ankles
- Very common, and very important that adequate healing is achieved if later problems are to be avoided.
- Plaster and sometimes pinning required.
- Three to four months' healing time.

Ribs
- Frequently broken – may even be broken following violent coughing.
- Held together well by the muscles and other ribs acting as a splint.
- Unless displaced into the lung, for example in a car accident, these usually heal well if left alone. Antibiotics may be necessary for any lung infection, which is more common in the elderly.

Neck or spine
- The importance of not moving someone, without professional help, if these injuries are suspected cannot be overemphasised. Incorrect movement can cause paralysis or even death.

Care of the plaster cast
- Don't get it wet.
- Don't walk on it or use it to lean on unless you are specifically told it is a weight-bearing plaster.
- If it cracks or becomes floppy and soggy have it replaced or repaired immediately. Not doing so may mean an even longer healing time, or at worst a permanent, unnecessary disability.
- Scratching down the inside of the plaster with a smooth ruler or shaking some talc down it is generally OK, provided there are no skin cuts or stitches below the plaster.

Bronchiolitis

Bronchiolitis is an infection of the small airways of the lungs of infants and young children. Many children are infected particularly during winter and early spring. It is most common between six months and two years of age. It is rare to have bronchiolitis after two years of age. Breathing becomes noisy and requires more effort. Children with mild infections can stay at home, but hospital treatment is needed for serious infections. The infection is usually over after about a week.

Symptoms
* Starts as a cold with cough, temperature and runny nose.
* After a few days breathing becomes noisy and difficult.
* Babies are noticed to be at their most breathless when feeding.
* Feeds are not finished, or are refused.
* The baby may appear to be 'working very hard' to breathe.
* Breathing is rapid. As the infection worsens, so the rate of breathing increases.
* Dramatic, rapid, noisy breathing may develop.
* Wheezing, or a high-pitched sound as in asthma, can sometimes be heard.
* Attacks of wheezing during colds are more common after a baby has had bronchiolitis. Permanent breathing difficulties are, however, rare.

Causes
- Several viruses cause bronchiolitis.
- One virus causes the majority of attacks.
- The same virus in older children may only cause a cold.
- Bronchiolitis may be followed by a chest infection caused by bacteria.

Prevention
- There is no vaccine available.
- Breast-feeding may give some protection.
- When anyone in your family has a cold avoid coughing or sneezing over small babies.

Treatment
- Usually there is no specific treatment, other than ensuring that plenty of fluids are taken.
- Paracetamol liquid should be given for high temperature.

The Doctor
- Consult your doctor, who will be able to judge the severity of the illness, but mild infections can usually be managed at home.
- Antibiotics are only given for an added bacterial chest infection.
- Call your doctor again if:
  - your baby's breathing becomes very fast
  - your baby looks miserable and exhausted
  - your baby is not taking plenty of fluids
- Serious infections are sent to hospital, where:
  - a chest X-ray will be taken
  - oxygen may be given
  - a feeding tube is often passed through the nose to the stomach; this stops the baby becoming exhausted trying to feed
  - drugs in spray form are sometimes used
  - very ill babies may be attached to a respirator
  - usually the baby completely recovers, with no lasting damage to the lungs

Bronchitis

Bronchitis is an inflammation of the air passages of the lungs. There are two main forms – acute and chronic bronchitis. Acute bronchitis is a sudden onset of chest symptoms in someone who is generally well. People with chronic bronchitus have symptoms much of the time, which may be worsened by infection. This is very much linked to cigarette smoking.

Symptoms
Acute bronchitis
* May start with the runny nose and sore throat of a cold.
* There is a chesty cough with coloured phlegm.

* Breathing may be noisy, with wheezing.
* You may be hot and cold, with a fever.
* You may have a dry, irritating cough for some weeks following acute bronchitis.

Chronic bronchitis
* There is a frequent productive cough.
* You may be short of breath all the time.
* You may catch infections which worsen your symptoms.
* The lack of oxygen may cause blue lips, and the illness may strain the heart, causing swollen ankles.

Causes
- Many different bacteria and viruses cause acute bronchitis. These include measles and influenza viruses.
- Dust, fibres and cigarette smoke cause chronic bronchitis.
- Early lung damage from measles or whooping cough may play a part.

Prevention
- Stop smoking, which is the main cause of chronic bronchitis. The damage depends on how long you smoke for and how many cigarettes you smoke.
- Dusts and fibres in the air contribute. Wear a mask if dealing repeatedly with fibres or dust.
- People with chronic bronchitis are recommended to have the flu vaccine each year.
- Vaccination against measles and whooping cough in children will reduce the risk of lung damage, making bronchitis less likely in later life.

Treatment
- The same principles apply to acute bronchitis as are described for pneumonia. (See **Pneumonia**.)
- Paracetamol will control fever and to some extent pain and discomfort.
- For relief of cough see **Cough**.
- Plenty of drinks will also soothe the cough. See your doctor if you have a chesty cough and coloured phlegm.

The Doctor
- Will listen to your chest for signs of bronchitis.
- Antibiotics will be prescribed if these signs are found.
- Chronic bronchitis may need constant treatment.
- There are pills and inhalers to open up the airways, as described for asthma. These may help to ease shortness of breath symptoms but are not always effective in chronic bronchitis because the lungs are damaged and cannot respond to the medicines.
- Some people need to have oxygen at home as the condition worsens.
- Take antibiotics at the first sign of an infection. It may be worthwhile asking your doctor if you can have a spare course of antibiotics to keep at home.

Bunions

In bunions the big toe joins the foot at an angle, rather than in a straight line. On your left foot, for example, the big toe would be pointing out to the left. It is on the angle created by this poor lining-up of the big toe with the foot that bunions occur. Each joint is surrounded by a structure like a plastic bag filled with fluid. In bunions this bag protrudes from the edge of the foot and causes problems, particularly when rubbing on footwear. Sometimes they can be very painful. They affect three times as many women as men and tend to run in families.

Symptoms
* Misshapen feet.
* Difficulty and discomfort wearing shoes.
* Pain, especially if the bag of fluid (bursa) mentioned above becomes inflamed (bursitis).
* Problems with the other toes caused by the big toe pushing against them.
* Hard skin or callus may form over the bunion. (See **Corns**.)

Causes
- The odd shape of the feet may be a family characteristic.
- Ill-fitting shoes can push toes into a position where bunions occur.
- Painful bunions are usually due to a bursitis (see above). This can happen after prolonged wearing of ill-fitting shoes or a lot of walking.
- The worst shoes are high heels with pointed toes; these aggravate the problem but are unlikely to cause it in the first place.

Treatment
- Wear correctly fitting shoes always.
- If a bunion is painful cut a hole in an old shoe over the bunion to relieve pressure.
- Rest painful bunions until inflammation settles.
- Chiropodists can often help, advising treatment similar for that described for corns.

The Doctor
- Rarely, surgery is undertaken to try and straighten out the angle of the big toe that is causing problems. However, this should not be done lightly and is only advised if the pain is unbearable and makes walking very difficult. The foot is normally in plaster for up to two months after surgery.

Burns

Burns should always be taken seriously. It is very easy to underestimate the extent of damage; there is little relation between severity and amount of pain. Very severe burns can be painless because nerve endings are destroyed. Whatever the type or extent of a burn it is the loss of body fluid that poses a real danger. This fluid can be lost below the reddened skin of what appears to be a superficial scald – see a doctor at once.

Symptoms
* Blisters formed by the loss of body fluid; these may not appear immediately.
* Red areas of skin.
* Raw, red, oozing, weeping areas.
* Blackened areas.
* Pus – generally an indication of infection.

Causes
- Hot liquids.
- Hot objects.
- Electricity.
- Chemicals.
- Friction.
- Hot gases.
- Fire.

Treatment
- Remove source of burn. *All* clothing must be removed unless actually stuck to the skin. Clothing soaked in hot liquid or chemicals will continue to burn until removed. Remove everything, as areas that may appear to be unaffected have often also been scalded.
- Cool the affected area immediately. Immerse the burn in cold water or running cold water for about ten to fifteen minutes. This must be done within five minutes to be effective. It stops burns penetrating to affect

deeper layers of tissue and causing more damage. It also helps to reduce fluid loss by making blood vessels contract.
- Never apply creams, ointments, butter, fat or other substances. Water only, as outlined above.
- Raise affected limbs to decrease swelling and loss of fluids.
- Cover with non-fluffy, clean material only. Clingfilm can be used to cover an area while travelling to hospital or surgery.
- Do not burst blisters; this only increases soreness and may cause infection.
- See a doctor: for almost any burn it is wise to seek advice. Failure to do so may at best lead to unnecessary scarring, at worst may lead to death from loss of body fluids.

Cancer

Everybody fears that they will get cancer. Most people know somebody who has died of cancer or been treated for it. Fortunately, the number of people who can now be cured of cancer is much greater than previously. It is important never to give in and think that cancer can't be treated; if you have symptoms you fear may indicate cancer, seek help now. Early treatment can lead to effective cure.

Cancer occurs in many different parts of the body. The word refers to a group of the body's cells starting to multiply and spread in an uncontrollable way. Some cancers spread more quickly than others. For example, nearly all men over eighty have cancer of the prostate gland, but it lies dormant in the prostate gland and seldom causes problems. (See **Prostate**.)

The word tumour refers to a collection of growing cells. Some tumours are malignant, meaning that they spread to other parts of the body and may be fatal; other tumours are benign, and although they grow in size they do not spread.

Cancer appears to be more prevalent in some families than others. It is not, however, inherited, nor is it contagious.

Symptoms
* There may be no symptoms of the cancer until it is well advanced. Symptoms may only occur as a result of the cancer spreading to affect another part of the body.
* Pain is not always a feature. Cancer can be present without causing any pain.
* Non-specific symptoms may occur, such as loss of weight, loss of appetite and tiredness.
* Some cancers are described elsewhere in the book. Particular signs that should alert you the possibility of cancer include:
  - bleeding after the menopause
  - unexplained bleeding from the back passage or urine passage
  - blood in the spit particularly in smokers, or persistent cough
  - alteration of regular pattern of urine or bowel habit
  - skin changes around a mole including changes in size, colour, number, itching and bleeding
  - appearance of an unexplained lump anywhere

If these signs do indicate cancer, early treatment can be effective.

Causes
- Smoking causes lung cancer. You should stop.
- Nearly 80 per cent of other cancers may be caused by what are called carcinogens found in the environment and some foods. These include asbestos, tar, chromium and nuclear radiation.
- Viruses are also implicated in causing some cancers.

□ Exactly how these cause cancer or why cancer should occur is not clear.

Treatment

- About a third of all cancers can be cured. Early detection is important. There are now screening programmes for cancer of the cervix and breast which can detect cancer early enough to ensure adequate treatment.
- Cancer of the lymph glands and some leukaemias can now be effectively cured where previously death would have been inevitable.
- Treatment may be by:

Surgical removal

- Many tumours can be completely removed. If the cancer has spread, or may have spread, additional treatment may be required. Some cancers do not need to be removed but can be treated by other methods such as:

Radiotherapy

- Some tumours shrink up and are satisfactorily treated by exposure to radiation. Your skin will be marked to indicate the area to be treated. You then have to attend a series of sessions at regular intervals to have the treatment, which lasts for a few minutes. Be prepared for the rooms where the treatment is given to be rather off-putting, being filled with machines, flashing lights and odd noises.

Chemotherapy

- This is the use of drugs to affect the cancer cells. Some cancers respond well to being treated with specific drugs, though many of the drugs have side-effects, including causing changes in the blood, nausea and hair loss.
- Your doctor or specialist can advise you on the need for, and potential benefit of, each type of treatment. Not every person, nor every cancer, can be treated in the same way. The importance of seeking medical help early if you fear you have cancer cannot be over-emphasised. Treatment can now be very effective and provide a cure for many cancers.

- ☎ Cancer Research Campaign, Cambridge House, 6–10 Cambridge Terrace, Regent's Park, London NW1 4JL. Tel: 071 224 1333.

- ☎ Imperial Cancer Research Fund, P.O. Box 123, Lincoln's Inn Fields, London WC2A 3PX. Tel: 071 242 0200.

- ☎ BACUP (British Association of Cancer United Patients), 121–123 Charterhouse Street, London EC1M 6AA. Tel: 071 608 1661.

Cataracts

This refers to the central part of the eye, gradually becoming misty. Many people are affected by cataracts causing some deterioration of vision, but not everyone requires treatment. There are often others in the family who have cataracts. It is not serious and the treatment, if it is necessary, is simple and the results dramatic.

Symptoms

* Gradual decrease and disturbance of vision. Objects, particularly distant ones, may appear hazy.
* The difficulty with vision becomes worse with time.
* Both eyes are usually affected, sometimes one more than the other.
* More difficulty with vision may be experienced in bright sunlight.

Causes

□ Normally it is a natural part of later life. The gradual clouding of the lens in the eye interferes with the reception of light by the eye, thus distorting it and producing poor images.

- Cataracts can be caused by diabetes. (See **Diabetes**.)
- They can occur in babies whose mothers have caught German measles while pregnant. (See **German measles**.)
- Iritis is an uncommon eye condition which is painful and, if longstanding, can cause cataracts.

Treatment

- Often spectacles and reading in a good light can provide satisfactory vision. Ensure that your optician is providing the most suitable glasses possible.
- Surgical correction will usually be done when vision has become so poor that it is interfering with daily living.
- It is the commonest eye operation and can be carried out under local or general anaesthetic.
- The operation involves removing the misty lens and replacing it with an artificial lens. Sometimes the lens is removed but not replaced and the vision is corrected by the use of spectacles or contact lenses.
- Occasionally, after the lens has been removed, despite the help of spectacles or a new lens, vision is still poor. This can be a result of the back of the eye no longer being able to pick up the light and convert it into images. Little can be done for this condition, known as macula degeneration.

Cervical problems

The cervix is the neck of the womb. It is about an inch in length and juts down into the top of the vagina. You can feel it easily if you put your finger into the vagina; it feels a bit like the end of your nose. The cervix is made up of firm muscle tissue with a canal passing through the middle of it. This canal not only opens up in labour to let the baby out but is used by sperm entering the womb and for menstrual flow to emerge during periods.

The lining of this canal is made up of a different type of skin from the inside of the vagina. It is at the junction between the skin inside and outside the canal that most of the cervical problems occur. When a doctor takes a smear test the cells on both sides of this junction are examined under the microscope.

In this section we will look at:

Abnormal cervical smear
Cervical cancer
Cervical erosion

Abnormal cervical smear

If you are told that your smear test needs to be repeated this does not necessarily mean you have cancer. Many normal processes in the body can lead to changes found on the smear test. The usual consequence of having an abnormal smear test is for it to be repeated after three or six months. Very often after this interval the changes first noted have disappeared. Sometimes they stay the same and can be watched by having regular smear tests. In some people the changes progress, but this still does not necessarily mean you have cancer. Treatment is now available for the changes found on smear tests, and is often used long before any evidence of invasive cancer is found.

Symptoms

* There may be no symptoms. It is therefore particularly important for women to have regular cervical smears (see below).
* Some discharge may be noted. There may be bleeding after intercourse (see **Cervical erosion**, below) or between periods.
* Bleeding after the menopause should always be reported to your doctor immediately.

Causes
An abnormal smear may be seen:

- In puberty.
- In pregnancy.
- At the menopause.
- If there is infection.
- When there is new cell growth around the entrance to the canal of the cervix. This can happen because of the more delicate cells in the canal coming in contact with vaginal secretions which are more acidic. (See **Cervical erosion**, below.)
- If the cells in this area between the inside of the canal and the vagina develop abnormally then dysplasia may be found. In its early stages this is not cancer. Cells showing the changes of dysplasia may revert to normal. The number of women who have dysplasia on their smear tests and then revert to having normal cell changes is not yet clear. Some specialists suggest that as many as 80 per cent of mild dysplasia (also called mild dyskaryosis or CIN 1) may revert to normal without treatment. Others feel that a much larger percentage will progress to more severe dysplasia. More severe dysplasia may be referred to as carcinoma in-situ or CIN 3. This means that abnormal cells are confined to the surface tissue, but have begun to show cancerous change. Treatment will cure the condition completely.

Prevention
- Cancer of the cervix can be prevented from developing by having regular smear tests, thus allowing early treatment of abnormal changes that are found.
- Smear tests every three years are recommended from when you first start having intercourse.
- If you have had a previous abnormal smear test or a viral infection (such as herpes or warts) you should have a smear test every year or as advised by your doctor. (See **Genital herpes** and **Warts, genital**.)
- See cervical cancer for those groups of people who are most at risk of developing abnormal cell changes.

Treatment
- The doctor who takes the smear test may contact you with the result; however, it is your test and if you have not heard the result within a few weeks you should ask for it.
- If you are asked to have another smear test, remember that this does not necessarily mean you have cancer. A repeat smear is very important to check the changes on the cervix.
- Treatment of infection or other causes may lead to your having a normal smear result subsequently.
- Your doctor may refer you for an examination of the cervix in more detail. This is called a colposcopy examination. An instrument similar to a microscope is inserted into the vagina and allows a closer study to be made of the cell changes on the cervix. Small scrapings and pieces of tissue can be removed to examine the extent and severity of the changes. Colposcopy is not painful and takes about ten minutes. You are awake and the doctor will be able to explain what is going on during the examination.
- If severe changes are found treatment may be given either by freezing the abnormal area or by using laser treatment. (Sometimes a burning technique called cautery is used.)
- Freezing treatment takes ten to fifteen minutes, laser treatment only two or three. Neither are very painful, although the discomfort felt varies from

person to person. It will help if someone goes with you to distract you during the treatment, which is usually done while you are awake.
- Treatment may be followed by a watery discharge which can be heavy at first and may continue for two to three weeks. Laser treatment leads to less discharge. Report any heavy bleeding following the treatment to your doctor; this could be a complication of the treatment.
- Treatment is usually complete in one visit.
- A cone biopsy refers to an operation to remove part of the cervix. This used to be the treatment for many of the abnormal cell changes on the cervix. Modern treatments have made it less frequently necessary. An advantage is that all the cells in the area at the entrance of the cervical canal can be examined in detail, any abnormal area being completely removed. A disadvantage is that it weakens the cervix and may lead to an increased tendency to miscarry. The operation is done under general anaesthetic and usually a stay of three to five days in hospital is required. Some rest for about two weeks after the operation is advisable as there is a small risk of bleeding.
- Following any treatment of the cervix, regular follow-up checks will be arranged. Usually these are done about every six months for two years, then yearly thereafter.

☎ Women's Health, 52 Featherstone Street, London EC1. Tel: 071 251 6580. (Send s.a.e. for information.)

☎ Women's Nationwide Cancer Control Campaign, Suna House, 128–130 Curtain Road, EC2A 3AR. Tel: 071 729 2229 (helpline), 071 729 1735 (leaflets).

Cervical cancer

This is most prevalent in women over forty years of age. Cervical cancer can be prevented by checking any changes on the cervix by regular smear tests. The number of deaths from cervical cancer has decreased in areas where regular smear tests are carried out on all women. The vast majority of women who die from the disease have never had a smear test. There is some increase in the incidence of cervical cancer amongst younger women.

Symptoms
* In the early stages there may be no symptoms, hence the importance of regular smear tests to detect and treat any changes. (See **Abnormal cervical smear**, above.)
* Discharge with or without bleeding.
* Bleeding after the menopause is always abnormal and should be reported to your doctor at once.

Causes
☐ The exact cause of cervical cancer is not clear. A number of factors may increase your chance of developing cervical cancer. These include:
  - early age of starting to have sexual intercourse
  - having a sexually transmitted disease, which is more likely if you have had several partners
  - having several children at a young age
  - there is some association between having viral infections such as herpes or genital warts and abnormal cell changes; the significance of this association is not yet clear

Treatment
- Is effective if the cancer is detected before spread occurs.

- The cervix and womb can be removed, and/or radiotherapy can be given. Radiotherapy can be given from pellets inserted into the vagina and placed next to the cancer.
- Treatment, providing the cancer has not spread beyond the womb and cervix, has a very high success rate – much higher than in most cancers. It will not be possible to have children following treatment.
- See addresses listed after **Abnormal cervical smear**, above.

Cervical erosion

As described above, the skin of the cervical canal is different and more delicate from the skin on the outside of the cervix and in the vagina. Where this canal skin is exposed to vaginal secretions a sore place or ulcer may develop. This is not painful and frequently clears up on its own. The cell changes found in an erosion are not necessarily abnormal. Sometimes, however, abnormal cell changes are found at the junction between canal skin and the skin outside the canal. These are described under **Abnormal cervical smear**, see above.

Symptoms
* Often no symptoms occur, a cervical erosion being found during a routine examination.
* Discharge may occur. This may be clear, yellow, white or brownish. Bleeding may occur after intercourse or between periods.
* Bleeding after the menopause is abnormal and should always be reported to your doctor.

Causes
▫ Some people appear to be more prone to developing cervical erosions than others.
▫ It may occur during pregnancy or while taking the Pill.

Treatment
- Provided you are having regular vaginal examinations and smear tests no treatment is necessary unless symptoms are severe. Usually any problems associated with the erosion fluctuate considerably in severity.

The Doctor
- Will take a smear test and swab tests to check for any infection.
- Infection will be treated with tablets or pessaries inserted into the vagina.
- It may be difficult to obtain a satisfactory smear test from an area of erosion on the cervix due to bleeding. This makes it more difficult to examine the cells found when the smear test is examined under the microscope.
- If the appearances of an erosion persist or smear tests are not satisfactory referral for further examination and treatment as described under **Abnormal cervical smear**, see above, may be arranged.

Chicken pox

Chicken pox most commonly affects children aged from two to eight years old. It is usually a mild infection, but adults and newborn babies are more unwell. It lasts for about a week and is highly infectious. It is caused by the same virus as shingles. A severe form affects children with weakened immunity caused by leukaemia, cancer treatment or having taken steroids by mouth.

Symptoms
* There is an interval of fourteen to twenty-one days between catching the disease and the rash appearing.
* The day before the rash appears your child may feel unwell, with sore

throat, headache, backache, tummy-ache and fever.
* Spots appear in crops over the chest, tummy and head.
* They turn into blisters which are very itchy.
* After a few days these crust.
* Fresh crops of spots appear for a few days.
* The spots may become infected.
* Pneumonia is a rare complication in children but more common in adults.
* Unborn babies are usually unaffected, but occasionally get a bad infection.

Causes
□ The virus *herpes zoster* or *varicella zoster* causes chicken pox.
□ After having chicken pox you cannot catch it again.
□ The virus may remain dormant and later cause shingles. (See **Shingles**.)
□ It is usually caught from someone with chicken pox, and rarely from someone with shingles.

Prevention
- Is usually unnecessary because it is a mild infection.
- There is no vaccine available, but a protective injection can be given to those with weakened immunity, e.g. women in late pregnancy and newborn babies who have contracted the virus.
- It is most infectious the day before the rash appears.
- It remains infectious until the last blister crusts.

Treatment
- You do not need to see a doctor if you are sure of the diagnosis, which is usually obvious.
- Paracetamol helps the temperature and pain.
- Calamine lotion, which can be bought over the counter, helps the itch.
- It must be applied frequently.

The Doctor
- May advise:
  - antihistamines by mouth if the itch is severe
  - a mouthwash if there are spots in the mouth
  - antibiotics, sometimes needed for infected spots or complicating chest infection

Chilblains

Too often the enjoyment of building a snowman is ruined by those painful feet. Chilblains are red, swollen, itchy areas of angry skin on fingers and toes particularly. They are more common in children but may also affect adults. They are not serious and almost always go away by themselves with simple treatment.

Symptoms
* Pain.
* Red swollen areas, particularly along the backs of toes.
* Itching, often intense.
* Reddish-blue discolouration.
* Become worse on repeated exposure to cold and damp.
* Pale numb areas on fingers.

Causes
□ The body protects us from cold by stopping our blood going to the skin; in chilblains this mechanism goes wrong. The shortage in the blood supply to the skin leads to the variety of unpleasant symptoms.

Prevention
If you have a tendency to develop chilblains you can often avoid them by taking the following precautions:

- Keep warm; it is important to keep all parts warm, not just the areas affected.
- Wear a hat and scarf.
- Kep your chest warm with woolly jumpers. This has the effect of sending more blood to where it's needed to stop chilblains.
- Gloves are useful, particularly ski gloves.
- Warming pads are available, some running on batteries, to wear inside gloves.
- Wear lots of socks.
- Avoid damp and change socks and gloves as soon as they are wet.

Treatment

- There is no cure; they will clear in a few days.
- It is best to practise the above precautions if affected.
- Talc patted on, not rubbed, may help.
- Ointments are of little value and the rubbing during application is likely to stimulate more itching and therefore risk of skin damage.
- If ulceration occurs see the doctor.
- Doctors may in very severe cases advise drugs to allow more blood to fingers and toes. These drugs are called vasodilators; an example is nifedipine.

Colds

The common cold which everyone experiences is caused by one of several hundred different viruses. As we catch a cold and get better we build up immunity to that particular virus, but because there are so many, and because the viruses themselves can change to infect us again, it is not surprising that we catch a cold so frequently. A baby in the first year of life is very prone to catching a cold, and a schoolchild may catch as many as half a dozen a year, whereas an older person will have some benefit from the immunity they have built up over the years and catch fewer. A common cold is not serious, but the same virus may produce more serious symptoms if the ears, sinuses, larynx or lungs are affected (see below).

Symptoms

* Runny nasal discharge, usually clear to start with, then becoming yellowy-green.
* Sneezing.
* Watering eyes.
* Sore throat.
* Hoarseness.
* Coughing.
* Headache.
* Mild fever.
* Catarrh, which is a general term used to describe the symptom of intermittent blocking of the nose which may be particularly troublesome on lying down to sleep. The nasal discharge causing catarrh may also drip down the back of the throat, causing coughing.
* Symptoms of a cold may persist and develop into sinusitis, earache, laryngitis, bronchitis, all covered elsewhere in the book.

Causes

- Viruses cause colds (see above).
- How they are transferred from one person to another is not yet absolutely clear. It is thought to be mainly by droplets spread from coughing and sneezing. Transfer may also take place by shaking hands with someone after holding your hand in front of your mouth to block a sneeze.
- Because immunity is built up to viruses quite quickly, the arrival of an outsider to a small community may bring new viruses in contact with people who have no immunity, thus

causing a widespread outbreak of cold symptoms.

Treatment
- Stay at home, keeping yourself to yourself.
- Keep the room warm but not too dry.
- Drying towels on radiators or boiling a kettle with the lid off can help keep the air moist.
- Drink plenty of fluids.
- Use steam inhalations (see **Cough**).
- Blow your nose frequently as this helps to clear the airways and prevent infection in other parts of the air passages, such as the sinuses and lungs.
- Medicines from the chemist such as aspirin or paracetamol are helpful in lowering temperature and relieving aches and pains.
- Various cold remedies are available to buy which contain products which may add to the *relief*, such as antihistamines, but these may have side effects and will not offer a *cure*.
- Vitamin C is widely used to help fight a cold, although there is no firm medical evidence to show that it makes a significant difference. There is no doubt that many people find great relief and benefit from taking it, but for others it has no effect.

The Doctor
- If cold symptoms persist for more than ten days or appear to be developing into a more serious infection you should consult a doctor.
- It is unhelpful to consult a doctor for ordinary cold symptoms as antibiotics have no effect on viruses.
- If you have a sinusitis, laryngitis, bronchitis or ear infection the doctor may prescribe an antibiotic. In many cases the infection is viral without a complicating bacteria, and in these cases the antibiotic will only serve to prevent a bacterial infection but may make no appreciable difference to the symptoms.
- If you have a tendency to recurrent severe infections, or have chest or ear problems, this may be an indication for antibiotics at the onset of cold symptoms.

Cold hands (Raynaud's disease)

These are often not just a result of being inadequately dressed, but can be caused by a problem first described by someone called Raynaud. The blood supply to the fingers, and occasionally the toes, becomes oversensitive to cold. Even putting something into the fridge can set off a spasm of the blood vessels in the hands, making them feel abnormally cold.

This is a common problem, particularly in women, who generally first notice it as young adults. It is not usually serious but can sometimes lead to a decreased sense of touch. Rarely, it is seen as part of another illness affecting other parts of the body.

Symptoms
* Cold hands.
* Affected areas go very pale, and then blue, before becoming pink again as the blood vessel spasm wears off.
* Pins and needles.
* Not generally painful.
* Comes on quickly.

Causes
- Sudden decrease in the blood supply to the affected areas.
- Can just develop by itself (Raynaud's disease).
- Can be brought on by certain jobs such as using pneumatic drills (Raynaud's phenomenon).

Treatment
- Keep hands and feet warm, using appropriate clothing.
- Stop smoking, as smoking impairs the circulation.
- Avoid cold situations as far as possible.

The Doctor
- Will try and find a cause related to your present or past job and encourage you to stop. Raynaud's phenomenon, caused by using vibrating tools, can increase in severity quite quickly.
- Will advise on the use of drugs to increase the amount of blood reaching affected areas (vasodilator drugs, e.g. nifedipine).
- Alcohol may be advised in moderation as this warms the extremities.
- Surgery can sometimes increase the circulation to fingers and toes, but it is not always successful and the effects may not last.
- (See also **Chilblains**.)

Cold sores

These are small blistering areas that appear around nostrils, lips and elsewhere on the face. They dry, scab over and clear, but may become infected. They are not serious but are infectious. They are caused by a virus called *herpes simplex*, which is not the same type of herpes virus as causes what is recognised as genital herpes. All age groups can be infected. They may reappear several times, very often, or only once and never again. Normally they have cleared by themselves in ten days.

Symptoms
* Burning feeling before the blister appears.
* Painful red areas sometimes crusting over.
* Itching.
* Weeping as the blisters open. The wet blisters are vey infectious.
* In children a first attack of this virus may appear as a crop of blisters inside the mouth and around the gums. Eating can be so difficult for a few days that fluids are all that can be managed. There is fever and the child is generally unwell.

Causes
- The virus is often present in the skin without producing symptoms. Symptoms may appear years after first contact with the virus.
- An outbreak of cold sores can be started by:
  - sunlight
  - cold
  - heat
  - wind
  - tiredness
  - being run down
  - other illness
  - periods
  - stress

Treatment
- Avoid touching, scratching or picking at the blisters.
- Vaseline can be soothing and is harmless.
- Prevent spread by keeping to one towel.
- Prevent recurrent attacks by trying to avoid any factors that produce the cold sores.

The Doctor
- Obtain your doctor's advice on how you can begin treatment early to avoid having a bad attack.
- Herpes near or in the eye should be reported to your doctor at once.
- There are now anti-herpes creams and paints which your doctor may prescribe. It is important that they are

used as directed and discarded afterwards.
- Infection with other germs may need antibiotic creams.

Colic

This occurs in very young babies under four or five months of age. It frequently occurs in the evening and is sometimes called evening or six o'clock colic. Exactly what causes colic and what is happening to the baby is unclear. It can be very distressing for both the baby and parents but does always get better on its own.

Symptoms
* After an evening feed or on waking the baby cries out loudly.
* May turn red and draw the legs up.
* Is difficult to settle.
* Appears to be suffering tummy pain.
* No usual soothing tricks seem to give lasting comfort.
* The baby is often contented and happy the rest of the day.

Causes
- Doctors don't agree about what causes colic.
- Muscular spasm in the gut, wind, hunger and indigestion may all play a part.

Treatment
- Every baby is different and colic may be very difficult to manage. It is helpful to remember that it will cease of its own accord.
- First check the baby is not wet, hungry, cold or needing to be more firmly wrapped to make him feel securely held as he was in the womb.
- Check there is no fever or other signs of being unwell. If the symptoms of colic have been coming on all day and the child has been difficult, restless and unhappy it is unlikely to be just colic.
- Try every method you know of soothing, such as walking around, carrying the baby in a sling, burping, rocking, and so on. Each method you try is likely to help for a little while.
- Nursing with the baby lying on his tummy on your knee, while gently patting his back, may help.
- Use a comforter or dummy, also called a pacifier. (see **Comforters**).
- Giving the baby a bath at this time is often helpful.
- Breast-feeding mothers should rest if possible during the day and eat and drink plenty. Waiting for a partner to return home before your main meal if you are breast-feeding often means that the evening feed you give the baby is unsatisfactory. You will be tired, have less milk, and be less able to relax. This may exacerbate colic in your baby.
- Tapes of womb noises are available from some large booksellers and record stores. These may help to settle a restless baby unless the baby is truly distressed by colic.
- Use of a lambswool fleece for the cot or pram can help some babies. It is unlikely to alter a colic pattern significantly, but is perhaps worth trying, available from large department stores.

The Doctor
- Will be able to check for any other causes of distress in the baby.
- If repeated bouts of colic are causing you and your baby great distress do see your doctor. Discussing the problem and ideas on what you might try is often helpful.
- Previously a medicine called dicyclomine, useful for spasms of the gut,

was sometimes prescribed. This is now contraindicated in children under six months because it has been found to affect some babies adversely.

What about gripe water?
It is advisable to consult your doctor before trying any over-the-counter remedies from the chemist. Gripe water is not generally recommended as a first resort in colic. The action of gripe water is poorly understood. It does contain alcohol so repeated doses should not be given. If you feel you really want to try it give it about one hour before feeds and only as directed on the bottle. Avoid repeated or prolonged use.

Colour blindness

In its commonest form this is a difficulty in distinguishing different colours or shades of the same colours; it is only in a very rare form that everything appears grey. It is a characteristic that runs in families, being ten times more common in men than women. It is not usually a serious problem.

Symptoms
* It is very often never discovered until a medical examination is carried out.
* There are no real problems in coping with daily life.
* Children may have difficulty at school, though they can manage by identifying objects by their name or shape rather than colour.
* Traffic lights and warning signals can normally be identified from their shape and the positioning of lights.

Causes
☐ This is present from birth.

Treatment
- None whatsoever is available.
- Just as we are born with a skin colour or a physical characteristic that runs in the family, so we can do nothing about an inability to distinguish colours.
- It can help your child if you remind each new teacher that he/she has this minor difficulty.

The Doctor
- You will be asked to identify numbers on special 'dotted' cards and trace different-coloured squiggles on cards.
- When diagnosed, it is important that the severity and type of the condition is explained.

Comforters

Most children at some stage adopt an object, or their own thumb, as a comforter. It is not a sign of insecurity, nor of any problem in a child. Thumb-sucking may start in the womb and has various advantages, including the fact that it doesn't get lost and parents don't have to worry about finding it at tense moments. If they have not done so long before, most comforting habits cease at around six years old.

Symptoms
* Often infants find an object to prize as their most intimate possession at around their first birthday. This may be a bottle, blanket, piece of cloth, scarf, tie, or a cuddly toy.
* This object usually needs to be kept by the child whenever they are left with someone unfamiliar or are put to bed.
* Great distress can occur, making everyone's life a misery, if the comforter is lost.
* The dirty or ragged appearance of the object often becomes increasingly embarrassing for the parent, but this has no effect on its importance to the child.

* They are most often needed at times of shyness, uncertainty, stress, and when mother is absent.

Causes
☐ Exactly why thumbsucking or treasuring certain objects occurs is not clear. Psychiatrists call them 'transitional comfort objects' as they may help the child to cope with gradual independence from mother.
☐ They provide security and give confidence.
☐ The object or thumb may be very important in enabling the child to be left alone for sleeping.

Prevention
- There is no real need to prevent use of a comforter.
- Teeth are not affected by the use of a comforter that is sucked until the age of six years old. Special orthodontic dummies are available from chemists if you are concerned, but the child may not accept them so easily. The stress involved in forcing a change to a supposedly more suitable dummy may not be worth while.
- Take the comforter to childminders, nursery school and on outings. Always tell babysitters of the importance of any comforter to a child.
- Avoid washing dirty, loved blankets more than necessary. The accumulation of days or even weeks of dirt and holes in a cloth seems to add to its importance to the child.
- Buy spare dummies or duplicates of other comforters. Some people cut a cloth that has become a comforter in half in the early days, before a child notices, in order to keep half for an emergency when the comforter is lost.

Treatment
- It is sad and generally unnecessary to discourage thumb-sucking. This usually ceases on its own in the second year of life.
- Don't try to stop the use of a comforter. It will not be possible and will only cause distress. Persistently trying to alter a comforting habit will only heighten insecurity and create friction.
- If the use of a dummy or other object has persisted to six or seven years old it is sometimes useful to give the child a target of a birthday to cease using the object. After this event they can try to keep it in a safe place but not use it for sleeping, for example.
- There is no established link between the use of a comforter and emotional difficulties or insecurity. There is therefore little need to discourage a young child from enjoying a comforter.

Confusion

Confusion may occur at any time of life, particularly in the elderly. It should never be accepted as an illness in itself as there is always an underlying cause. If confusion occurs in people of any age, particularly if it is of sudden onset, seek medical help without delay.

Symptoms
* Mixing up times, places or people.
* Accidents may occur.
* Drugs may be taken in incorrect dosage and add to confusion.
* Underlying causes may produce associated symptoms such as fever, cough or headache.
* Hearing or visual difficulties may make confusion worse.

Causes
* Infection is a common cause of confusion. This may be due to the illness

itself or the fever it produces; particularly common in the elderly.
- chest infection (see **Pneumonia**)
- urine infection (see **Urine infection**)

☐ Heart problems or problems with the circulation may cause confusion.
- heart attacks (see **Heart attacks**)
- heart failure (see **Heart failure**)
- strokes (see **Strokes**)

☐ The brain itself can be affected by many factors, with subsequent confusion.
- head injury (see **Head injuries**)
- dementia (see **Dementia**)
- brain tumours

☐ Other problems which may cause confusion with or without symptoms are:
- hypothermia
- low blood sugar (see **Diabetes**)
- vitamin deficiency (see **Vitamin deficiency**)
- thyroid problems (see **Thyroid problems**)
- excess alcohol (see **Alcoholism**)
- prolonged use of excessive alcohol (see **Alcoholism**)
- alcohol (see **Alcoholism**)
- drugs prescribed and abused (see **Drug abuse**)
- glue-sniffing (see **Glue-sniffing**)
- fits (see **Epilepsy**)

Treatment
- Any sudden confusion should be treated with some urgency and attempts made to find the cause.
- Long-standing confusion may be due to dementia, but other causes should be excluded before this diagnosis is made.
- Appropriate spectacles and a hearing aid can help elderly people enormously.
- If possible an elderly person should be nursed at home in familiar surroundings. Confusion is then much less likely than if admitted to hospital.

The Doctor
- Will try and establish the cause of confusion through examination and tests. Hospital admission may be required if the cause of confusion is not immediately clear or management at home is not feasible.
- Many of the tests and treatments required are described elsewhere in this book.

Conjunctivitis

The eye is covered with a thin film or membrane. This also extends to cover the inside of the eyelid. In conjunctivitis this membrane becomes red and 'angry'. Doctors describe this as an inflammation. It is not serious if caused by infection but, because of the danger to the eyes if not correctly diagnosed or treated, a doctor's advice should always be sought. Most types of conjunctivitis clear quickly and do not recur.

Symptoms
* Red eye.
* Weeping.
* Pain.
* Itching.
* Light can be irritating.
* Yellow pus.

Causes
☐ Bacterial infection.
☐ Virus infection.
☐ Foreign body in eye. (See **Eye problems**)
☐ Hayfever.
☐ Other allergy.
☐ Part of an illness, e.g. measles.

Treatment
Infectious
- Antibiotic drops and ointment can be used, but if not responding rapidly a viral infection may be present and an eye specialist should be seen.

- Avoid touching the eyes or sharing face cloths/towels as this can spread any infection.

Foreign bodies
- These must be removed and the eye treated while it heals. (See **Eye problems**.)

Allergies
- These can be due to make-up or contact with soaps or perfumes, which should be avoided subsequently.

Hayfever
- Symptoms can be well treated with eye drops and medication from the chemist and doctor.

Note
- For babies, see **Eye problems – sticky eyes in infants**.

Constipation

Constipation indicates a difficulty or delay in passing a stool. It is a myth that it is necessary to pass a stool every day. Some people may pass anything from three to five stools a day, while others may only have only one stool each week. It is certainly not unusual to pass only two stools each week and this would not be described as constipation. Constipation has a good outlook and is only very rarely a sign of more serious disease. A change of the pattern of regular stools from your normal habit is of more concern than a brief episode of constipation owing to the causes below. If you do notice an unexplained change, particularly if you are middle-aged or elderly, it is advisable to see the doctor.

Symptoms
* Pressure and distension in the tummy.
* Discomfort and pain. This can be colicky, i.e. coming and going in waves.
* Tiredness sometimes develops.
* Stools, when they are passed, tend to be small and hard. They may resemble rabbit pellets.
* Breast-fed babies are not necessarily constipated if they pass no stool; they normally digest and absorb all the breast milk they are given. The stools of breast-fed babies may range from an appearance of frothy milk shakes to normal firm stools.
* There may be what is called over-flow diarrhoea if constipation is severe. In this case such a blockage has occurred that only liquid stool can ooze out.

Causes
- Lack of fluids and roughage in the diet causes constipation.
- Over-strong artificial feeds may cause constipation in babies. Breast-fed babies do not get constipation but may pass very infrequent stools (see above).
- Illness may lead to constipation – through fever and fluid loss, coupled with poor diet, for example. It is also common in bedridden patients and the terminally ill.
- Pregnancy has an effect on the intestines and constipation is common.
- Piles, either occurring in pregnancy or at other times, lead to constipation (see **Piles**). This is because of the discomfort of passing a stool. Straining to pass a hard stool may exacerbate the piles.
- Anal fissures may also cause constipation because it is painful to pass a stool (see **Piles**).
- Drugs, particularly painkillers and iron tablets, are a common cause of constipation.
- Emotional troubles can lead to constipation. This is more common in children; there may be a fear of sitting on school toilets, or worries

about 'parts of the body falling out'. A battle may develop over the child's ability to produce a stool as the child moves towards independence or seeks attention. This is more common if toilet-training has taken place early, or there have been many battles over it.

☐ Rarely, in infants there is an abnormality of the intestine which allows it to become grossly distended with stool, and little or no stool is passed. This is called Hirschsprung's disease. Usually the child is unwell and a doctor should be consulted.

Prevention
- Fluids should be taken, particularly if there is fever, you are travelling, working in a hot environment or sweating a lot.
- Roughage in the diet is important, e.g. fresh fruit and vegetables, bran cereals, wholemeal bread.

Treatment
- Laxatives are one of the most commonly taken medicines. It is important that these are not taken regularly unless on your doctor's advice. Incorrect or over use can lead to a lazy bowel and even worse constipation.
- A change in your pattern of going to the toilet should lead to your seeing the doctor.
- If constipation is severe or very troublesome, not responding to fluids and increased roughage, see the doctor.

The Doctor
- The doctor may prescribe one of several different types of medicine to help the problem:
  - medicines that increase the size of the stool, stimulating the gut to contract and push out the stool, e.g. methylcellulose or ispaghula husk granules
  - stimulant drugs that make the gut contract more, e.g. senna or bisacodyl; these should not be used repeatedly as they can adversely affect the gut if used excessively
  - medicines that soften the stool, making it easier to pass, e.g. lactulose
- The doctor may prescribe suppositories or an enema to clear severe constipation. You may then need to use one of the above medicines, combined with increased fluids and roughage, to prevent the problem recurring.

Convulsions, febrile

This refers to the convulsions many children experience due to a raised temperature. Seeing your own child in the middle of a convulsion is one of the most frightening experiences for any parent. Fortunately, the vast majority of children suffering a febrile convulsion suffer no harm. If there are repeated or prolonged fits the risk of harm increases.

The tendency to have febrile convulsions does run in families, but any child under about five years old is at risk of having a fit if their temperature is not controlled. After a first convulsion immediate steps should be taken to lower the fever, and all children should be seen by the doctor. About a third of children having a febrile convulsion go on to have further febrile convulsions when they have fever on another occasion.

Symptoms
* The convulsion generally takes place soon after the first rise of temperature.
* The child becomes unconscious.
* Arms and legs go stiff momentarily before starting to twitch and jerk in rhythmic movements. The face may also twitch.

* The movements are often violent.
* The fit usually lasts less than five minutes.
* Urine and faeces may be passed during the fit.
* Consciousness is slowly regained over the next three or four minutes. There may be irritability, headache and drowsiness.
* The fit is often followed by a period of sleep. The child is all right on waking, other than continued symptoms of the illness causing the fever.

Causes
- Fever causes febrile convulsions.
- Epilepsy is more likely to be an explanation if fits are recurrent or if they occur in the absence of fever. Other rare causes of fits are mentioned below.
- A child's brain is still developing, and it is thought that this makes it more sensitive to disturbances than that of an adult.

Prevention
- Lowering the fever early in an infection is particularly important as it is often in the early stages of fever that fits occur.
- For methods of lowering temperature, see **Temperature**.
- If there has been a previous febrile convulsion it is even more essential to lower the child's temperature to avoid further convulsions.

Treatment
- Prevent injury to the child by removing nearby dangers. Do not restrain the child, and there is no need to force anything between the teeth.
- Avoid inhalation of vomit by lying the child on his side with the head lower than the body.
- The fit usually passes off within five minutes. If the fit appears prolonged call an ambulance to get the child to hospital immediately.
- One fit in the presence of a fever does not necessarily require hospital admission or any treatment beyond lowering the temperature. The doctor should, however, be consulted to establish the cause of the fever, if this is not already clear. The doctor should always be consulted when the first fit due to fever occurs.

The Doctor
- Immediate treatment for a prolonged fit may be given by the doctor by injection of a drug called diazepam into the child's vein. Alternatively, a solution of the same drug can now be given into the back passage. Injections into the muscles tend to be slower to have an effect.
- Will identify the reason for the fever and commence treatment, if not already done.
- Whether the child should be admitted to hospital will be decided partly on the basis of the length and severity of the convulsion. If there is a possibility of meningitis, or the cause of the fever is not clear, hospital admission may be required.
- Much less common conditions which may cause fits will be considered, such as: brain tumour, low blood sugar, head injury, poisoning with drugs or lead, brain inflammation, or raised blood pressure.
- Investigations in hospital for fits will include blood tests, X-rays, recordings of the brain's electrical activity called EEG, and possibly a CAT scan (see **Epilepsy**).
- Children with febrile convulsions do not normally need to take medicine to prevent further convulsions. This will, however, be considered if:
  - the febrile fit occurs under one year of age

- there is a family history of epilepsy
- there is evidence of nerve damage either before or after the fit
- if the fit is particularly prolonged or localised to one part of the body
• The medicine given to prevent fits with fever is called phenobarbitone. Although it is effective, there may be problems with side-effects including irritability and hyperactivity. The medicine, if started, is normally continued for around two years and for one year after the last fit has occurred.

Corns

Corns are extremely common. They are small hardened areas, generally on the toes. Larger areas on the foot which are caused by a similar process are called calluses. They do not normally cause a lot of trouble and doctors are rarely consulted about them. They are harmless, unless you have other foot problems which impair the circulation, such as diabetes. They are not infectious.

Symptoms
* Area painful on pressure.
* Absence of black dots or splinters, which are signs of a wart. (See **Warts, Verrucas**.)

Causes
□ Pressure.
□ New or ill-fitting shoes.
□ People with 'bony' feet, and therefore less soft padding around the foot, are more prone to corns.

Treatment
• Comfortable shoes may lead to a previously painful corn disappearing.
• Corn plasters ease pressure and pain.
• Softening agents are available from chemists which can make it easier to file away the corn carefully.

• Chiropodists can help to pad a corn for for comfort and to cut it away correctly.

Cough

Coughing is a protective mechanism to keep our lungs clear for breathing. Any substances entering our air passages, from nose discharge to peanuts, will produce a coughing reaction in order to guard against damage to the lungs. In various illnesses coughing can be persistent and troublesome. Often it is not at all serious and will clear of its own accord as symptoms improve; on other occasions a worsening or persistent cough can be a sign of lung cancer or TB. It is much more common in childhood.

Symptoms
* Dry cough.
* Wet cough.
* Wheezy cough.
* Associated fever and flu symptoms.
* Aching chest.
* Painful tummy muscles.
* Runny nose.
* Other symptoms of more severe disease such as TB or cancer.

Causes
□ A dry cough is usually associated with colds, and is unimportant unless persistent or worsening.
□ A wet or productive cough can be more important, particularly if you are unwell and have fever. If it persists after antibiotics, an X-ray may be necessary. Associated with acute and chronic bronchitis, pneumonia, TB, cancer.
□ Wheezy cough: a spasm of the airways leads to wheeze and cough. This may be episodic and worse at night. It may indicate asthma. (See **Asthma**.)
□ Fumes from chemicals or cigarettes, both your own and others', can cause coughing.

- ☐ Inhaled dust or larger foreign bodies such as biscuit crumbs trigger coughing.
- ☐ Laryngitis produces secretions that irritate the airway, causing coughing.
- ☐ (See also **Whooping cough**.)

Treatment

- Propping a child up with pillows so nasal secretions don't trickle downwards to irritate and cause coughing.
- Blowing the nose is a much forgotten and underestimated way of clearing the upper air passages so less can trickle downwards and cause coughing. Useful at night when a child wakes coughing.
- Hot drinks moisten the air and help to decongest air passages.
- Steam inhalation can clear airways of sticky mucous and decrease coughing.
- Paracetamol or aspirin can help fever and flu symptoms.
- Pharmacists can often advise.
- Cough suppressants generally consist of one or more of the following types of medicine (their effect is variable):
  - antihistamines – decrease allergic and inflammatory reactions
  - antispasmodics – relax the airways and help breathing
  - sedatives – suppress the cough reflex; not always helpful, as nasal discharge is better out than in

The Doctor

- If after three to four days a cough is persistent and not improving the doctor may advise antibiotics after checking your chest for any obvious signs of specific problems such as pneumonia or bronchitis.
- Antibiotics are not always given, and more importantly do not always work, because the infections causing coughs are commonly viral.
- May measure how your lungs are working. Using a peak-flow meter, it is possible to gauge whether your lungs are in spasm and 'tight'. If your flow of air, breathing out, is limited you score poorly blowing into the meter. This can be an indication of asthma.
- May advise an X-ray if he considers the cough could be an indication of a more serious illness which antibiotics either cannot, or have not as yet, managed to treat.
- May suggest codeine linctus, which is one of the more effective cough suppressants but, because it does suppress the cough, should be used only with advice in case it allows more germs to enter the lungs by suppressing the cough.
- Generally doctors have little faith in cough mixtures available over the counter, knowing there is little evidence to show they are effective. However, they often give them to their children . . .

Crabs

Pubic lice are also called crabs as their shape is similar to that of a crab. They are tiny 2mm-long brown or white insects with little claws at the front. They live by sucking blood, and lay eggs which stick firmly to the pubic hair. The eggs can be seen with the naked eye and ordinary washing does not remove them.

Symptoms

* Itching, often very intense and most unpleasant.
* Sores and scabs follow the scratching and may be severe as infection sets in.

Causes

- ☐ Lice are usually transferred during sexual intercourse.

- Time interval between catching crabs and itching developing may be as long as three to four weeks. It may take this long for the lice to breed in sufficient numbers to cause symptoms.
- Crabs can also be caught from infested clothing and bedding which has been recently infested.

Treatment
- Lotions are available from chemists; follow instructions carefully.

The Doctor
- It is usually advisable to see the doctor to ensure effective treatment. He is best placed to advise on choice of lotion and/or shampoo.
- May check for other sexually transmitted diseases.

Cradle cap

This term refers to brownish-yellow scales on a baby's head, which can be very closely stuck to the scalp. It can vary from a dandruff-like appearance to a thick carpet of light, brownish-yellow scales which join together. It can look as if a thick paste has been smeared on the head and left to dry. It is very common in babies, but much older children can have thick scaly patches on their scalp which need the same treatment. It is never serious and always responds to treatment, usually in a few days.

Symptoms
* Flaky scalp.
* Scales, looking rather like splattered dried yoghurt.
* Red spots around edges of 'cap' area.
* If it becomes weeping, red and more widespread it can spread on to face and neck. This is known as seborrhoeic eczema.

Treatment
- Regular shampooing at least daily. Oil the scalp, starting with olive oil applied four times daily before shampooing. Arachis oil from the chemist can also be effective.
- These measures often loosen and soften the scales to allow gentle rubbing with a towel to remove scales. Do not be afraid of the soft spot. (See **Soft spot**.)
- Repeated, frequent applications and shampooing may be required.

The Doctor
- If the above has not solved the problem your doctor may advise:
  - a cream, such as aqueous cream, containing 1% sulphur and 1% salicylic acid; apply at night and shampoo off in the morning
  - a stronger shampoo, e.g. containing 1% cetrimide

Cramp

Most people experience cramp from time to time, caused by the muscles going into spasm. It is most commonly felt in the calf muscles of the legs. Elderly people are usually more severely affected. It is not serious and normally lasts for a few minutes only. The severity of the pain is sometimes extremely distressing, particularly as it may occur in the middle of the night. Cramps may occur in the legs on walking, if there is poor circulation of blood to the muscles.

Symptoms
* Sudden onset, passing off quickly.
* Muscle affected feels hard and cannot be used effectively.
* Pain is severe and unrelenting until the spasm wears off.

Causes
- Most cramps are not serious, and

exactly why they occur is never clear.
- Cramp may also occur after exercise has subjected a muscle to more work than it is able to cope with, or has strained it.
- Sitting or lying in an awkward position can also cause cramp.
- Prolonged sitting or standing without movement may lead to cramp.
- Elderly people may be more liable to cramp because their muscles are not exercised so frequently.
- If the cramp occurs on walking you may have a narrowing of the blood vessels supplying the muscles of the legs. This is caused by arteriosclerosis (see **Angina**) and is made worse by smoking. This leg cramp is called claudication by doctors.

Prevention
- Raising the foot of the bed by four inches is reported to help some people with night cramps.
- Some people drink hot milky drinks before going to bed to prevent night cramps. Exactly why this should have an effect is not at all clear.
- The variety of remedies for preventing a cramp reflects the little understanding there is of why a cramp should occur.

Treatment
- Massaging the affected muscle may help.
- Stretching the muscle, for example standing on the ball of your foot or pressing hard down on it, may help. You can also stretch the calf muscle by sitting on the floor with legs straight and pulling up on the toes and front of the foot.
- If cramps are persistent or very troublesome see your doctor.

The Doctor
- Usually there is no obvious cause.
- If night cramps are the problem the doctor may prescribe a drug called quinine sulphate to try and reduce the frequency of attacks. This is usually taken each night for seven to ten days, then stopped for a time. It may, however, be necessary to take it continually. It is dangerous if too much is taken and, as with any drugs, should be kept well away from children.
- By making an examination of the pulses in the blood vessels of the legs, and by checking the appearance of the skin of the legs, the doctor may discover if there is narrowing of the blood vessels affecting the circulation (see above).
- If there is blood-vessel narrowing this can be confirmed by a special X-ray examination when a substance is injected into the blood vessels so they show up clearly under X-ray. An operation can then replace narrowed blood vessels with synthetic pipes, or narrowings can be cleared by the passage of an instrument down the blood vessel. It is essential to stop smoking, which causes further narrowing of blood vessels.

Croup

This is a term doctors use to describe hoarseness, barking cough and noisy, strained inward-breathing. This group of symptoms has been given a special name because it is a particular combination which is very common in children. Typically, a child between six months and five years old who has had a cold for a day or two wakes with an alarming, noisy sound on breathing and a violent cough. The noisy breathing usually subsides over a few hours but occasionally goes on to cause more difficulty with breathing, and hospital admission may be necessary.

Symptoms
* Creaking noise, worse on breathing in.
* Hoarseness.
* Cough.
* Symptoms of a cold.

Causes
☐ Croup is a viral infection of the larynx. In older children it would be described as laryngitis.
☐ Much less commonly, inhaling a foreign body such as a peanut can cause croup. See a doctor at once if this is suspected.

Treatment
- Try not to add to the child's alarm by revealing your own. Distress will only make the child's breathing worse and the noise more marked.
- Immediately create a steamy atmosphere so that the child breathes moist air
  - run a bath or shower
  - leave a kettle boiling with the lid off to fill the room with steam

The Doctor
- If there is high fever, and especially if the child does not improve with steamy air, call the doctor while keeping the child in a steamy room with you.
- The doctor may prescribe antibiotics if there is an associated ear or chest infection, but usually croup is caused by a viral infection so antibiotics are not always given.
- If the breathing difficulty is not controlled it may be necessary to admit the child briefly to hospital for oxygen and the use of a 'steam tent'. Very rarely, a tube needs to be passed down the wind pipe to help breathing.
- If there is a sudden deterioration, with the child becoming bluish or grey, call an ambulance immediately.

Cuts

The bleeding seen when you have a cut actually helps to clean the wound. The natural process of healing starts with the bleeding, the blood then clots, a scab forms and healing continues. Nature heals well, and interfering with cuts as little as possible is a good rule. Ointments or creams prevent air getting to the wound and often hinder healing. If a cut is clean and the edges are not gaping a protective dressing is usually all that is required. Dirty cuts need more attention but, once clean, healing should be left to take place undisturbed.

Specific points on cuts and grazes
- Stitches are usually required where a wound is gaping. Special thin strips of adhesive dressing are now widely used on small wounds, and may avoid the need for stitches. If a wound gapes it will cause much worse scarring than if the edges are closely aligned.
- Dirty cuts must be cleaned. Running water, and lots of it, is usually best. Pick grit and dirt out if necessary; if left in a wound they will leave stained scarring which can be very ugly. Dirt is also likely to cause infection.
- Facial cuts bleed a lot due to the skin being tightly pulled over the face and a good blood supply. Cuts to face and head are often dramatic. See a doctor to see if stitching is necessary, as scars can be greatly reduced by good positioning of the cut edges.
- Never leave dirt in a graze on the face, or pigmented, stained scars will appear.
- Puncture wounds, such as a needle prick, often don't bleed very much. This causes more risk of infection, particularly as air cannot reach the wound. Do not hesitate to make the

wound bleed if you can. Watch for swelling, pain or redness developing, which may point to a need for antibiotics.

Treatment
- Bleeding from grazes usually stops by itself.
- Bleeding that does not stop by itself can be stopped by pressure. A clean dressing or handkerchief applied firmly is usually sufficient. If bleeding continues despite pressure, do not remove the wet dressing but apply another on top, more pressure and seek help.
- Blood normally clots in around six minutes. Do not stop pressing too soon.
- Cleaning the wound is best done under running water.
- Apply a clean dressing over the top, only if necessary to protect from dirt or further injury.
- Leave grazes open to the air if possible.
- Allow air on to all wounds. Taking off a protective plaster at night can often promote healing.
- If a cut has a complicated dressing on it and no signs of infection, leave it alone rather than peel off the healing tissue every day.

The Doctor
- It is not usually necessary to see the doctor for attention to cuts and grazes.
- He can give advice on the need for stitches and provide antibiotics for infection if necessary.
- He will advise on tetanus prevention, which should be given for any cuts or grazes:
  - as a course of three injections if there is inadequate previous immunisation against this illness
  - as a booster injection if it is more than ten years since your last tetanus injection
  - you should have a booster injection every ten years to keep up your protection

Cystitis

This is an inflammation of the inside of the bladder. Normally we are not aware of urine sitting in the bladder, but in cystitis the lining of the bladder is angry and produces a variety of symptoms to let us know that it is irritable. More than half of all women experience cystitis at some time; some are troubled with it recurrently. It is not usually serious, clearing up with self-help measures or with treatment from the doctor if persisting. Men are not usually affected as their urine passage is situated further away from their back passage, which is a common source of germs.

Symptoms
* Feeling that you need to pass urine often.
* Feeling of burning or scalding as the urine is passed.
* Feeling that you are bursting to go, but very little comes out.
* A need to rush to the loo to avoid urine passing without control.
* A dull ache in the lower tummy after passing urine and sometimes persisting.
* Fever.
* Backache.
* Cloudy, smelly or bloodstained urine.

Causes
- Germs. There are normally no germs in the bladder or in the urine passage. If germs get into the urine from outside they grow rapidly and irritate the lining of the bladder, leading to symptoms of cystitis and urine infection.

- Germs enter as a result of contact with the urine-passage opening through:
  - wiping your bottom from back to front (should always be the other way round)
  - inserting tampons
  - sexual intercourse
  - tight trousers can lead to friction, which introduces germs in much the same way as can happen during sexual intercourse (see also **Thrush**)
- Sensitive bladders: undoubtedly some people have a tendency to develop cystitis easily; exactly why is often not clear.
- Other factors that can cause cystitis are given below when we look at measures that can be taken to prevent it.

Prevention
- Wipe your bottom from front to back, helping to prevent germs spreading from the back passage.
- Wash the genital area twice daily.
- Drinking plenty of liquids (see below).
- Don't hold on to your urine for ages – go when you feel the need. Stagnant urine sitting in the bladder is a lovely breeding ground for germs.
- Passing urine after intercourse can flush out germs.
- Using a lubricant during intercourse can prevent bruising the urine passage, which can sometimes set off an attack of cystitis (see **Thrush**).
- Wear loose clothing, preferably cotton, so the clothes allow your skin to breathe.
- Avoid too much coffee or alcohol if you find these start cystitis attacks.
- Avoid antiseptics, disinfectants (never put these in the bath), perfumed soaps, bubble baths and deodorants. All these can sensitise your urine passage and lead to cystitis symptoms.

Treatment
- At the first sign of symptoms drink plenty. A guide is one pint immediately, then half to one pint every twenty minutes for at least three to four hours – or longer if you can manage it! This may seem a lot, but it is a very important means of flushing out the germs and is often enough to stop an attack developing after the first symptoms.
- Simple painkillers such as aspirin or paracetamol, taken early, can often ease discomfort.
- Hot-water bottles wrapped in cloth or towels placed behind the back and between the legs can be helpful.
- Bicarbonate of soda taken as one teaspoon in a tumbler of water makes the urine less acid, and thus less irritating to the angry bladder lining. Do not take repeatedly, particularly if you are on other tablets, without consulting your doctor.
- Potassium citrate mixture is available from chemists or on prescription and may be similarly helpful.

The Doctor
Despite drinking so much that you are never out of the loo, you may have to seek a doctor's advice.
- He will take a urine sample to look for germs causing cystitis symptoms.
- He may prescribe an antibiotic to clear the germs.
- It is important that the urine sample is taken before any antibiotics are taken as only a small amount of antibiotic can make it impossible to test the urine properly.
- The urine test is important as there are many different germs, and different antibiotics are sometimes needed for unusual germs. The test can

identify exactly what type of germ is causing your problem.
- If you have symptoms of cystitis following intercourse, particularly with a new partner, the doctor may advise a swab test taken from the vagina. Germs passed from one person to another during intercourse can cause cystitis symptoms (see **NSU**, **Pelvic infection**).
- (See also **Urine infection**.)

Deafness

Being born deaf is comparatively rare, though most people have hearing difficulties at some stage in their lives. The commonest ages at which problems with hearing occur are during childhood and in later life. There are two main types of hearing difficulty leading to partial or total deafness. Conductive deafness refers to the inability of sounds to reach the inside of the ear. Nerve deafness occurs when the sounds reach the ear satisfactorily, but the message created by the noise is not adequately transmitted to the brain.

Symptoms
* In children symptoms of hearing difficulty may include:
    - speech problems
    - behaviour problems
    - slow development
    - lack of response
* In adults hearing difficulty can lead to accidents. Deafness may add to confusion. It may lead to frustration and anger as people mistakenly consider a deaf person to be stupid or bad-tempered. See below for how to help those who have difficulty hearing.

Causes
Conductive deafness
☐ Wax blocking the ear canal.
☐ Infection in the ear.
☐ Foreign body in the ear.
☐ Glue ear.
(The above problems are considered separately in the section on ear problems.)
☐ Otosclerosis – one of the tiny bones on the inside of the eardrum becomes fixed instead of vibrating. Normally the movement of this bone transmits messages to the inner ear for onward transmission to the brain.

Nerve deafness
☐ May be present at birth.
☐ German measles in pregnancy may cause deafness. (*See* **German measles**.)
☐ Brain injury at birth can cause deafness.
☐ Meningitis can affect hearing permanently. (See **Meningitis**.)
☐ Exposure to noise. Prolonged periods of exposure to loud noise, especially high-pitched noise, damages the ear and its nerves.
☐ In old age there is frequently a deterioration in hearing, due to less efficient transmission of sounds to the brain.

Treatment
- Conductive deafness can often be helped by treatment of infection or insertion of grommets for glue ear (see **Ear problems**). Otosclerosis can sometimes be treated by an operation to replace the little bone that has become fixed and is blocking conduction of sound. There is a small risk of total deafness from this operation. A hearing aid may help partial deafness from otosclerosis.
- Use of a hearing aid can often help nerve deafness. Unless hearing loss is complete, it can be used to amplify the sounds reaching the ear. This is not always as effective as it might appear. Sound is distorted by a hearing aid and background noise can be a great problem. Hearing aids

may be helpful in a carpeted room but hopeless in a busy public place.
- Nerve deafness may be complete from birth and no help can be given using hearing aids. Being deaf does not affect intelligence and many deaf people learn to lip-read and use sign language in order to lead a full and normal life.
- For both the totally deaf and partially deaf the following advice may be helpful.

How to help the deaf
- To help lipreading:
  - face the deaf person clearly
  - make sure the light is bright
  - no cigarettes, pipes or pencils in the mouth while talking
  - move your lips clearly, articulating each word more slowly than usual; raise your voice slightly
  - remember – no other activities can be carried out while the deaf are trying to lipread; everything has to stop to enable them to concentrate on what you are saying
  - don't hold anything up in front of your face
  - use gestures while talking
- It is usually easier for deaf people to avoid noisy functions or public meetings where their disability is going to appear worse.
- Even if using a hearing aid, a deaf person needs to lipread, too, in order to comprehend fully.
- Remember the deaf may not be able to tell where the dog is, if the door bell rings, whether someone is approaching them from behind, or if the kettle is boiling.
- Always have pen and paper ready so repeated attempts to say difficult things can be avoided.

☎ British Deaf Association, 38 Victoria Place, Carlisle, Cumbria CA1 1HU. Tel: 0228 48844.

☎ British Association of the Hard of Hearing, 7–11 Armstrong Road, London W3 7JL. Tel: 081 743 1110.

☎ Royal National Institute for the Deaf, 105 Gower Street, London WC1E 6AH. Tel: 071 387 8033 (voice), 071 388 6038 (Qwerty).

Dementia

There are two main kinds of dementia. One is called senile dementia and occurs in the elderly; the other is called pre-senile dementia, or Alzheimer's disease, and occurs in people well under sixty years of age (see below). This article is primarily about senile dementia, which is extremely common and can affect any elderly person. It is rare under sixty-five years of age. The main characteristics are a tendency towards being forgetful, confused and out of touch with reality. This dementia has a slow onset and is not caused by any underlying treatable problem. The older people become the more likely they are to develop senile dementia.

Symptoms
* Loss of memory; this particularly affects memory of recent events. Details covered in the first part of a visit to someone with dementia may be forgotten by the end of the visit. The whole visit may be forgotten by the evening and you may receive a phone call asking why you haven't visited. Past events may be recalled with total clarity.
* Reasoning and understanding may diminish over a period of months.
* There is a gradual loss of interest in usual activities, friends, and in watching television or keeping up with events.
* There may be considerable personality change, sometimes involving emotional and physical instability.

* There may be uninhibited behaviour, which sometimes becomes anti-social.
* There is a general deterioration in personal hygiene, nourishment and well-being. Incontinence may occur.

Causes
- Wasting of the brain cells, which cannot be replaced.
- Hardening and narrowing of the arteries to the brain.
- Symptoms may be made worse by hearing or visual difficulties.
- Other causes of confusion may lead to symptoms similar to dementia. In these instances, however, the onset is usually more rapid and treatment can alleviate symptoms. (See **Confusion**.)
- Dementia symptoms may also be seen in depression, long-standing alcohol abuse, vitamin deficiency, thyroid illness, syphilis or brain trouble, for example caused by a tumour or bleeding following a head injury. Treatment of these problems often leads to an improvement in symptoms.

Treatment
- True senile dementia not caused by an underlying treatable disorder is progressive and incurable.
- Anyone suffering symptoms of dementia should be checked by a doctor to exclude any treatable causes.
- There is considerable risk of accidents in the home, and when out and about, for someone with dementia. Common sources of accidents are cookers, electrical appliances, fires, kitchen tools and medicines. Neglect may lead to ill-health and exacerbate the problems of incontinence.
- It is advisable for anyone with dementia to have their name and address clearly marked on a coat, handbag or bracelet perhaps. It is not uncommon for people with dementia to forget their way back home or even where they parked the car. (It is not advisable for people with dementia to drive or operate machinery if this can be avoided.)

The Doctor
- The family doctor is often in a good position to evaluate to what extent someone has begun to be affected by dementia. The slow, insidious onset of dementia may have been noted during visits, and reflected in difficulties managing medicines or housework.
- The doctor will look for a treatable cause and may be able to advise on ways of helping, such as preparation of lists, building up a routine and ensuring food and warmth.
- People with dementia generally do better at home in familiar surroundings. It may be possible to arrange a regular home help or meals-on-wheels service. Attendance at a day centre for the elderly is often very beneficial in creating a routine and provides supervision, companionship and a satisfactory diet.
- If necessary the help of a doctor specialising in the treatment of the elderly will be arranged. The hospital may agree to admit an elderly person for a short stay while relations involved in care take a holiday.
- In the long term, the best interests of the elderly person may be served by admission to a home or hospital. While often regretted, it may be the only way of managing the increasing problems caused by the dementia, and providing sufficient care and attention.

Pre-senile dementia or Alzheimer's disease

This is an illness affecting people well under sixty years of age which causes rapid deterioration of mental functioning. The capacity to think clearly, as well as respond with appropriate emotions, is lost. Unlike senile dementia, which progresses slowly and insidiously, this type of dementia tends to progress rapidly. Death may occur within five years.

As when any symptoms of confusion or dementia appear, it is important to exclude any underlying cause. In Alzheimer's disease the cause is not clear and deterioration may be so rapid, and the dangers to the affected person so great, that hospital admission is frequently required.

☎ Alzheimer's Disease Society, 158–160 Balham High Road, London SW12 9BN. Tel: 081 675 6557.

Depression

Most people feel depressed from time to time. The difference between just feeling depressed, and being ill with depression, is that in true depression you cannot lift yourself above it and the depression starts to interfere with your normal life. You may become depressed at any age, but it occurs most frequently around late adolescence, middle age and after retiring. There is a family tendency towards certain types of depression. Doctors distinguish between a reactive depression occurring in certain difficult situations, and an endogenous depression which may occur on its own or be precipitated by an illness. In any severe depressive illness there are chemical changes in the way the brain works, but the type of depression is less important than its effects and any possible treatment.

Symptoms
* Overwhelming feeling of sadness.
* Loss of energy.
* Loss of appetite.
* Loss of interest in sex.
* Sleep disturbance.
* Variation in severity of depression during the day. It may improve in the evening or gradually worsen during the day to make the evenings the worst moment.
* Tendency to lose touch with reality.
* Irrational guilt feelings.
* Hallucinations.
* Agitation and symptoms of anxiety.
* You may become increasingly withdrawn and reluctant to communicate with others.
* Many of these symptoms only occur in severe depression. Early treatment can prevent a more severe depression developing.

Causes
□ Often no obvious cause of depression is found.
□ Events and prolonged stress may cause depression.
□ It may follow childbirth. (See **Baby blues and post-natal depression**.)
□ Drugs can be a cause.
□ Glandular fever, shingles and other illnesses may be followed by depression. Depression is also part of an increasingly recognised problem called post-viral syndrome.
□ Depression may also occur in schizophrenia or mania. (See **Manic-depression, Schizophrenia**.)

Treatment
● It is always important to seek early help if you have persistent feelings of being depressed. Depression does become more severe until it interferes with your normal life.
● Take threats of suicide in others seriously. As many as one in five

people who are seriously depressed may attempt suicide.
- If you consider that someone you know is becoming depressed, try and persuade them to seek medical help. In true depression a change of scene or holiday treat is usually not helpful.

The doctor
- Will consider the type and severity of the depression before starting treatment. Often the way a depression progresses helps to indicate the best kind of treatment.
- Psychotherapy over a number of sessions may help depression, but may have to be combined with drug treatment.
- There are now many different drugs available to help depression. Tricyclic anti-depressants are a group of drugs, including some which may be suited to depression with agitation and anxiety symptoms, or to depression where there is no agitation but you are withdrawn and quiet. Other drugs, such as a group called monoamine-oxidase inhibitors (or MAOI for short), may be particularly good in some special cases. While taking MAOI drugs certain foods have to be avoided.
- The beneficial effect of drugs may take several weeks to appear and the dose may have to be adjusted for the best effect. Any drugs used for depression are dangerous if taken incorrectly or in overdosage.
- Severe depression may require hospital treatment. This usually involves a stay of several weeks. While in hospital there is likely to be individual and group psychotherapy, drug treatment and encouragement to join in activities to help you adjust back to normal living.
- The outlook for depression which is treated is good. Further attacks may, however, occur and treatment should be sought early. Long-term use of drugs can decrease the frequency of attacks.

Winter depression

This is a distinct pattern of depression that occurs over the winter months. It is a true depression with many of the above symptoms which occurs over more than one winter. To be diagnosed as suffering from winter depression certain fixed features to the depression must be noted, such as its natural lifting in the spring or summer and its recurrence. Research in America and at the Maudsley and Charing Cross hospitals in London has shown that exposure to special lamps for several hours a day may be of help. These lamps are very different from sun lamps, which should never be used to attempt treatment of depression.

☎ Samaritans (24-hour confidential free service for the suicidal and despairing. Phone numbers of local branches are listed in the telephone directory.)

Diabetes

Diabetes mellitus is a condition which affects more than a million people in this country. Normally the way you use up sugar is controlled by a hormone called insulin. In diabetes the body has difficulty controlling the amount of sugar in the blood stream, because insulin is either not produced, or produced in inadequate quantities.

There are two main types of diabetes mellitus:

Insulin-dependent diabetes
- Most common in younger people.
- Little or no insulin is produced and insulin injections are required. (Insulin cannot be taken by mouth as it

is not absorbed from the stomach.)
- Diet control helps to keep the sugar level correct.

Non-insulin-dependent diabetes
- More common in middle-aged or older people.
- The amount of insulin is inadequate for the body's needs and the body cannot use sugar correctly.
- More than a third of people with this type of diabetes have a history of the disease in the family.
- Control of the sugar may be possible using diet and tablets. Insulin may be required as the disease progresses.

Symptoms
* Both types of diabetes typically start with symptoms such as:
    - excessive thirst which cannot be satisfied
    - passing large amounts of urine during the night, as well as during the day
    - loss of weight
    - tiredness
    - visual disturbances and pins and needles
    - recurrent skin infections
* Most diabetics using insulin experience the symptoms of too low a blood sugar at some stage. This is called a 'hypo' and must be corrected immediately by taking sugar. Symptoms include:
    - sweating
    - unsteadiness, feeling faint
    - irritability
    - loss of consciousness if the low sugar level is not corrected; emergency medical treatment is then required

Causes
☐ The exact cause of diabetes is unknown.
☐ Genetic and environmental factors, such as eating too much refined sugar, play a part.
☐ Recent research suggests that a viral infection might trigger a problem with the body's own defence system possibly causing diabetes.

Prevention
- Diabetes cannot be prevented.
- Eating a healthy diet low in refined sugars and animal fats, and controlling your weight, will certainly help you if you have diabetes.
- If you have diabetes, maintaining a near-normal sugar level correctly is important in order to prevent long-term complications. The eyes, kidneys, heart and feet are particularly affected.

Treatment
- There is no cure for diabetes but treatment can be effective in maintaining your normal lifestyle.
- Losing weight can have very beneficial effects in non-insulin-dependent patients and may delay the need for tablets or insulin treatment.
- Diet is an essential part of treatment. It is no longer considered necessary for this to be as restrictive as it used to be. Potatoes, pasta and bread are no longer taboo. The most important foods to avoid are sweets, cakes, biscuits and animal fats.
- In non-insulin-dependent diabetes tablets work in one of two ways, either by leading to more insulin production or by increasing the amounts of sugar absorbed by the body. Insulin injections may become necessary.
- In insulin-dependent diabetes insulin is given by injections under the skin. Even children quickly learn to give the injections themselves. The dose can be adjusted according to changes

in sugar level depending on what you eat, exercise and results of quick testing of your blood and urine. Special sticks are dipped in the urine or a drop of blood and change colour according to the amount of sugar present. Doctors and other health workers can inform and advise, but ultimately you are the one who is best able to manage your diabetes.

New developments in insulin treatment include:
- The use of tiny pumps that strap to the body and inject a small amount of insulin continually under the skin.
- Insulin can now be given from a device shaped like a pen, with a needle point. Doses can be easily adjusted and given while travelling or keeping to a busy schedule. This is likely to be very helpful if you have frequently changing insulin requirements.

☎ The British Diabetic Association, 10 Queen Anne Street, London W1M 0BD. Tel: 071 323 1531.

Diarrhoea

In adults
This is when very loose and frequent bowel motions are passed. It is rarely dangerous in adults, but can be infectious. The severity may vary from one or two loose motions to catastrophic explosive trips to the loo with abdominal pain. It generally clears completely with simple measures.

Symptoms
* Loose motions.
* Liquid motions.
* Cramp-like abdominal pain which comes and goes in waves.
* Associated vomiting.
* Sometimes fever.

Causes
- Stress: for example, before examinations people may not infrequently have a bout of diarrhoea.
- Over-indulgence: eating or drinking to excess.
- Travel: changes of diet and drinking habits on trips abroad is one of the commonest causes.
- Infection with bacteria or viruses. This is common in summer when flies spread infection on to uncovered food. Partially cooked or re-heated foods are often culprits.

Treatment
- Stop eating.
- Drink clear fluids, water preferably; if it must have flavouring, *very* dilute fruit juice. This should be continued until diarrhoea stops or improves considerably.
- Eat only when symptoms are greatly improved. Food should then be confined to a starting diet of: boiled rice, boiled chicken, stewed apples (without sugar), bananas and bread.
- Avoid dairy products, coffees, fizzy drinks.
- Medicines for diarrhoea include:
  - kaolin mixture, available without prescription
  - bowel-calmers, such as loperamide they stop the overactive bowel and help reduce the frequency of motions; available without prescription
- Avoid antibiotics, as they may make the condition worse.
- The doctor should be seen if:
  - it persists or becomes increasingly severe despite the above measures after 24–48 hours
  - pain is continuous, not coming and going
  - following a visit to a foreign country you have persistent diarrhoea

- attacks are repeated and/or do not clear completely between attacks.
- there is any blood or slime in the motion
- (See **Gastroenteritis**.)

In babies
- If severe, diarrhoea can be dangerous.
- Consult your doctor.
- Fluids can be lost faster than they can be replaced. Continue giving clear fluids, trying to give more than is lost.
- Continue breast-feeding.
- Watch for fever or vomiting.
- (See **Gastroenteritis in infants**.)

In toddlers and children
- They can become ill quickly, particularly if diarrhoea is accompanied by vomiting.
- Again, it is important to replace more fluid than is lost.
- Consult your doctor if they are not taking adequate fluids or are unwell in other ways.
- Give clear water at first. Sachets, e.g. Dioralyte, available at the chemist or on prescription, are often more acceptable to children and replace the minerals and salts the body requires.
- Stop feeding until condition improves.
- When the child starts to feed, stick to boiled rice, chicken, stewed apples (without sugar), bread and bananas. A mixture of some of these can be quite palatable.
- Don't give sweets and dairy products until symptoms improve.
- Don't give anti-diarrhoea medicines, which can keep the infection in the stomach and make the illness worse.
- Red or black motions should be reported to your doctor at once.
- Diarrhoea can sometimes be a sign of infection elsewhere in children, and complaints of earache or discomfort elsewhere should be taken seriously.
- (See **Gastroenteritis, Gastroenteritis in infants**.)

Dislocation

This term refers to the displacement of a joint, when the two joint surfaces are separated, usually as a result of injury. The separated ends of the adjoining bones break out of their surrounding capsule, which damages the various muscles, ligaments and blood vessels surrounding the joint. Ligaments normally hold the joint firmly together, but if they are weakened or stretched a joint may dislocate recurrently. This is common in the shoulder joint.

No dislocated joint can function properly. There may also be a broken bone near the joint, as the forces necessary to dislocate a joint are often sufficient to cause a fracture. Hip joints can be dislocated at birth (see **Hips**), and are also commonly dislocated when an elderly person falls, perhaps also breaking the thigh bone.

Most dislocated joints can be easily replaced, and return to normal function is usually achieved unless damage to surrounding structures is considerable.

Symptoms
* Misshapen joint.
* Severe pain.
* Swelling.
* Discolouration of skin.
* Loss of movement.
* Numbing or even paralysis, particularly if the vertebrae are dislocated.
* There is an increased likelihood of osteo-arthritis in any joint that has been dislocated. (See **Arthritis**.)

Causes
□ As mentioned above, injury or

accidents are the usual cause of dislocation.
- Also congenital dislocation of the hip. (see **Hips**.)

Treatment
- Some people with recurrent dislocation of the shoulder or jaw learn to replace it themselves. In order to check for damage to surrounding structures a doctor should, however, be consulted.
- Avoid eating and drinking after the injury, as a general anaesthetic may be required to restore the joint.

The Doctor
- The swelling is usually so great that a general anaesthetic may be necessary to replace the joint.
- The joint will then be splinted so it cannot move. This may be left in place for a variable amount of time, depending on the joint involved. It allows healing of the injured structure and helps the swelling to resolve.
- Physiotherapy can be very helpful, and both doctor and physiotherapist should be consulted before normal activities or sports are resumed.
- Recurrent dislocations may be prevented by surgery to the ligaments to tighten up the joint. This is followed by a prolonged period of immobilisation of the affected joint.
- Surgery may be required if moving the bones around under anaesthetic does not restore them satisfactorily to a useful position.

Drug abuse

Drugs may be abused in many different ways, and their effects can vary enormously from person to person. Many people may try a drug once or twice only; fortunately far fewer go on to become addicts. As addiction develops the amount of drug required, and the debilitating effect it causes, increases. Drug abuse occurs more commonly in families where the parents appear to be dependent on tobacco and alcohol. (See also **Glue-sniffing**.)

Symptoms
* Loss of appetite and loss of weight.
* Unpredictable mood changes with bouts of irritability and aggression.
* Schoolwork, hobbies, jobs and even friends may be neglected.
* Longer spells of sleeping or being drowsy.
* Dishonest behaviour, including telling lies, stealing money or valuables.
* General deterioration in appearance, performance and ability to cope.
* Unusual tablets, powders, capsules, tinfoil or syringes may be found around the house.
* Marks or smells on the body may be noted. Puncture marks at the elbow or elsewhere on the arm are signs of drugs being injected into veins.

Causes
- Many different factors may lead to drug abuse. Curiosity, boredom, a desire to experiment, depression, anger and resentment may all play a part.
- What may start as a way of spending spare pocket money may develop into an addiction through finding the company of other addicts exciting or the drug a means of escaping briefly from everyday problems.

Dangers
– Dependence on many drugs develops rapidly. This not only means that more is required to produce the same effect, but also that coming off the drug becomes increasingly difficult. It also becomes more difficult for drug users to recognise their own deterioration as their needs increase.

- Confusion and frightening hallucinations may occur. These may lead to serious or even fatal accidents.
- Mental disorders, sometimes persisting for years and recurring years later, may be brought on or exacerbated by drug abuse.
- Sickness and vomiting may occur.
- Death from using a drug may not only occur from the drug itself, but may also follow inhaling vomit while unconscious.
- Periods may be upset and constipation is common. These symptoms may accompany more serious physical symptoms due to general deterioration.
- Infected sores, abscesses, boils, may occur, particularly after injection of drugs.
- AIDS, hepatitis and other infections may be transmitted through shared-needles and equipment used by addicts.

Prevention

- Avoid making drugs a 'no-go' subject of conversation in your family. Work out your attitudes towards drugs and discuss your feelings before a problem arises. Think about how you would react if your child started to use drugs regularly, or if they just tried them once or twice.
- Make time to talk to your child about what they think of drugs. Try and inform them of the dangers without filling them with exaggerated horror stories. Hearing such tales is likely to be unhelpful; it may make them disbelieving of what you say and more interested in experimenting with drugs.
- Be available and supportive if your child or a friend comes to you with a drug problem. Help them to seek professional help if necessary.

Treatment

- There are now many agencies working to help drug-abuse problems.
- It is best to seek help early rather than allowing what starts as an occasional habit to become an addiction.
- Much can be done, and much depends on the individual's desire to succeed in coming off drugs. There is an enormous sense of personal achievement in ceasing a drug habit. The restoration of pride in oneself and having money and energy for other activities can help in many ways, as well as helping to prevent further drug use.
- Agencies may have a waiting list and it is often necessary to support someone through what may be an extremely difficult and distressing period before the drugs can be reduced under supervision.

The Doctor

- Can discuss a drug abuse problem either with the person concerned or with a relative or friend.
- Will be able to provide addresses and phone numbers of local agencies involved in helping drug abusers.
- May be able to draw up a plan of reduction of a drug and support the drug user as they come off the drug. Often a deal will be made with the drug user to provide specific help if he keeps to his side of the bargain. Failure of such a contract usually indicates a lack of resolve or ability to come off the drug at that time, or in that way.

☎ SCODA (Standing Conference on Drug Abuse), 1–4 Hatton Place, London EC1N 8ND. Tel: 071 430 2341. (Can inform you of local services throughout the country.)

☎ Families Anonymous, Room 8, 650 Holloway Road, London N19 3NU. Tel: 071 281 8889. (Useful for parents of drug users and can provide you with a contact group in your area.)

☎ ACCEPT (Addictions Community Centres for Education, Prevention, Treatment and Research), 724 Fulham Road, London SW6 5SE. Tel: 071 371 7477.

Ear problems

Ear problems considered here are:

Ear ache
Ear wax
Ear-piercing
Ears, protruding (bat ears)
Foreign body in the ear
Glue ear
Infection of the middle ear
Inflammation of the outer ear (canal)

Deafness, tinnitus and vertigo are considered as separate entries.

Ear ache

Ear ache is a very common problem in adults and children. Two frequent causes are infection of the middle ear, and inflammation of the outer ear. Pain may also come from teeth, tonsils, sinuses and jaw.

Symptoms
* The pain may be dull and constant, throbbing or sharp.
* It may affect one or both ears.
* There may be a discharge or deafness.
* Young children may pull, poke or rub the affected ear.

Causes
☐ Ear ache may be caused by a problem in the ear itself:
  – infection of middle ear (see below)
  – inflammation of outer ear (see below)
  – boil in ear canal (see **Boils**)
  – glue ear (see below)
  – shingles can affect the ear
☐ Ache may be felt in the ear but caused by a problem elsewhere:
  – tonsillitis, sinusitis, toothache, laryngitis (see these items under appropriate headings)
  – painful, tense neck muscles
  – pain from the spinal column in the neck

Ear wax

Ear wax is a normal product of the ear canal, and the flow of wax helps keep the canal clean. It is normally unnecessary to remove wax. Attempts to remove wax, or clean inside the ear canal may cause wax to become wedged inside. This can set up a vicious circle, making artificial removal necessary and wax reaccumulate. Hard wax may affect hearing and then it may be removed by drops or syringing. People produce different amounts of wax, some producing very little indeed.

Symptoms
* Wax is normal and usually causes no symptoms.
* Hard, caked wax may interfere with hearing.
* It is more commonly a problem with the elderly.
* You may feel a sensation of the ears being bunged up. This may feel unpleasant, but it is not usually painful. If the wax is pressing on the eardrum, fiddling with a cotton bud may cause earache and even dizziness.

Treatment
● Ear wax is often blamed for unrelated problems. As a consequence there are

often unnecessary demands for its removal.
- The main reason for removal is if it is causing deafness.
- Hard wax must first be softened. This can be done at home with warm oil, e.g. olive oil. Pour several drops or a small spoonful into the problem ear. It can be kept in by applying a small cottonwool ball or pad just at the entrance to the ear canal. Tilt the head on to the other side for a few minutes. Do this two or three times a day for five days.

The Doctor
- Can prescribe ear drops to soften the wax.
- These are used in the same way as described above.
- Once the wax is softened, the ear can be syringed if necessary. Often, softening the wax is sufficient to restore hearing, the wax being removed as it appears at the entrance to the ear canal.

Ear-piercing

Ear-piercing only hurts for a few seconds. It is then important to keep the ears clean, and to wear sleepers to stop the hole closing. The ears may be infected at piercing or later when wearing earrings. The skin may react against the metal of some jewellery. Some serious infections can be caused by ear-piercing, so it is important to visit a reputable clinic.

Symptoms
* For a few days after piercing there is usually some inflammation and discharge.
* Bacterial infection will cause hot, red, painful, swollen earlobes.
* An allergic reaction produces skin which is itchy; there may be crusting and yellow discharge which indicate that an infection may be complicating the allergy.
* Hepatitis B has been spread by contaminated instruments during ear-piercing. The importance of carrying out the procedure correctly is therefore obvious. AIDS could also be spread in this way.

Causes
Problems with ear-piercing may be due to:

□ Bacterial infection caused by *streptococci* and *staphylococci* (see **Boils**).
□ An allergy will be more common in someone who has other allergies, or eczema/dermatitis problems.
□ Nickel is often the cause of such metal allergies.

Prevention
- Ensure that you go to a clinic which properly sterilises its equipment.
- If you are carrying either the hepatitis or AIDS virus, tell the clinician, who may prefer to discard used items.
- Use antiseptic solution or wipes to prevent bacterial infection.
- People who have other allergies should choose pure metal earrings, e.g. gold and silver.

Treatment
- A mild bacterial infection can be treated with locally applied ointments from the chemist.
- Painkillers may also be needed. If symptoms do not settle in five days see the doctor.

The Doctor
- May prescribe antibiotics, and take a swab test.
- Allergic reaction will require a mild steroid cream. Then try gold or low-allergen earrings.

- Do not wear earrings during treatment for infection or allergy.

Ears, protruding (bat ears)

Bat ears is an unpleasant term to describe prominent ears in children which stick out at an angle from the head. At their most extreme the ears may stick out at right angles. Whether minor abnormalities need to be corrected depends largely on the child's and parents' feelings about the appearance. They can be corrected by an operation, which is best performed around the age of four to six. Most people are untroubled by having prominent ears, and may disguise them beneath long hair. There is no effect on hearing, but they may cause emotional upset, especially if a child is teased.

Treatment
- If the problem is severe it is worth while consulting a doctor. Strapping the ears back does not help.

The Doctor
- If the bat ears are very prominent, it may be best to seek early treatment to prevent emotional problems. This should ideally be done before the child goes to school.
- Less severely protruding ears may need correction if either the child or parents want it.
- A plastic surgeon can perform the operation, which is done by removing a small piece of skin and cartilage from behind the ears. The ear is then sewn back to give a normal appearance. The head is covered with protective bandages like a turban until the scar has healed. Normally you are only in hospital one or two days. Any scars are well hidden behind the ears.

Foreign body in the ear

More damage is done to the ear by inexpert attempts to remove an object than is ever usually caused by the object itself. Although a bead, for example, entering a child's ear is very frightening, it can usually be removed without too much difficulty.

Cotton buds or other devices pushed into the ear either to remove wax or a foreign body may:

- push the object further in and make it less accessible
- injure the eardrum
- injure the ear canal which runs from outside the ear up to the eardrum; once injured, irritation and infection may develop.

The Doctor
- Will remove the object either by grasping it with special tweezers under magnified vision, or by using a special suction microscope.
- May prescribe antibiotic eardrops if the ear canal is injured.
- Ear-syringing for wax is not normally necessary in children or adults as the ear is self-cleaning and the wax moves to the outer ear. Here it can be cleaned away easily. Repeated use of cotton buds or ear-syringing may cause more problems than they solve.

Glue ear

This term refers to the build-up of fluid behind the eardrum. The fluid is thick and sticky, hence the name 'glue'. A common problem in children aged two to eight years old, it is often mild and gets better quickly. Glue ear is important because it is a common cause of deafness at a vital age for learning language. It may follow an ear or throat infection. Sometimes the ears have to be drained of the 'glue' by a simple procedure in which a grommet is inserted in the eardrum (see below).

Symptoms
* There may be no symptoms because deafness is easily missed.
* You may notice that your child does not turn as you come into a room. (Not coming when called is usually not caused by deafness!)
* See if your child turns to a bang, clap or more subtle noises, but make sure any movement necessary to make the noise cannot be seen.
* There may be earache which comes and goes.

Causes
- The deafness is caused by thick secretions in the ear.
- These are unseen behind the eardrum.
- They follow a blockage of the tube which leads from the ear into the throat.
- This may happen:
  - when the adenoids are too big
  - after a throat, ear or sinus infection
  - to an infected child after air travel
  - to children with frequent infections
  - to those with cleft palates or Down's syndrome.

Prevention
- Decongestant medicine may help. It is not usually given for ordinary ear infections but can be given to children with an infection who have to travel by air, or to children who are known to be at risk.

The Doctor
- See your doctor if you suspect poor hearing because deafness can delay your child's development.
- Your doctor will perform a simple hearing test.
- The ears will be examined with a special torch.
- The doctor may wait for a few months before starting any treatment, as this condition may clear on its own.
- Decongestant medicines and antibiotics for a few weeks may open the blocked tube.
- You may need to see an ear, nose and throat specialist.
- If the glue in the ear persists it is usually necessary to make a small slit in the eardrums which allows the glue to discharge and be drained off.
- Sometimes grommets are inserted to help keep the ear clear of glue and fluid. These are very small plastic tubes shaped like a thimble. They are placed through the eardrums while the child is under anaesthetic, and left in place for a few months.
- Grommets usually work their own way out over the following six to eighteen months.
- Unless advised by the ear specialist, it is usually best not to place the head under water while grommets are in place. Swimming may still be possible if your specialist gives you the all-clear.
- Tell your doctor that there are grommets in place if eardrops are prescribed.
- The specialist may notice that the adenoids are too large and there may be signs of repeated tonsil infection. In this case the adenoids and/or tonsils may be removed. This is a bigger operation, but the child is often home the next day. (See **Tonsillitis**, **Adenoids**.)

Infection of the middle ear

The term middle ear refers to the part of the ear found behind the eardrum. Looking at the eardrum gives important information about the middle ear. Infection of the middle ear is very common in children, partly because they suffer many throat infections and colds. An episode is usually followed by complete recovery. It may, however, cause a perforation of the eardrum, or glue ear with deafness.

Symptoms
* There is an intense throbbing pain in one or both ears.
* It is a common cause of children waking, screaming.
* It is common at the age of six to twelve months.
* The child is miserable and feverish.
* There is no discharge unless the eardrum perforates, when there is a thick, yellowy-green discharge.
* There is deafness during the episode, which usually clears up quickly unless the child develops glue ear.

Causes
- It usually happens during a head cold. (See **Colds**.)
- It may occur as part of measles or scarlet fever.
- Many different germs, both viruses and bacteria, infect the ears.
- Infection may spread from adenoids or tonsils.

Treatment
- Give paracetamol for the pain and fever.
- A warm cloth applied to the outer ear is soothing.

The Doctor
- Will examine the ears with a torch, looking for red eardrums which are a sign of infection.
- May take a swab test of any discharge.
- Antibiotics are usually prescribed, which will treat bacterial infections but have no effect on viral infections. It is not possible to tell just by looking at the ear whether the infection is viral or bacterial.
- Decongestant nose drops or medicines are sometimes given.
- If the ear infections recur frequently your doctor may refer you to a specialist to consider whether removal of the adenoids might help, or to check for glue ear. (See **Glue ear**.)

Inflammation of the outer ear (canal)

The term outer ear refers to the tube that runs from the side of the head to the eardrum. It is also called the ear canal. Its average length is three-quarters of an inch. Inflammation of the ear canal is commonly seen in adults and children. It causes itchy, painful discharging ears. Despite the unpleasant symptoms, it is not a serious condition and usually clears up quickly. An intense throbbing pain with fever may be caused by a boil in the ear canal (see **Boils**), and is not typical of an ear-canal infection.

Symptoms
* The canal is itchy.
* The whole ear feels painful.
* There may be a clear or yellowy discharge.
* There is no fever.
* There may be deafness, usually due to the accumulation of cells and tissues blocking the ear canal.

* It may hurt to pull on the ear lobe.

Causes
- Commonly follows swimming.
- People with eczema are more often affected than others.
- There is often a combination of inflammation and infection.

Prevention
- Avoid poking objects into the ear, which sets up irritation or causes infection.
- Earwax automatically cleans the ear canal.
- Clean the outside of the ears with towels or cotton buds. Do not poke these into the ear canal. As well as causing irritation, it is possible to perforate the eardrum.
- During treatment keep water out of the ears.
- If you have many attacks, wear a cap to swim or when taking a shower, and be careful when washing hair.

The Doctor
- Your doctor will examine your ears with a torch, and may attempt to clean them. A swab test may be taken.
- Eardrops consisting of a combination of antibiotics and mild steroids are usually prescribed. After inserting the drops, tilt the head to the other side for a few minutes. Alternatively, the doctor may give antibiotics by mouth.
- If the problem is severe or persistent you may need to be seen at hospital, where special suction microscopes are used to clear out the ear canal so eardrops can more easily treat the infected skin.

Eczema

Eczema is an itchy, sore condition of the skin which can blister and look dry, scaly and cracked. It is extremely common, affecting millions of people. Babies and adults can have eczema, but the most common form is seen in children. There are often other members of the family affected. It is not infectious and should not prevent you from leading a normal life. Most children with eczema do improve as they get older. Adults may have long periods when they are clear or less severely affected. People with eczema may develop asthma and commonly suffer hayfever symptoms.

Symptoms
* Blistering of the skin.
* Dry skin.
* Flaking of the skin.
* Cracking of the skin.
* Red, angry areas.
* Crusty, weeping areas (can be a sign of infection).
* Pain and discomfort.
* Soreness in skin creases (where eczema is often first seen or becomes worse).
* Sudden flare-ups of itching and skin irritation on contact with certain things (see below). In adults this is called contact dermatitis.

Causes
- No one knows exactly why eczema appears.
- There are undoubtedly allergic factors that cause eczema to become worse, but these are not necessarily causes of eczema in the first place.
- If you have eczema avoid:
  - biological powders
  - perfumed soaps
  - bubble baths
  - strong chemical cleansers

- tight clothing with rough zips or scratchy buttons
- nylon and other synthetic fibres
- scratchy wool
- feather and horsehair bedding
☐ Dietary factors are sometimes found to aggravate the condition in some people, e.g. eggs, cows' milk, fish, cheese, chicken, wheat, food colourings and preservatives.

Treatment
- There is no cure, but it often improves with time.
- It may be helpful to:
  - use cotton clothes and sheets
  - wear mittens at night
  - wash bedding and clothes regularly
  - rinse clothing very thoroughly after washing
  - keep dust levels down by cleaning regularly
  - not be so keen to look for and avoid aggravating factors that the eczema takes on an exaggerated importance; this can spoil the enjoyment of a pet, or make mealtimes a nightmare, for example
- Moisturing treatments are of prime importance, particularly between flare-ups. Keep the skin moist, lubricated and soft, e.g. using E45, unguentum merck, aqueous cream and emulsifying ointment – useful as a soap substitute in the bath. Oilatum emollient is a softening oil to add to baths.
- Steroids can be used, always starting with weak preparations, e.g. 1% hydrocortisone (available without prescription). Stronger preparations should not be used on the face, and used only with careful attention to instructions.
- It is better to use 1% hydrocortisone generously for a short burst to get the situation under control, than sparingly now and again. When the situation has improved, it can often be controlled by continued use of moisturisers.
- Failure to respond to steroids may be due to another germ infecting the eczema and making it worse. An antibiotic cream or antibiotic/hydrocortisone mixture is then called for. Occasionally tablet antibiotics are necessary.
- Some useful tar-based preparations exist but are, unfortunately, messy.
- Bandages: creams and pastes applied beneath these can often have good effects. Do not use steroid creams in this way, however. Icthopaste bandages applied to legs or arms at night are messy but can be very effective.
- Antihistamines can help reduce itching and help with sleeping.
- Special preparations exist to help with eczema on the scalp, but this can often be kept clear by using Catavlon or Polytar shampoo.

☎ National Eczema Society, 4 Tavistock Place, London WC1H 9RA. Tel: 071 388 4097.

Elbow pain

Repetitive use of the elbow joint or a minor injury may lead to discomfort at the elbow. This has come to be known as tennis elbow, if it occurs on the outside edge of the elbow, and golfer's elbow, if found on the inside. It may have very little to do with either golf or tennis, but the process causing the pain is the same. It is called a tendonitis. Muscles are attached to bones by tendons; if these tendons become inflamed the resulting pain can be severe. Tendonitis is also a cause of pain at the shoulder (see **Shoulder pain**). This type of elbow pain usually settles quickly, but various treatments may be required if it persists.

Other causes of elbow pain include injuries and also bursitis (described under **Elbow, swollen**). Pain felt at the elbow may also in some cases be coming from a problem at the shoulder or neck. (See **Neck problems**.)

Symptoms

* Gradual onset of pain and discomfort.
* There may be acute tenderness on the bony lump on the outside of the elbow, or on the inside. The side affected depends on how the joint has been used.
* A minor pulling injury can produce symptoms which develop more quickly than the usual slow build-up.
* Ability to lift pots and pans is reduced and can become increasingly difficult.
* Pain and difficulty using the elbow may recur after symptoms have ceased.
* Pain may be felt further down the arm.

Causes

- Any chronic or long-term strain to the muscles where they are attached to the bones can lead to the above symptoms of tendonitis.
- Sometimes an injury causes a small tear in the tendon leading to a tendonitis.
- Unaccustomed use of the elbow joint in DIY or sports activities are common causes of tendonitis.
- Working with a lathe can also cause tendonitis at the elbow.

Treatment

- Resting the elbow, with the use of a sling if necessary, is often enough to let the tendonitis settle down. An improvised sling can be made from a scarf; if possible open out a large square scarf so that the elbow is supported as well as the wrist.
- Strapping the elbow and the arm above it is helpful. An elasticated stockinette bandage is available from chemists which slides over the arm. This is both comfortable and convenient.
- Simple painkillers such as aspirin or paracetamol should be taken regularly for maximum effect.
- After a few days' rest, exercise the joint to avoid stiffness. If you are aware of any activities that provoked the pain these should be avoided.
- If symptoms are severe, recurrent or persistent see your doctor.

The Doctor

- May request an X-ray to exclude other bone or joint problems.
- Can provide a stronger painkiller, but before doing so may inject the joint with a steroid and possibly a local anaesthetic. This may initially cause more severe pain but often provides dramatic relief. It can be repeated. (See **Shoulder pain**.)
- Physiotherapy can help to make symptoms settle more quickly.
- In severe cases, not responding to any other treatment, the elbow and upper arm may be put in plaster. This is not often necessary.

Elbow, swollen (olecranon bursa)

An injury may cause swelling around any joint; this may be due to a broken bone, sprain or dislocation, all described elsewhere. Arthritis or infection may also cause swelling, but usually there is pain and other symptoms of the illness. (See

Arthritis.)

A painless swelling often appears at the elbow called an olecranon bursa. This can be quite large and cause considerable concern. If it becomes inflamed it is known as student's elbow. The olecranon is part of one of the bones making up the elbow joint; an olecranon bursa is common in anyone whose elbow presses persistently on a firm surface.

Symptoms

* Swelling appears at the elbow, slightly further up the arm from the joint, when the elbow is bent. It varies in size from around ½–2 inches across.
* It may gradually increase in size.
* It may become tender and painful, in which case there is a bursitis.

Causes

☐ As mentioned above, students or other people whose elbow is pressed for long periods on a firm surface may develop a bursa.
☐ It may also appear without any obvious explanation.
☐ Inflammation causing a bursitis may be caused by increased use or injury.
☐ Bursitis may also cause pain at the shoulder or in bunions. (See **Shoulder pain**, **Bunions**.)
☐ Housemaid's knee is a bursitis which may occur in anyone often working on their knees, e.g. electricians and plumbers.

Treatment

● A painless swelling at the elbow should always be shown to a doctor to exclude other problems which could be more serious than a bursa.
● If the swelling is an olecranon bursa, as described here, many people choose to leave it alone. This is perfectly acceptable.
● If it is troublesome or recurrently inflamed you should see your doctor.

The Doctor

● May refer you to an orthopaedic surgeon if simple measures have not helped.
● If the bursa is troublesome, it is usually best to have it removed by operation, under anaesthetic.

Epilepsy

Epilepsy is the tendency to have repeated fits, convulsions or seizures. Anybody may suffer an occasional fit, as seen with fever in children (see **Convulsions, Febrile**) or following a head injury or brain infection (see **Meningitis**). This is not epilepsy.

Children with epilepsy may suffer fits over a few years which they then grow out of, e.g. *petit mal* or absence seizures. The average length of time during which people suffer epileptic fits is about ten years. People may only suffer from mild epilepsy with an occasional fit. At the other extreme are severe forms which begin in infancy and delay development. Modern treatment can control epilepsy in many people, although some fits may still occur. People tend to be frightened of epilepsy because it is unpredictable, but those affected can usually lead normal lives and go to a normal school.

Symptoms

* The most common type of epileptic fit is the *grand mal* or major type.
* The sufferers suddenly go stiff, lose consciousness and fall to the ground.
* They may cry out as air is suddenly expelled from the lungs.
* The lips may go purple and saliva may come out of the mouth. This looks very worrying, but lasts only a matter of seconds.
* The next phase is repeated jerking of the head, arms and legs. This usually

goes on for two or three minutes.
* After the fit sufferers feel drowsy, with a muzzy head for up to an hour.

Causes

- In most cases there is no obvious cause. The brain is otherwise normal and intelligence is normal.
- Epilepsy which begins early in childhood or in old age is more likely to be brought on by an illness such as a brain tumour.
- There are inherited conditions which cause brain damage. Although epilepsy runs in families, the risk to a new baby if one parent or child is affected is very small.
- There may be damage to a baby from viruses while in the womb.
- Lack of oxygen during birth is called asphyxia and may cause fits.
- Meningitis at any age may be followed by epilepsy. (See **Meningitis**.)
- Brain tumours are rare at all ages, but less so in children and elderly people.
- A stroke is sometimes followed by fits.
- Flickering lights on TV or at a disco can cause some people to have a fit.

Prevention

- Some viral infections can be prevented by vaccination, e.g. measles.
- Good care during childbirth reduces the chances of asphyxia.
- Early treatment of meningitis reduces the chance of brain damage.
- Reduction of high blood pressure reduces the chance of a stroke.
- There are some sensible restrictions designed to protect people with epilepsy from harm:
  - they should only swim if a friend or teacher is nearby
  - they should avoid cycling on a busy road
  - epileptic mothers should have someone around when bathing their babies
  - epileptics can do most jobs, but would be better to avoid scaffolding or dangerous machinery
  - you can get a driving licence if you have not had a fit for two years, or had only fits at night for the last three years
  - you cannot get an HGV or public vehicle licence if you have an attack over the age of five years

Treatment

You may come across someone having a fit. The most important thing is to stop them harming themselves.

- Turn them so they lie halfway between lying on their side and face down, with the head lower than the body. In this position the tongue comes forward and they do not choke. Do not put any hard objects into their mouths. It is common for the tongue to be bitten and, although it bleeds and hurts, it is not serious as it heals quickly. Put a cushion or pillow under the head.
- It is only necessary to get medical help if the fit is prolonged.
- If a fit has lasted for five minutes you should call for urgent help, but a fit lasting less than fifteen minutes is very unlikely to cause brain damage. A mother of an epileptic child may be trained to give medicine in the back passage.

The Doctor

- Can give an injection into a vein or the bottom to stop the fit.
- A specialist opinion from a neurologist may be arranged.
- A brain-wave test called an EEG will be done. This is a painless test which lasts a few minutes. Sometimes a

brain scan called a CAT scan is done.
- The doctor will prescribe drugs to be taken each day to prevent fits. These drugs may have side-effects which must be balanced against their benefit. Side-effects include acne, enlarged gums, and increased body hair. The dose is adjusted according to the results of blood tests. This is especially important in pregnancy or when certain other drugs are given.
- Drugs which interfere with epilepsy drugs include the contraceptive Pill, some antibiotics and cimetidine used in ulcer treatment. Do not suddenly stop taking epilepsy drugs, because this can cause fits.
- There is a very small risk of damage to a baby in early pregnancy from the drugs; this is usually less than the risk from the mother having a fit.
- Breast-feeding is usually quite safe while taking drugs for epilepsy.

☎ British Epilepsy Association, Anstey House, 40 Hanover Square, Leeds LS3 1BE. Tel: 0532 439393.

Episiotomy

An episiotomy is a cut made, normally under local anaesthetic, through part of the skin between the vagina and anus towards the end of childbirth. It is done to protect either your skin or your baby, but should not be done as a routine. The cut allows the head to be born more easily and prevents tearing of the skin. It also allows a quicker delivery when the baby is distressed. A local anaesthetic is given, when needed, before the cut is repaired. Discomfort after the cut may last some weeks but should not be severe. Problems are less likely if the wound is not sewn too tightly and is kept clean.

Reasons for the episiotomy
To prevent tearing of the skin
- A large tear is much harder to repair than a cut.
- There is a risk that the tear may extend into the back passage.
- The midwives can see if the skin is becoming very thin and a cut is needed.
- A cut will be done if there has been bad tearing at a previous delivery.
- A cut is more likely, but not always necessary, when forceps are used.
- The skin is more likely to tear if the baby is born face-up rather than in the more common face-down position.

To protect the baby
- If there are signs that the baby is distressed, a cut may be made to speed up the delivery; similarly, if there is a delay in the delivery and the head is stretching the skin.
- When the baby is very small or premature.
- At breech delivery – when the baby is born bottom first. As well as making this type of delivery easier, it helps to protect the head, which is born after the body.

What is done
- You will need a local anaesthetic (unless you have had an epidural anaesthetic). When the local anaesthetic is injected you will get the same numb, tingly feeling as you would from a dental anaesthetic.
- Usually the cut is made as the skin is stretched. The aim is then to deliver your baby at the next contraction.
- After the baby and afterbirth have been born the cut is repaired. Another injection of local anaesthetic is given. After waiting for this to work, the doctor or midwife will start the repair. Internal stitches, which dissolve, are placed inside the vagina.

The outside skin is then repaired. This can be done with soluble stitches, or ones which have to be removed.

Prevention of problems
- The cut will be examined each day for signs of infection.
- You should have a salt bath each day. Dissolve a handful of salt in the water.
- Change your sanitary towels frequently, several times a day if necessary.
- Contact your midwife or doctor if you have renewed pain or a temperature. If there is a discharge, swabs will be taken and antibiotics started.
- Occasionally the wound is very painful at first. It helps to sit on a bag of ground ice cubes or a rubber ring, frozen peas make a useful icepack (but don't eat them after use). Painkillers will also help.
- You can expect some discomfort for a few weeks, and when you first have intercourse. Lubricating jelly such as KY jelly from the chemist may help.
- You will be examined at your six-week check to see that everything has healed satisfactorily.
- If pain continues, or you cannot have intercourse, see your doctor. It is only extremely rarely that the repair has to be redone.

Eye problems

Eye problems considered here are:

Foreign body in the eye
General swelling of the eyelid
Sticky eyes in infants
Swellings amongst the eyelashes (styes)
Swellings inside the eyelid
Swellings on the skin outside the eye

Cataracts and conjunctivitis are considered as separate entries.

Foreign body in the eye

The importance of any particle touching or resting in the eye is the danger of damage to the eye's delicate surface. A foreign body can very easily scratch the surface, set up infection and impair vision by scarring the eye. If a camera or binocular lens is scratched its use is permanently affected; the same can apply to the eye.

Symptoms
* Watering of the eye.
* Itching.
* Pain.
* Gritty sensation.
* Not wanting to open the eye.
* Speck may be visible on the eye's surface.
* After a few hours redness may develop.
* (See **Conjunctivitis**.)

Causes
- Dust.
- Sand.
- Chemicals.
- Chips from hammering masonry or ironwork without protective goggles.

Treatment
- Avoid rubbing the injured eye, but rubbing the other one will lead to watering of the affected eye which may flush out the object.
- Crying is helpful and this is a good occasion to encourage a child to have a good weep.

Objects
- Using a good light, inspect the eye to see if you can see anything.
- If the foreign body is over the coloured or black part of the eye do not attempt to remove it, as this can scratch the eye and interfere with

vision. See the doctor.
- Pull down the lower lid to look for the particle.
- Pull down the top lid over lower eyelash and let it ride back up; this may dislodge the particle.
- If you can see the particle remove it with a clean tissue or cloth; do this by dabbing gently, avoid rubbing if possible.
- Someone may be able to help you by pulling out the top lid and if necessary bending it over a matchstick to inspect the under side.

Chemicals
- Any chemicals in the eye should immediately be flushed away, using lots of running water. This can best be done lying down with the head on one side pouring water from a jug. It may be necessary to hold the eyelids apart firmly while water is run over the eye.
- Seek advice after any chemical has injured the eye; cover the affected eye and consult a doctor.

The Doctor
- Should be consulted if any particle appears to be embedded in the eye or is not dislodged by the above methods.
- May numb the eye with local-anaesthetic drops and remove the particle.
- May use a coloured stain to reveal any scratches on the eye's surface.
- May prescribe antibiotic drops to treat any infection and cover the eye with a soft bandage.
- May plan to review the eye over the next few days to ensure that healing is taking place.

General swelling of the eyelids

The eye lies in a padding of soft tissue which encircles it. This soft tissue can become infected, causing a dangerous eye problem called orbital cellulitis. It usually only affects one eye. Treatment should be sought immediately, as there is a danger of the infection spreading to cause meningitis.

Symptoms
* Swelling of the eyelids.
* It may be so severe that the eye appears to close, or there may be difficulty in closing it.
* Redness in the eye.
* Fever.
* The eyeball may be pushed forward.
* The symptoms may be similar to those of severe conjunctivitis. (See **Conjunctivitis**.)
* Sometimes pus is visible.

Causes
□ Germs can enter the space around the eye from a nearby infection such as a stye, or from sinusitis. (See **Sinusitis**.)

Treatment
- This should be started as soon as possible with high doses of antibiotics from your doctor.
- Usually the swelling subsides quite quickly and there is no long-term effect on the eye or vision.

Sticky eyes in infants

Most sticky eyes in babies are not serious and clear up very quickly. Some may progress to conjunctivitis if a germ has been picked up either at the time of delivery or subsequently. The importance of sticky eyes lies in distinguishing between the simple condition which will go, the infected eyes that need treatment and the recurrent sticky eyes caused by blocked tear ducts.

Symptoms
* Mild sticky eyes in the morning, not persisting for more than one or two days. Eyes are not red.
* Red inflamed eyes and copious pus; this indicates that conjunctivitis has developed and treatment is necessary.
* If eyes are watery without necessarily being sticky, the tear duct may be blocked.
* Recurrent sticky eyes, often over many months despite treatment.

Causes
☐ Blood or amniotic fluid entering the eye briefly at delivery can set up a reaction leading to sticky eye; this clears easily.
☐ Germs from the vagina can enter the eyes at birth (see **Gonorrhoea**, **NSU**). This may cause severe conjunctivitis, which must be treated.
☐ Blocked tear ducts are a common cause of recurrent sticky or watery eyes.

Treatment
● Mild sticky eyes can be wiped with cottonwool dipped in cooled boiled water. Wipe outwards away from the other eye. This should be done in the morning and repeated during the day as the eyes become sticky. This is often enough to solve the problem.

The Doctor
● Consult the doctor if the eye does not clear on washing, and particularly if it becomes worse.
● He will take a swab to establish the germ, if any, responsible.
● Antibiotic eye drops and ointment will be given. Eye ointment is easier to use and more likely to remain in the eye for longer to treat the infection. Occasionally, antibiotics may be required for severe infections.
● If sticky eyes are a recurrent problem, or the eye is watery, this suggests a blocked tear duct. The doctor will show you how to empty the tear sac, which is below the inner lid at the inner corner of the eye. This can be done easily by massaging this area gently, which dislodges the contents of the sac and will lead to less sticky or watery eyes for the rest of the day.
● The blocked tear duct normally clears itself during the first year of life.
● If the problem persists after the child is one year old, it is usual to see an eye doctor, who will attempt to open the duct by probing under general anaesthetic.
● (See also **Conjunctivitis**.)

Swellings amongst the eyelashes (styes)

A spot like a small boil may appear on the eyelid, in amongst the lashes. This is a stye, which is not serious and usually clears on its own within about seven days. It may be recurrent and can cause considerable discomfort.

Symptoms
* Gradual increase in size of red spot around an eyelash.
* Yellow head appears on the spot.
* Discharges and settles down.
* Vision not affected.

Causes
☐ A bacterial infection at the bottom of an eyelash, in the hair follicle, causes a stye.

□ The process of infection and germs involved are similar to that described for **Boils**.

Treatment
- They usually go on their own.
- They can be brought to a head more quickly by applying hot compresses three or four times daily. Use a large wad of cottonwool soaked in hot water applied directly over stye.
- Pulling the eyelash out when a head appears on the stye releases pus, causing relief.

The Doctor
- May prescribe antibiotics if styes are severe or recurrent.
- Swabs may be taken from the nose to see if you are carrying a particular bacteria which often causes styes. If you are, nose ointment may be given. (See **Boils**.)

Swellings inside the eyelid

This is likely to be a chalazion. Also called a meibomian cyst. These are small, often painless, lumps that appear just beyond the line of lashes on the red, inner surface of the eyelid. They may intermittently become infected, causing pain and swelling.

Symptoms
* Visible swellings or distortion of eyelid.
* It may feel like a small piece of gristle in the eyelid.
* It may reach the size of a pea and press on the eye.
* Swelling and redness when infected.
* They often go on their own.

Causes
□ The inside of the eyelid contains glands which produce a lubricant for the edge of the eyelid. These are called meibomian glands. If the gland is blocked, it swells up and causes the chalazion.

Treatment
- It may be possible by massaging the gland in the direction of the eyelash to make it discharge.
- If it is infected and painful it is usually necessary to see the doctor.

The Doctor
- Will prescribe an antibiotic if there is an infection.
- If the chalazion persists the doctor will arrange for you to have it removed under local anaesthetic in an out-patients clinic. A small cut inside the eyelid allows it to be removed easily.

Swellings on the skin outside the eye

May be:

1. Harmless fleshy pink papilloma.
   - No problem apart from appearance.
   - Can be removed at a small operation with local anaesthetic if required.

2. Yellow fatty lumps called xanthelasma.
   - Flat or slightly raised.
   - May indicate a family problem of high body fats. Ask your doctor to check your lipids by a blood test.

Fainting

A faint is a temporary loss of consciousness. Faints are much more common than more serious causes of collapse, and are especially common in adolescent girls. No treatment is required providing the person does not hurt themselves in the fall.

Symptoms
* You turn pale.
* You may feel sick or dizzy.
* Your vision is affected.
* You fall down.
* The loss of consciousness usually lasts for a few seconds or minutes.
* You are likely to be confused when you come round, but recovery is usually rapid over about five to ten minutes.

Causes
- A simple faint does not mean anything is wrong with the body.
- It is caused by a brief drop in blood flow to the head. This may happen on standing up suddenly after sitting or lying down. It may happen after prolonged standing on parade or in school assembly.
- This is more likely if you have had no breakfast or a very light breakfast.
- Having to wear inappropriately warm clothing on a hot day may be the cause.
- People sometimes faint on standing up after a hot bath.
- An emotional upset or the sight of blood may cause a faint.
- Other important causes of collapsing are:
  - epilepsy (see **Epilepsy**)
  - low blood sugar (see **Diabetes**)
  - kinking of blood vessels in the neck (see **Neck problems**)
  - a minor stroke (see **Stroke**)

Prevention
- Loosen clothing on a hot day.
- Keep wriggling your toes if you have to stand still for a long time. This helps the circulation.
- Do not stand up suddenly if you are prone to fainting.

Treatment
- No treatment is needed if there has been no injury.
- Do not try to keep someone upright if they have fainted. It is important to make them lie down, keeping their head lower than the rest of the body. If possible raise the feet off the ground, e.g. on a chair.

Fibroids

These are benign growths that occur either in the wall of the womb or on stalks inside and outside the womb. There is usually more than one present at any one time. The extent to which they grow and cause problems is variable. Over three years some may only grow to the size of a pea, whereas others reach the size of a tangerine. They are very common indeed, occurring in almost a third of all women over thirty-five. Their size decreases after forty-five years of age.

Symptoms
* Often none, being discovered during a routine check.
* Heavy, prolonged periods.
* Painful periods.
* Pain on intercourse.
* Vaginal discharge.
* Felt as painless lumps in the lower part of the tummy.
* Interference with passing urine.
* Difficulty conceiving.
* Pain in pregnancy when they often grow rapidly but do not normally interfere with the growth of the baby.
* Sudden pain if a fibroid twists on its stalk may lead to admission to hospital.

Causes
- It is not fully understood why fibroids should develop.

The Doctor
- Will watch the growth of the fibroids by regular examinations.
- If symptoms are troublesome may refer you to a gynaecologist.
- The gynaecologist may do a 'scrape' of the womb (also called a D and C) to check for any other diseases of the womb lining.
- Fibroids can be removed surgically. This may be necessary, particularly if they are interfering with conception.
- They can be removed individually or the womb may be removed at hysterectomy taking the fibroids with it.

Flat feet

This expression refers to the position the sole of the foot takes up when you are standing. If you have flat feet the inside edge of the foot will be touching the floor instead of the usual upward curve or arch on this edge. All of us have flat feet at birth, and a toddler walks with what is described as a flat-footed gait. The foot develops as we grow and continues to do so until around sixteen years of age. Although a common worry, the flat feet of an infant usually are normal by six years of age.

Symptoms
* In adults can sometimes lead to foot pain.
* Walking with unusual gait.
* Difficulty running fast.

Causes
- Failure of the arch to develop as a normal part of growth, particularly in the first six years of life.
- Ill-fitting shoes can damage feet and should always be avoided.

Treatment
- Encouraging children to walk barefoot or in socks is thought to help foot development.
- Foot muscles should be made to work, and you could try the following exercises:
  - walking on tip-toes
  - picking up objects with toes
  - using a skipping rope
- Walking on different surfaces without shoes makes the foot work harder. It is harder, for example, to walk barefooted on sand than on a road.
- Foot inserts or adapted shoes should not be worn without a doctor's or foot specialist's advice.

Flu

An infection affecting people of all ages which is caused by a virus lasting anything from twenty-four hours to several days. It is not serious in the young and healthy but can be in the elderly. Those with bronchitis, asthma or heart conditions are particularly at risk. It is infectious like a common cold, being spread by droplets from nose and throat. For babies and young children see **Viral illness**.

Symptoms
* Feeling shivery.
* Aching head.
* Temperature.
* Sweating.
* Loss of appetite.
* Feeling sick.
* Aching joints, limbs and back.
* Cough, sometimes persisting when other symptoms have cleared.

Causes
- There are many different types of flu virus.
- A flu epidemic is usually caused by one virus becoming dominant over all the others.

- Different viruses may produce different symptoms and illnesses of different severity.
- Having had one type of flu, your body develops a defence to that particular virus, but you may catch 'flu' again from a different virus.

Prevention
- This is particularly important for the elderly and those with chest conditions.
- Avoid crowded places if flu is about.
- Avoid others with flu.
- Ask your doctor for advice about flu vaccinations.

Treatment
- There is no magic medicine.
- Antibiotics do not help flu because it is a viral infection. Only your own defence system can clear you of flu, so look after yourself:
  - stay indoors.
  - keep warm
  - take regular aspirin or paracetamol four times a day for aches and pains.
- The simple preparations aspirin BP and paracetamol BP are usually just as effective as more expensive special brands in fancy packaging.
- Rest in bed if you feel shivery or feverish. The same medicine as taken for aches and pains will lower your temperature.
- Avoid too many blankets or clothes, which keep your temperature up.
- Drink plenty. Cool drinks can not only make you feel better but keep you well topped up on body fluids lost in sweating. You are then more able to fight the infection. Four to six pints daily is not unreasonable.
- Do eat well and treat yourself; it all helps to keep up your defences.
- It is usually not necessary to see the doctor unless the symptoms persist for more than four days or you get suddenly worse.
- Many people take vitamins during flu, though there is little evidence to suggest that you recover any more quickly. (See **Vitamin deficiency**.)

Flu vaccination
- Doctors are often not enthusiastic about giving flu vaccination because it only protects against a few different viruses. There are many flu viruses around each winter and the vaccination cannot guarantee to protect you from them all.
- It is only recommended for those especially at risk. As well as those with bronchitis, asthma and heart conditions mentioned above, diabetics and chronic kidney disease patients should be considered. In elderly people's homes and children's homes it may also be given.
- Young, fit people are not normally vaccinated because they will get better immunity by catching the flu. There is no reason why they should not get over flu without serious effects.
- The vaccination itself is not without risk of your having quite a nasty, but short, flu-like reaction to it.
- Vaccination needs to be repeated each year, as new viruses appear and our protection generally only lasts around one year.

Foreign body in the nose

Quite often a bead or piece of cottonwool a child has been playing with gets stuck up the nose. It is usually unhelpful to ask why or how it got there as the distress of having it removed is more than enough to deter a child from doing it again. It is only serious if the object is inhaled, and because this is a real danger medical advice should always be sought.

Symptoms
* Foul-smelling nasal discharge, usually on one side only (unless there's something up both nostrils).
* Irritation.
* Bleeding (very often does not occur).

Causes
- See above.

Treatment
- Unless the object is protruding from the nostril and can be easily removed, seek medical help.
- Trying to make a child blow the object out can be dangerous, as it can very easily be sniffed further in to the air passages by accident.

The Doctor
- Will attempt removal using special instruments which allow the nostril to be gently opened so the object can be grasped.
- Occasionally it is necessary for the object to be removed under general anaesthetic.

Foreskin problems

The foreskin is the piece of skin which covers the top of the penis. Although it should be easily pulled back in men, this is only true for about half of all newborn boys. No attempt should be made to force back the foreskin. Gentle attempts at bath-time may sometimes be needed, but are usually unnecessary. The foreskin will naturally become mobile by the age of two to three years of age.

Foreskin problems considered here are:

Balanitis (infection of the tip of the penis)
Circumcision
Para-phimosis (foreskin stuck behind the tip of the penis)
Phimosis (tight foreskin)

Balanitis (*infection of the tip of the penis*)

Symptoms
* Most common in baby boys and toddlers.
* The tip of the penis is red, swollen and sore.
* It hurts to pass urine.
* Yellow pus may come from the tip.
* The foreskin may be stuck down.

Prevention
- Regularly clean and dry the area, but do not force back an infant's foreskin. (See **Phimosis**.)
- Do not leave infants for long periods in unchanged nappies.

Treatment
- You can give paracetamol solution for the pain.
- Take your child to see the doctor.

The Doctor
- Will prescribe antibiotics, either to be applied locally to the penis or taken by mouth.
- Your child may need a circumcision if there are repeated attacks.

Circumcision

This is the name of the operation performed to remove the foreskin. Newborn Moslem and Jewish babies must have it done according to religious law, usually by their religious leaders. In some circumstances it may be carried out under the NHS for medical reasons. There are risks of damage and bleeding after a circumcision. These are greatest with small babies.

Causes

- It is rarely necessary for newborn babies to be circumcised. Their foreskins are often normally adherent to the end of the penis (see **Phimosis** below). This gives some protection to the urine passage from contact with urine in nappies.
- Rarely, the hole through which urine passes is incorrectly placed, in which case the foreskin is needed for the corrective operation and must not be removed.
- The medical reasons for circumcision include:
  - a foreskin so tight that urine can hardly be passed
  - a foreskin which cannot be returned to the tip of the penis by pressure; do not force back an infant's foreskin (see **Phimosis**)
  - repeated infections of the tip of the penis

The operation

- A circumcision done for medical reasons is a delicate operation which requires a general anaesthetic.
- Children usually recover quickly from the operation.
- Young children are often home the next day.
- An alternative operation is to make a small slit in the underside of the foreskin. This may be done if the above conditions are not too severe.

Para-phimosis

In para-phimosis the foreskin cannot be drawn forward over the penis tip following an erection.

Symptoms

* The foreskin has been pulled back, e.g. during sexual intercourse.
* It cannot be returned to cover the tip of the penis.
* A ring of swollen skin forms around the penis.
* It becomes increasingly painful.

Treatment

- You may be able to return it yourself by placing both thumbs on the tip of the penis. Then put your index and middle fingers around both sides. Slowly bring the fingers up to meet the thumbs. This may take some time, but if there is progress, continue.
- If this does not help, contact a doctor urgently. The longer you leave it the worse it will become.

The Doctor

- A local anaesthetic cream may make it bearable, and usually the foreskin can be returned without a general anaesthetic.
- Sometimes an operation is needed to free the foreskin, or a circumcision may be carried out straight away.

Phimosis (*tight foreskin*)

This is most common in infants and toddlers, but it also affects young men.

Symptoms

* The tight foreskin cannot be pulled back, and covers the hole through which urine is passed.
* Only a thin, weak stream of urine can be passed. Passing urine may be painful and difficult.
* The foreskin may balloon out when passing urine.

* It interferes with sexual intercourse.

Causes
- Usually present at birth, it may improve with time.
- The foreskin is often stuck to the tip of the penis at birth. These adhesions normally disappear by the age of two.
- Abnormal adhesions may develop following repeated infection.
- They may also develop after forceful attempts to pull back the foreskin.

Prevention
- Do not force back the foreskin.

Treatment
- Small children may improve with time.
- You can help the problem by *gently* pulling the foreskin back in the bath, but do not pull it back further than it will go.
- If there are no problems with passing water it is not necessary to pull the foreskin back.

The Doctor
- If the foreskin fails to loosen naturally the doctor will send your child to a surgeon and an operation may be required. Circumcision is usually required in young men.
- The foreskin can be removed, which is called a circumcision, or a slit can be made in the foreskin.
- Both operations are done while the patient is under general anaesthetic; admission to hospital is seldom for longer than twenty-four hours.

Ganglions

These are generally harmless swellings which may appear quite suddenly or develop slowly. They are traditionally made to disappear with a firm blow from the family bible. Fortunately, such drastic measures are rarely necessary as ganglions are neither serious nor very troublesome. Usually only seen in adults.

Symptoms
* Pea-sized (or larger) swellings.
* The wrist is most commonly affected.
* They may appear on the top side of the foot and, much less commonly, elsewhere.
* Painless.
* Vague discomfort usually caused by a difficulty with the ganglions position interfering with clothes, shoes or work activity.
* May be hard or soft.
* Can be unsightly.

Causes
- The swelling is caused by the accumulation of a jelly-like substance between tendons and their covering. This build-up causes a ballooning of the cover.
- The amount of fluid in the ganglion will determine whether the lump is hard or soft.
- Sometimes a ganglion will form around a joint. Joints are covered in a lining which can bulge out, forming a ganglion.

Treatment
- Usually none is required.
- They can occasionally be dispersed by applying pressure.
- If troublesome or very unsightly they can be removed surgically. (The surgeon won't usually use a bible.)
- They often disappear without treatment.

Gallstones

The gallbladder is a small purse-like structure tucked under the liver. In the gallbladder the bile is concentrated and gallstones may form. The gallbladder is connected to the intestine by channels which allow the bile to flow into the intestine. Gallstones may cause problems in the gallbladder itself or in the channels leading to the intestine. Only about half of all those people who have gallstones ever have any symptoms caused by the stones. As many as one in three of those aged over sixty-five years have gallstones.

Symptoms

* Often gallstones cause no symptoms.
* If the gallstones move from inside the gallbladder they may block one of the channels leading from it to the intestine; this causes severe pain on the right side of the abdomen. The pain may spread through to the back and may be felt up to the right shoulder-blade. It may come and go in waves – hence the term gallstone colic.
* The pain may cease after a few hours, when the gallstone moves on from where it is causing a blockage.
* If the stone does not move on it can cause an obstructive jaundice by preventing the bile from reaching the intestine. (See **Jaundice**.)
* If germs enter the bile passages and the gallbladder, infection will occur with pain in the area of the gallbladder. (This is called acute cholecystitis.)

Causes

☐ Cholesterol is a fat which, if present in excess, contributes to the formation of gallstones. Butter, solid packet margarine and animal fats contain a lot of cholesterol.

☐ If the gallbladder is diseased, or does not contract well, gallstones are more likely to form.

☐ Some blood disorders such as sickle cell anaemia and thalassaemia cause gallstones. (See **Anaemia**, **Jaundice**.)

The Doctor

- You will have to see a doctor for control of the pain if your gallstones give you trouble.
- The use of painkillers and antibiotics to treat any infection may lead to relief of symptoms in the short term.
- In the long term you will be offered the possibility of having the gallstones removed, particularly if the pain is recurrent and very troublesome.
- Ultrasound tests, as used in pregnancy, can reveal the number, size and position of the gallstones. Only about one in ten of gallstones can be seen on X-ray. Special X-ray tests, using a dye which concentrates in the gallbladder, can also be used.
- The size, type and position of the stones affects the choice of method used for their removal.
- Stones mostly composed of cholesterol can be dissolved using medicines. This treatment has to be taken over several years and the stones may recur following treatment.
- Stones near the intestine, at the lower end of the bile channels from the gallbladder, can sometimes be removed from inside the intestine. This is done via a tube passed down the oesophagus through the stomach and into the intestine. It is like a long bendy telescope with an instrument for removing the stone attached to the end.
- An operation may be performed called a cholecystectomy. This removes the gallbladder and any gallstones. It is done under general anaesthetic and you will normally be in hospital for about seven to ten days following the operation. A cholecystectomy can be done either when symptoms occur or after a delay of several weeks. This usually cures the symptoms, although in a few cases they continue.

Gastritis

This is a term which doctors use to describe symptoms that may seem to you very similar to severe indigestion. It is not uncommon to have an attack of gastritis from time to time; those who are heavy smokers or drinkers are most at risk. Gastritis normally settles quite quickly on its own, without requiring treatment from the doctor.

Symptoms
* If caused by a viral infection there may be:
  - vomiting
  - pain in the stomach or back
  - cramping stomach pains coming in waves
  - diarrhoea
* Gastritis caused by other factors will produce symptoms resembling those listed under **Indigestion**.

Causes
- In gastritis the lining of the stomach becomes inflamed.
- This can be caused by:
  - viral infection: this may be severe and affect other parts of the intestine causing diarrhoea
  - drugs, particularly aspirin and drugs used for arthritis (see **Arthritis**)
  - food which you tolerate poorly, though others may cope with it, perfectly well
  - heavy smoking or drinking
  - overeating

Treatment
- This is aimed at giving the stomach time to settle down and return to normal.
- Drink only water for the first twenty-four to thirty-six hours.
- Try taking an antacid medicine, available from chemists.
- Eat small quantities of food which is likely to settle well on your stomach. Mashed bananas or stewed apples without sugar may be possibilities.
- Stop smoking.
- If you seem to have recurrent bouts of gastritis try and find out if the episodes are linked to heavy drinking or overeating and make the necessary adjustments.

The Doctor
- If pain or vomiting persist, or if there is blood in the vomit, see your doctor.
- The doctor will prescribe an antacid medicine if gastritis seems likely. You may also be asked to try a change of medicines you are already on.
- If symptoms are persisitent or the diagnosis is not clearly gastritis, the doctor may wish to carry out simple tests and investigations. These will be as described for **Ulcers, stomach**.

Gastroenteritis and food poisoning

This refers to a generalised inflammation and irritation of the intestines. In its commonest form this is sometimes referred to as gastric flu. It is one of the most frequent reasons for people to contact the family doctor, but there is little in the way of specific treatment beyond self-help measures. Gastroenteritis is usually caused by a viral infection and it may spread very easily to other people, causing small epidemics. Food poisoning may also cause symptoms of gastroenteritis (see below). Gastroenteritis in infants is considered separately.

Symptoms
* Great variation in severity from:
  - mild nausea and later diarrhoea to
  - one or two bouts of vomiting with

three or four runny stools to
- prolonged repeated vomiting and copious watery diarrhoea
* There may be pain and cramps coming and going in waves in the stomach; fever and weakness may also occur.
* Rarely, symptoms are so severe that it is difficult to get up and about.
* Recovery is usual within forty-eight hours.
* (See Gastroenteritis in infants.)

Causes

- Usually a viral infection.
- Also occurs as part of food poisoning. This is a general term used to describe contamination of food with either a germ or a chemical of some sort. Germs most commonly causing food poisoning are the *salmonella* and *staphylococcus* bacteria. *Salmonella* is in many foods already and is normally destroyed by cooking. *Staphylococcus* may reach food from a food handler's cut or boil (see Boils). Both these germs are more likely to cause infections when food has been left warm for several hours, or has been inadequately cooked.
- Some people may suffer an allergic reaction to certain foods, thus causing a severe gastroenteritis.
- Certain drugs, including antibiotics, may upset the normal balance of the intestine and cause gastroenteritis.

Treatment

- For infants see Gastroenteritis in infants.
- Rest as much as possible during gastroenteritis.
- Take care to wash your hands, particularly after visiting the toilet or before handling food, as gastroenteritis is easily passed on to others.
- Take plenty of fluids to avoid dehydration. Take only water for the first twenty-four hours with no food at all. Take sips of water every fifteen or twenty minutes. Avoid sugar, dairy products, coffees, teas and alcohol, as well as painkillers such as aspirin or paracetamol.
- Useful foods to start on when symptoms have started to settle include:
  - boiled rice, perhaps flavoured with a small amount of lemon juice or beef extract
  - boiled chicken
  - stewed apples (without sugar)
  - bananas
  - bread

The Doctor

- There is no specific treatment for viral gastroenteritis and the doctor is unlkely to do anything beyond confirming the above self-help measures, unless the symptoms suggest an alternative diagnosis such as appendicitis. (See Appendicitis.)
- If vomiting is severe an anti-vomiting drug may be prescribed, or a drug such as loperamide may be recommended for the diarrhoea. This is available without prescription and should be discontinued as soon as the diarrhoea ceases. It should not be used for infants or young children.
- (See also Vomiting, Diarrhoea.)

Gastroenteritis in infants

This stomach upset, described above for adults, which causes generalised inflammation of the intestines, can have much more serious consequences in babies and young children. The loss of body fluids through vomiting and diarrhoea can rapidly lead to dangerous dehydration. Gastroenteritis is more likely to occur in bottle-fed babies since feeding on breast milk tends to protect the intestine from infection.

Symptoms
* Frequent loose runny stools. These may be greeen, but the colour is not always important. (Note that breast-fed babies' stools may range in consistency from frothy milk shakes to normal stool. (See **Constipation**.)
* Irritability.
* Feeding may deteriorate.
* Vomiting may occur.
* Signs of dehydration include a dry mouth, sunken eyes, sunken soft spot on the top of the head (see **Soft spot**), lethargy and irritability. See your doctor at once if these signs occur.
* Severe signs of dehydration include refusing to feed and loss of skin elasticity; the baby's temperature may not necessarily be raised. See the doctor at once if these signs occur, as this can lead to brain damage or death.

Causes
See **Gastroenteritis and food poisoning**.

Treatment
- Mild gastroenteritis in a baby may settle quickly on the following regime. If symptoms become worse or fail to settle it is important not to delay in seeking help.
- If you are breast-feeding you should continue to do so, although the frequency of feeds may have to be increased. If additional fluids are required give fluids as described for bottle-fed babies. See the doctor if you are unsure or worried.
- If you are bottle-feeding, substitute cooled boiled water for the milk and give no more milk until symptoms settle. Sachets such as Dioralyte, available from the chemist on prescription, should be added to the water as instructed on the sachet as soon as you are able to obtain them. (Several 'feeds' of plain water will usually be fine.) If you are unable to obtain these sachets, a solution made up of five level teaspoons of glucose in 500 mls of previously boiled water can be used for the first twenty-four hours.
- Give at least the child's usual amount of fluid, but this should be given in small amounts every hour if necessary.
- Symptoms will normally improve within twenty-four to forty-eight hours. As symptoms improve milk should only be reintroduced slowly. Start by giving a quarter of the usual amount of milk powder in the usual amount of water. After twenty-four hours give half the amount of milk powder in the usual amount of water and so on, until feeding is back to normal.
- If a young child is eating all foods then it is quite reasonable to reintroduce foods as described for adult gastroenteritis; however, this should only be done when symptoms are settled.
- Precautions such as washing hands after visiting the toilet, changing nappies or preparing food are important.

The Doctor
- If you are worried about a young baby or infant call the doctor.
- Mild cases may only require the use of fluids as above and the doctor may prescribe the sachets. If the doctor is either unclear about the reason for the gastroenteritis, or the infection is severe, hospital admission can usually settle the problem quickly.
- In hospital fluid intake and fluids lost will be very carefully checked. If fluids are not being tolerated because the stomach and intestine are too

unsettled they can be replaced via a small tube inserted into a vein. This is called an intravenous infusion or drip. This enables the replacement of vital body fluids and chemicals, without which the child could be in great danger. Normal feeds can usually be reintroduced by following a gradual regime as described above, quite soon after symptoms settle.

Genital herpes

This is an infection in the genital area caused by a virus. It is painful, makes you feel unwell and may recur. It is commonest in young adults. There is usually freedom from the virus between attacks and it does not mean the end of your sex life. When you have an attack you are, however, infectious. Although very uncomfortable and distressing, it is not dangerous except at childbirth. The attacks may cease altogether in time; about half of those infected never have another attack.

Symptoms

* Stinging, tingling or itching around the genital or anal area.
* Flu-like symptoms of feeling unwell.
* Blisters which weep and leave red ulcers. Some of these ulcers are more painful than others and may take longer to heal.
* There can be an infection with symptoms but no visible ulcer, the ulcer being out of sight inside the vagina or back passage.
* Men may have blisters on the penis or in the back passage.
* Women passing urine can have pain when urine touches the sore areas.
* Lymph glands can be enlarged in the groin area.

Causes

- It is caused by the *herpes simplex* virus. This is type 2 of the virus. Type 1 causes cold sores. (See **Cold sores**.)
- Infection with type 2 virus is usually transmitted by touch.
- What may seem to be a first attack may be a recurrence of the virus caught years before, when symptoms did not suggest the diagnosis.
- Occasionally, cold sores on the face can infect the genital area during oral sex. If this happens the herpes attack in the genital area is usually less severe than from the type 2 virus.
- The exact type of virus can only be identified by laboratory testing, and very often it is not identified. It is not absolutely necessary to do so.

Treatment

- Anything which soothes the area may help, such as:
  - salt solution – 1 tablespoon to 1 pint water
  - calamine lotion
  - anaesthetic cream from the chemist – do not use for more than a few days or a reaction to the cream may develop!
  - salt baths – add a handful of salt to bath
  - ice packs
  - witch hazel – can keep sores dry; dab on a small amount
- Mild painkillers such as aspirin and paracetamol can help and make you more comfortable.
- If passing urine is uncomfortable try doing so in a warm bath.
- Avoid:
  - hot baths
  - sunbathing
  - sunbeds
  - becoming overtired
  - intercourse when you have an attack
  - tight clothing

- nylon underwear

All these may worsen or bring on an attack.

- It can be useful to keep a careful diary of attacks to try to identify and thereby avoid factors that bring on an attack.
- It is very unusual to be infectious between attacks. You can normally have intercourse a few days after an attack.

The Doctor

- Doctors may provide help to treat the attack, but cannot provide a long-term cure. They may prescribe anti-viral cream, paint or tablets. The tablets are useful on a first attack but less worth while on the often less severe subsequent attacks.
- All anti-viral medicines are strong and expensive and should only be used exactly as directed by the doctor or clinic.

Note

In pregnancy inform your doctor and midwife if you have genital herpes. The baby in the womb is not affected, but special care needs to be taken during childbirth if you have an active herpes sore in the birth passage.

German measles

German measles (rubella) is similar to ordinary measles, in that it causes a rash, but it is usually a much milder infection. Measles can be serious but German measles is only serious for unborn babies. If a pregnant woman has neither had German measles, nor been immunised against it, her baby may be affected if she comes in contact with German measles during pregnancy. Girls aged around eleven years old are normally immunised against German measles.

Symptoms

* It usually starts with the symptoms of a cold, coming on two to three weeks after contact.
* Headache, fever and red eyes may be the first sign.
* The rash starts soon afterwards.
* Small red spots spread from the face to cover the body.
* The rash lasts from only a few hours to as long as five days.
* Children do not usually have a very high temperature.
* The lymph glands in the head and neck are swollen and may be tender.
* There may be painful joints, especially of the hands; this is more common in adults.

Prevention

- Keep an infectious child away from pregnant women. The period of infectivity lasts from up to a week before to two weeks after the rash appears.
- All girls should be vaccinated at around eleven years old.
- Your doctor can do a blood test to see if you have protection against rubella. It is sensible to see your doctor before you become pregnant.
- The hospital also does this blood test routinely on all pregnant women.
- Ask them the result so you know if you are protected.
- In America the rubella vaccine is given with mumps and measles vaccines.
- It is planned to introduce the mumps/measles/rubella combined vaccine here. This will be given at around fifteen months old.

Treatment

- Take paracetamol.
- You do not have to consult your doctor if the illness is mild.

Pregnancy

You may be worried because you have been in contact with German measles or have developed a rash. Firstly, what stage of pregnancy are you at? If you have passed four months it is a lot better than contracting the disease in early pregnancy; any serious harm usually occurs earlier in pregnancy. Secondly, you are likely to be protected, see above. Thirdly, the rash may not be German measles; other viruses can appear very similar.

If you are at risk, especially in early pregnancy, see your doctor at once. He or she can do two blood tests, a couple of weeks apart, to see if you have caught German measles. If you have, in early pregnancy, you will be offered a termination.

You may be found to be unprotected as a result of routine blood tests in pregnancy. You will then be offered the vaccine after you have given birth. It is advised that you do not become pregnant within three months of this, although there is little evidence to suggest that the vaccine can harm a pregnancy.

Glandular fever

A throat and flu-like infection caused by a particular virus. It is also known as infectious mononucleosis, common in young people between their mid-teens and mid-twenties. How badly the virus affects you varies enormously – from a sore throat over in days to a severe illness with jaundice and rash lasting several months. Although infectious it is unusual to find it in more than one member of the family at the same time.

Symptoms
* Fever.
* Sudden onset of sore throat.
* Gradual onset of sore throat.
* Aches and pains in joints and muscles.
* Tiredness.
* Loss of appetite.
* Glandular swelling:
  - in neck
  - under arms
  - in groin
  - inside stomach, sometimes even giving symptoms like appendicitis.
* A rash, similar to German measles in appearance and made worse or brought on by ampicillin often prescribed for the sore throat.
* Jaundice: in some cases the liver is infected sufficiently to give temporary jaundice, which is usually not severe.
* An enlarged spleen.

Treatment
- Rest.
- Ice cream, ice, cold drinks, gargles. (See **Tonsillitis**.)
- No kissing, as the illness is passed through saliva. It is sometimes called the 'kissing disease'.
- No strenuous activity until you are fully recovered, and particularly in case you injure the enlarged spleen.

The Doctor
- If sore throat symptoms persist for longer than expected or are unusually severe, the doctor may:
  - look for red spots on your palate which are often seen along with white patches on the tonsils (see **Tonsillitis**)
  - take blood for a glandular fever test (monospot test)
  - examine your tummy for an enlarged liver and spleen, an organ designed to help with infections
  - rarely, give steroids to shrink down the swollen glands, help swallowing and relieve discomfort; steroids given in a short course do not have very serious side-effects

How long does it last?
- It varies in duration.
- Children are usually better in three to four weeks.
- Most people are back to normal after eight weeks.
- Rarely, can last for many months of tiredness and malaise.

Glue-sniffing

Breathing in the vapours of a number of different solvents may cause you to become 'high', rather like having too much alcohol. This is called glue-sniffing and is common among children and adolescents. It is not against the law but may lead to your breaking the law because you are intoxicated. It is against the law for anyone to sell solvent-based products to someone under eighteen if they know or suspect that they may not be used for their normal purposes. Solvents that are contained in glues, and cause this effect, are also present in many household and industrial products. Accidents, hallucinations, unconsciousness or even death may occur as a result of glue sniffing.

Symptoms
* Chemical smell on breath or clothes.
* Used containers of glue, firelighter fluid, aerosols. These may be found in unusual places in the house, garden shed, or hidden away.
* Soreness around the mouth, eyes or nose.
* Persistent cough.
* Loss of appetite, loss of weight.
* Slurred speech and intoxicated behaviour.
* Irritability and mood changes. Telling lies or increasing secretiveness.
* Poor school attendance, start of truancy and poor performance at school.
* Loss of money.

Causes
- Why people sniff glue varies from person to person. Young people often find it more easily available than alcohol. It is also cheaper.
- Unhappy children may turn to glue-sniffing to seek attention or to try and forget about problems they have.
- Boredom amongst a group of children may lead to games involving glue-sniffing from which it may be difficult for an individual to escape. It may be presented as the latest craze by older children to younger ones to see the effects it has on a child who has not done it before.

Treatment
- Many children may sniff glue as part of a phase which they soon grow out of, the child realising it is often unpleasant and can be very dangerous.
- If you suspect your child may be glue-sniffing it is usually unhelpful to react violently or aggressively.
- Give children time to talk to you and support them through any difficulties they may be having. It is often helpful to talk to teachers, parents of your child's friends, or your doctor, health visitor or social worker.
- If your child seems to be mixing with a crowd of youngsters who sniff glue it is better to inform your child of the dangers. The child will often be pleased to find it is all right to talk about it and share anxieties with you.
- Unfortunately, glue-sniffing often brings a child into contact with people selling or giving away other kinds of drugs, which are then abused. (See **Drug abuse**.)

The Doctor
- If you are worried, discuss things with the doctor. It may be helpful to take your child with you. A trip to

the doctor may have several effects. It can impress upon a child how seriously you take the problem and let him know you are concerned and supportive. It may also allow children, depending on their age, to feel this is something they could do themselves, if they were to get into difficulties later.
- Leave the child alone for a few minutes with the doctor. This can often allow him to share things he feels unable to tell you. The doctor may be able to help the child to share anxieties with you.

Gonorrhoea

Gonorrhoea is a sexually transmitted disease. It is an infection which can be caught through oral, anal or vaginal sex. It is rarely caught by other close bodily contact. Men with penile infections experience symptoms, but women or men with throat or anal infections may not. It causes pelvic inflammatory disease in women. It can be easily treated.

Symptoms
* A man may have a thick milky discharge from the penis.
* There is pain or burning on passing urine, which begins about two to five days after catching the infection.
* This is similar to the symptoms of non-specific urethritis (see NSU) but the symptoms of gonorrhoea develop after a shorter period.
* The infection may spread to the testicles, making them red, swollen and painful.
* Women and homosexual men may have throat or anal infections. There may be a sore throat, or anal discharge, but commonly no symptoms.
* A woman may have a vaginal discharge, or pain on passing urine.
* The neck of the womb is inflamed, and the infection may spread to the vagina or rectum.
* It may spread to the fallopian tubes, causing PID. (See **Pelvic infection**.)
* A blood-stream infection causing fever, joint pains and a rash can occur.
* Babies born through an infected birth canal may have a serious eye infection.

Prevention
- Use a condom or a diaphragm (cap).
- Early investigation and treatment of symptoms will help to prevent problems developing due to the infection.
- Do not have sexual intercourse until you and your partner are both treated.
- Inform any sexual contacts of your infection.

Treatment
- Most cities and large towns have a clinic where expert help is available. This is known as a genito-urinary or venereal disease clinic. The address is in the phone book.
- You may prefer to visit your doctor.
- Swabs will be taken from the infected area.
- Treatment may be given before the results are known.
- A single dose of penicillin is usually enough; a second drug may be given to increase its effects. A different antibiotic is given if you are allergic to penicillin.
- If you have picked up the infection from a Far Eastern or American contact there is a greater risk of resistance to treatment with penicillin; a different antibiotic will be required.
- If you continue to have symptoms after treatment you must see the doctor again.
- You can resume intercourse once you and your partner have both been

- given the all-clear.
- Infection which has spread from the original site, to involve joints for example, needs prolonged treatment.

Gout

Gout is an extremely painful condition, usually affecting the big toe joint, which comes on suddenly. It is much more common in men than women. The tendency to have gout runs in families, although not everyone in the family will be affected. Fortunately, although perhaps the most painful joint disease, it is the easiest to treat. Two hundred years ago a doctor wrote that 'more rich than poor, more wise than fools' suffered gout – so you are in good company!

Symptoms
* A typical attack starts at night in the big toe joint.
* A red, swollen, tender joint, which can appear like a large boil.
* Pain is very severe, often worsened by the slightest move or knock.
* Other joints sometimes affected are the knee, elbow and wrist.

Causes
- An acid, called uric acid, is a waste product of the body's chemical processes. This acid builds up to high levels in gout.
- The acid forms crystals, and it is these crystals collecting in the joint that cause the attack.
- A high level of this acid in the blood does not lead everyone to have gout attacks. Those with others in the family affected are much more likely to suffer.
- Those prone to gout can trigger an attack by over-indulgence in food and drink.
- Other factors leading to attacks include exhaustion, other illness, operations – even tooth extractions.
- Water tablets can lead to a build-up of acid and make gout more likely.

Treatment
- Drinking plenty of fluids can help to wash the acid out of the body.
- Diet is felt to be less important now there is good treatment available, but excessive protein and being overweight are worth avoiding. Most people with gout can eat and drink moderately, but should avoid excesses or anything that starts an attack.

The Doctor
- A visit to the doctor is usually necessary – to confirm that you have gout, by measuring the level of uric acid in the blood stream, and to obtain treatment.
- The doctor will usually prescribe one of a large family of drugs which are not steroids, stop the inflammation and quickly relieve the pain (non-steroidal anti-inflammatory or NSAI drugs), e.g. indomethacin. Taken as a short course, the side-effects are not usually too bad, but taken for longer indigestion in particular may be a problem. Take with or after food.
- Colchicine is another useful drug (derived from the autumn crocus!).
- To prevent further attacks you can take a drug called allopurinol. This has few side-effects but is generally taken for life once started. When starting this drug, one of the other drugs should also be taken for about the first month.

Hair loss

There is a much greater general turnover of hair than most of us realise. At times this can be much more marked, such as after pregnancy. Men and women are both affected by hair problems. It is never serious, but the effect on appearance is often distressing. With general hair care much can be done to help. In most conditions leading to hair loss regrowth can be expected with time.

Patchy loss

In babies
- Hair is much less firmly attached.
- It is normal to get a bald patch on the back of the head. Not a sign of neglect – merely a result of rubbing against cot sheets.
- In the first weeks of life some downy hair is lost. This is replaced by normal hair, but a period of baldness may occur.

In children
There are three main causes of patchy hair loss in children:

Alopecia

Symptoms
* This leads to clear, smooth, white, often round, areas of complete hair loss.
* It is not itchy.
* It occurs suddenly.
* Regrowth always takes place over a period of months.
* Regrowth starts with fine white hairs, replaced later by darker hairs.

Causes
- It happens usually as a result of severe illness, when hair growth stops for a time and patches of hair fall out as a consequence.
- It can be seen after severe upset or stress such as a relative dying.

Treatment
- There is none.
- Sometimes dermatologists may give a course of steroid injections to try and encourage regrowth. Results are rather variable.

Fungal infection

Symptoms
* Patchy areas of hair loss.
* Itching.
* Base of 'patch' is often scaly and can be reddish, pink or grey.
* Other signs of fungal infection elsewhere (itchy redness).
* It is infectious; children should not be at school until treated.

Causes
- An infection with a fungus (ringworm, similar to that in athletes' foot) damages the scalp.
- This prevents hair growth.
- Skin infection on the scalp then provides the itch and scaly appearance.

Treatment
- Anti-fungal creams, ointments and, if severe, tablets are available.
- A doctor's prescription and advice should be sought.
- General hair care (see **Hair problems – Dandruff**) will help to prevent recurrence.

Hair-pulling
Some children, particularly when concentrating, develop a nervous habit of actually pulling out their own hair. Hair loss is generally widespread, but may be in particular patches on the scalp.

Watch the child while he is concentrating, to see if twisting and pulling of the hair has become a habit. The treatment involves distraction and the co-operation of parent and child to try and prevent the problem.

In adults
- Patchy hair loss is usually due to alopecia (see above). The symptoms, causes and treatment are as for children.
- Although fungal infection can occur, it is much less common.

General loss

This includes thinning of the hair, which mainly affects women, and baldness, which mainly affects men.

Thinning

Symptoms
* May be quite marked and sudden.
* brushing or washing hair vigorously can lead to a severe hair fall, causing surprise and alarm.

Causes
- Most common after having a baby. Starts three months after the birth and regrows over following six months.
- Ageing – there is a progressive thinning of the hair that occurs naturally. It starts in young adulthood and continues throughout life. The speed with which it takes place varies enormously.
- Rarely, severe illness such as iron deficiency or thyroid problems (see **Thyroid problems**) can be a cause.

Treatment
- Nothing can be done to prevent thinning with age.
- After childbirth simple hair care is the only treatment needed.
- If another illness may be a cause, the doctor should be consulted, and will usually do a simple blood test.
- Hair growth returns after recovery from the illness.
- Nothing can be done to prevent natural thinning with age.

Baldness

Symptoms
* Men are mainly affected.
* It starts as a receding hair line at the top of the forehead, or the crown may thin.
* The whole scalp may be affected.
* There is often a family history of baldness.

Causes
- Baldness is a natural process.

Treatment
- There is no treatment commonly available for natural baldness.
- Hair transplants can be attempted, but are not always successful.

Hair problems

Hair problems considered here are:

Dandruff
Greasy hair
Unwanted hair

Hair loss is considered as a separate entry.

Dandruff

Causes
- This is caused by abnormal production of flakes of dead skin on the scalp. Although the hair itself is not affected, hair care is the prevention and treatment.

Treatment
- Choose an anti-dandruff or tar-based shampoo.
- Shampoo every two to three days.
- One application of shampoo is usually adequate.

- Massage scalp with fingertips for about five minutes, concentrating on areas worst affected.
- Leave shampoo on for one or more minutes.
- Rinse very thoroughly.
- Wrap towel around hair.
- Comb out gently to avoid hair fall.
- Avoid too-hot rollers or tongs as this damages the hair.

The Doctor
- If persisting, doctors can provide stronger scalp lotions, e.g. steroids.
- The scalp may have a condition such as eczema or fungal infection complicating the situation, and this may need treatment.

Greasy hair

Causes
- Frequent shampooing removes the natural oils from the hair.
- The hair produces an excess of oils to compensate for those lost by excessive shampooing.

Treatment
- Greasy hair can be best managed by a carefully controlled reduction in the frequency of shampooing. Gradually decrease shampooing from daily to once every two or three days.
- The choice of shampoo is important. An anti-dandruff shampoo used continually may be too strong. It can be helpful to alternate with a milder shampoo.
- Your hairdresser can often give much better advice than your doctor.

Unwanted hair

Unwanted hair is a common problem.

Treatment
This includes:

- Shaving – does not in fact make hair grow back more thickly, but needs to be repeated very frequently.
- Creams and sprays – effective, but irritate sensitive skin.
- Abrasives – can be effective but tend to cause areas of soreness. Not suitable for the face.
- Plucking – long-lasting and effective.
- Waxing – long lasting. It works in a similar way to plucking, but the wax allows many hairs to be removed at once.
- Electrolysis – should only be done by an expert. Can be used on the face.

Hayfever

Hayfever symptoms are due to an allergic reaction and are concentrated around the nose and eyes. It is an extremely common problem which may affect you at any age. In some people hayfever may only last a few years; in others, it is a lifelong nuisance needing elaborate preventive measures. It is of no danger but may be associated with asthma, which can be serious. Eczema is also frequently found in people with hayfever and there are often others in the family who have been affected. The peak time for symptoms is June and July, but the hayfever season runs from May to September. Some people have year-long symptoms of hayfever which is called perennial rhinitis.

Symptoms
* Intermittent blocked nose.
* Repeated sneezing.
* Watery nasal discharge.
* Itchy and watery eyes which may be sore.
* Difficulty with taste and smell.
* Dry throat.
* Wheeze.
* Swollen eyes often made worse by rubbing.

Causes

- Seasonal hayfever is caused by your being sensitised to pollen. This is carried in the wind and comes particularly from grasses and weeds. Pollens of trees, shrubs and flowers also cause symptoms.
- Other substances such as feathers and hair of household pets may cause problems for people with perennial rhinitis. (See **Allergies**.)
- Contact with the substance which is irritating causes the release in the body of a chemical called histamine. The histamine makes the cells of the nasal passages and eyes swell and release fluid causing the symptoms.
- There is a hereditary factor. More than three-quarters of people with hayfever have others in the family who have had the symptoms.

Treatment

- Because the symptoms are due to a reaction with something outside the body, a great deal can be done by avoiding contact with the substance concerned. Those affected by pollen should:
  - keep windows closed while driving in cars
  - sleep with windows closed
  - avoid country walks through long grass
- There are a variety of treatments available which decrease the severity of reactions when contact occurs, and help symptoms if contact has taken place. These include:
  - antihistamines, many of which are available without prescription; they decrease symptoms, particularly those of runny nose and sneezing; it is well worth while trying several different preparations because the extent to which one drug or another may be effective is very variable; do not drive or operate machinery after taking antihistamines
  - nose drops – not generally helpful as they can lead to the nose secreting even more discharge as soon as their effect wears off

The Doctor

- May prescribe further antihistamines, some of which are only available on prescription. It is not unusual for a doctor to prescribe three different preparations for you to try, one each week over three weeks, to see which is most effective.
- Sodium cromoglycate which is a drug used in asthma may help in hayfever.
- There are spray forms of steroids available which can be used in the nose to great effect in hayfever. For maximum benefit they should be used regularly. Because they are used in the nose they do not have the side-effects of steroid drugs taken as tablets by mouth.
- Allergic testing can be arranged by the doctor. This involves small needle pricks over a patch of skin; these inject a very small diluted quantity of various possible allergens. This may reveal that particular substances cause a more severe reaction, and hence avoidance action can be taken.
- Desensitisation injections to decrease your body's response to a substance causing hayfever symptoms help in about three-quarters of patients. The injections have to be continued over three years and are by no means a complete cure. There is a small risk of dangerous shock reactions to these injections and they should only be carried out where there is adequate medical supervision at the time of the injection and for a short while following it.

Headaches

In any one year nearly everyone in the population will experience at least one headache. Despite the fact that they are extremely common, there is very poor understanding of the exact mechanism that leads to the sensation of a common headache. There are a few serious causes of headache, outlined below, but nearly all headaches are temporary and do not indicate serious illness.

Symptoms

* Symptoms of a common headache are:
  - a feeling of pressure in the head, or of a band around the head
  - both sides or the front or back of the head may be affected
  - sleep is not generally affected
  - no association with vomiting
* The presence of other symptoms, such as vomiting, may indicate migraine (see **Migraine**). If there are symptoms of neck and head pain on moving the head, drowsiness, dislike of light or recent head injury a doctor should be consulted.

Causes

- Most of the common headache symptoms above are caused by pain brought on by muscle tension around the neck, face and scalp.
- If you feel your neck or scalp during a headache you can often notice the tension.
- The muscle tension is brought on by many factors:
  - poor posture
  - straining eyes
  - working hard over a desk
  - stress and worry
  - smoky or stuffy atmospheres
  - noisy or 'busy' atmospheres
  - lack of sleep
- Headaches are also extremely common when there are symptoms of a cold. Fever adds to the headache brought on by a cold.
- Fever from any illness can cause headaches.
- Pain may also be caused by a problem around the face, head or neck whose only symptom is a general headache. For example:
  - sinusitis
  - increased pressure in the eyes (glaucoma)
  - dental problems
  - jaw-joint problems
  - trapped nerves from the neck
  - facial neuralgia
- Hangover headaches are thought to be caused by the blood vessels in the head dilating. Alcohol makes the blood vessels bigger and this triggers pain signals which cause the classic 'morning after' headache. There are many tricks to try and avoid a hangover but alcohol is a powerful drug and there is usually no escaping it having its effects.
- High blood pressure does not usually reveal itself as a headache. In fact high blood pressure is usually discovered when it is checked for other reasons. Rarely, it may cause headaches.
- Serious causes of headache arise from:
  - infection, such as meningitis or encephalitis
  - bleeding internally (subarachnoid haemorrhage)
  - inflammation of a large artery running over the temple (temporal arteritis)

These illnesses are usually associated with more complex symptoms than those listed above for common headaches. If your headache is persistent or is complicated by the presence of other symptoms, see your doctor at once.

- Head injuries not only cause pain at the time, but a headache may develop some time after the injury or persist over a long period. See your doctor. (See **Head injuries**.)
- Brain tumours are very rare and do not usually cause a simple headache as described above. Tumours may cause a headache that is present on waking, associated with nausea and vomiting. Often there are other symptoms such as visual difficulties, unsteadiness or personality change. They may cause fits.

Treatment

- For common headaches treatment is very limited and does not really extend beyond the removal of the provoking factor and the use of painkillers such as aspirin or paracetamol.
- It may be useful to:
  - exercise or massage neck and shoulders
  - relax in a hot bath
  - apply hot or cold compresses
  - lie down in a darkened room
  - have a good night's sleep
  - drink plenty of fluids

The Doctor

- Will discuss with you possible causes and make specific enquiries which can usually quickly exclude serious causes of headache.
- May prescribe stronger painkillers not available from the chemist.
- May look into your eyes to examine the back of the eye; this reveals information about the brain and blood vessels.
- May take your blood pressure, although this is very often done in order to reassure you rather than in the expectation of finding it raised.
- If your headaches cannot be satisfactorily helped or explained the doctor may refer you to a neurologist.
- The neurologist will arrange tests and X-rays of the head to check for any serious illness.

Head injuries

Any blow to the head should be taken seriously, both because of the immediate consequences and because of the possibility of further problems arising subsequently. The brain is like a very firm collection of porridge inside a shell. If the shell is shaken or hit hard the porridge will not only be displaced where the blow strikes, but will be pushed hard against the other side of the shell. The brain moves in a similar way during a head injury, and the damage can be much greater than expected.

A skull fracture greatly increases the risks of brain injury, not only because there may be physical damage due to displaced bone but also because of the risk of infection entering the brain and causing meningitis. A skull fracture may also lead to the loss of brain fluid (a colourless liquid called cerebro-spinal fluid). (See below.)

Symptoms

* These obviously depend on where and how hard a blow strikes.
* Minor injuries may only lead to a headache which clears over one or two days.
* More severe injuries may lead to:
  - loss of consciousness for a few seconds (concussion)
  - loss of consciousness for days or longer (coma)
* As well as effects on consciousness there may be:
  - memory upset, also called amnesia, which can lead to difficulty in assessing the severity of a head injury as it may not be possible to

find out how it happened
- weakness
- paralysis
- speech difficulty

* These symptoms often improve with time. Some may, however, persist, leading to permanent disability.
* Late symptoms of head injury occurring days or even weeks after the event should be taken seriously.
* Headache, drowsiness, vomiting or weakness occurring days or weeks after a head injury may be caused by an internal blood clot producing symptoms as it swells and presses on the brain. Report symptoms to a doctor immediately.

Causes
□ Most head injuries are caused in road accidents, particularly motorcycle accidents, although the compulsory wearing of crash helmets has helped to reduce the severity of injuries.

Treatment
Immediate
- Consult a doctor early for advice.
- Watch for blood loss and treat as for cuts. (*See* Cuts.)
- Watch for clear fluid loss from ear or nose. This may indicate a fracture, causing cerebro-spinal fluid (CSF) to escape.
- Hospital admission will usually be necessary for any head injury with loss of consciousness. If there is a fracture, or CSF loss, it is essential.
- While in hospital careful checks will be made of blood pressure and consciousness to ensure that any more serious effects of head injury are discovered immediately.

Subsequent
- If you are either discharged from hospital or kept at home after consulting your doctor, simple instructions may be provided to alert you or your family to signs which should be reported. These include:
  - changes in consciousness
  - vomiting
  - headache
  - weakness, numbness or signs of nerve injury developing
- As mentioned above, symptoms returning some time after an injury should always be discussed with a doctor.

Long-term outlook
- A simple head injury usually has a good outlook with complete recovery. Any more complicated or severe injury may lead to:
  - persistent disability such as partial paralysis
  - recurrent headaches over the next one or two years, even in the absence of lasting disability

Headlice

The horror of finding lice in your hair, or more commonly your child's hair, can be memorable. It is helpful to know that headlice infestation has reached such widespread proportions that it is now unusual for children not to be affected at some stage. It takes two to three weeks for the eggs of the louse to hatch; the louse then emerges, bites the scalp, and causes itching. You may have been carrying lice around for some weeks before making the discovery. They are tiny two-millimetre-long brown or white insects that lay their eggs on hair. It is the eggs that are referred to as nits. They are harmless unless left untreated, when the scratching may lead to infection. The treatment is simple and effective.

Symptoms
* Scratching; a child scratching his or her hair should lead to your checking

for lice and nits.
* Widespread scalp irritation, often concentrated behind ears.
* Also commonly seen on back of neck, crown and below fringe.
* Eggs (nits) seen as shiny white drops on hairs.
* Eggs stuck to hairs, unlike dandruff which shakes off easily.

Causes
- Headlice survive by sucking blood. It is this action that causes the irritation.
- The nits hatch, then lay more eggs, leading to increasingly heavy infestation.
- Spread is by lice literally walking from head to head. Any rough-and-tumble and close contact with other children can lead to spread.
- Infestation has nothing to do with being dirty. Lice are as happy on clean, glossy hair as they are on dirty hair.

Treatment
- Lotions and shampoo kill the lice and render the nits inactive so that no more can hatch.
- These are available from chemists.
- The treatments usually contain malathion.
- Do not use a hairdryer after applying treatment as this renders it useless.
- Schools should be informed and can advise on the best treatment.
- Take care, as with all medicines, that the lotions are kept out of the reach of children.
- Combing out all the nits is not only extremely difficult (fine-toothed nit combs are available from chemists), but is not strictly necessary. If the lice and nits are treated correctly they will be killed and rendered harmless.
- Repeating the treatment after about a week is advisable.

The Doctor
- Can prescribe lotions or shampoos, and will advise on the best one to avoid the increasing problem of headlice becoming resistant to some available treatments.
- Will treat any infection that has affected the scalp through vigorous scratching.

Note
Combs and brushes will not harbour the lice if free of hair, as they will only lay eggs where there is hair. It is a wise precaution not to share combs or brushes, as a louse crawling on to a brush could easily be transferred.

Heart attacks

Only one in three heart attacks are fatal. Despite this, it is the commonest cause of death in the Western world. Nobody knows exactly why one person should suffer a heart attack and another not. Most deaths due to heart attacks occur within two hours of the attack, death being due to the inability of the heart to continue its job of circulating the blood round the body. With every month that passes following a heart attack your future health prospects improve (Coronary thrombosis is the medical description of a heart attack, a thrombosis forming in one of the coronary arteries supplying the heart muscle. (See **Thrombosis**.)

Symptoms
* Crushing central chest pain, which may vary in severity from a mild tightness to a crushing bear hug accompanied by a bursting sensation.
* Pain may also be felt in the neck, jaw or arms.
* There may have been worsening angina prior to the attack.
* There is usually no warning; the

attack may occur at any time. If occurring during exercise or at times of emotion the pain does not improve when this ceases – as it would if due to angina. (See **Angina**.)
* Shock may develop. (See **Shock**.)
* Heart failure may develop. (See **Heart failure**.)
  Other associated symptoms which may occur are:
  – dizziness and feeling faint
  – sweating and chills
  – nausea
  – shortness of breath
* In the elderly only very mild symptoms may occur. This is sometimes referred to as a 'silent' heart attack.

Causes
- Heart attacks are generally caused by a blood clot forming in one of the blood vessels supplying the heart muscle.
- If the blood vessels supplying the heart are narrowed, a clot is more likely to form. The vessels may be narrowed due to arteriosclerosis. (See **Angina**.)
- When one of these blood vessels is blocked the heart muscle is starved of blood and oxygen. Consequently it cannot function properly and is damaged. The damaged area is called an infarct.
- Whether or not the damage leads to death, heart failure, or recovery depends on the extent of damage caused by the blockage. A small area of damage may not interfere with the activity of the heart and recovery may be complete. Greater damage may stop the pumping action of the heart from being effective and heart failure may develop. At worst the heart can no longer function and death occurs.

Treatment
- A heart attack is a medical emergency and medical help should be sought at once.

The Doctor
- Will give a painkilling drug such as morphine, usually combined with a drug to stop the sickness which morphine may provoke.
- Heart tracings will be taken to record the electrical activity of the heart. This gives information on the extent and position of the damaged area of heart muscle. Several tracings may be required, or continuous heart tracings may be recorded on a machine with a small screen.
- Blood tests will be done to monitor the heart chemicals which are present in increased amounts after a heart attack occurs.
- The changes following a heart attack may vary over the first few hours and days. It is often only after several tests, and watching how you feel, that a full picture can be built up of what happened and the likely future consequences.
- A number of drugs may be given to control blood pressure, heart rate and activity, and also to treat any heart failure that may develop. Some of these drugs may be discontinued as you improve following the heart attack.
- The outlook is good; more than 90 per cent of people who are all right six hours after a heart attack survive that attack satisfactorily.

After a heart attack
– You are not, and need not be, an invalid.
– Hearts heal in much the same way as other injured parts of the body.
– Your future prospects improve as time passes.

- If angina occurs it can be treated. (See **Angina**.)
- You should be able to return to your work as normal. There is no evidence showing that taking a part-time job improves your chance of survival.
- Stop smoking.
- Keep your weight down and eat a fat-free diet.
- Take regular exercise, but do not start too vigorously. Start gently, doing something you enjoy; in this way you are much more likely to continue it. It is much better to take a walk every day than to start doing twenty-minute bouts of exercise and give up after only a month or so.

☎ British Heart Foundation, 14 Fitzhardinge Street, London W1H 4DH. (Regional offices listed in the telephone directory. Send s.a.e. for publications list.)

☎ CORDA (Coronary Artery Disease Research Association), Tavistock House North, Tavistock Square, London WC1. Tel: 071 387 9779.

☎ Coronary Prevention Group, 60 Great Ormond Street, London WC1. Tel: 071 833 3687. (Please send s.a.e. for information.)

Heart failure

Heart failure sounds as though death should occur imminently. This is not at all the case. Heart failure refers to the pumping action of the heart becoming less efficient, causing the accumulation of blood in the veins leading to the heart. If the veins are overloaded, and the blood is not being moved on sufficiently quickly by the heart, body fluids accumulate. These fluids build up in the lungs and other parts of the body, leading to the symptoms of heart failure. Treatment is effective and, depending on the underlying trouble affecting the heart, normal life can usually be continued.

Symptoms

* Accumulation of fluid in the lungs leads to:
  - shortness of breath which is worse after exercise
  - shortness of breath may occur on lying down; you may waken at night struggling for air and feel the need to open the window; night attacks can be quite frightening, lasting for an hour or more (sleeping propped up on pillows may help)
  - severe symptoms include bubbly chest noises, chest pain, and frothy blood-specked sputum
* Accumulation of fluid elsewhere in the body leads to:
  - tiredness
  - swelling of ankles, if you are up and about; if lying in bed, swelling may appear over the coccyx
  - congestion of the liver may lead to pain
  - loss of appetite
  - confusion

Causes

☐ Heart failure may arise as a result of anything which decreases the efficiency of the heart's pumping mechanism.

☐ Faulty valves in the heart may make it more difficult to move blood forward out of the heart.

☐ Weakened heart muscle due to disease or following a heart attack makes the heart less efficient.

☐ The accumulation of blood in the veins leading to the heart because it is pumping less efficiently causes increased pressure in the veins. This increased pressure in the veins forces fluid out of the veins into body tissues such as the lungs and around the ankles, as mentioned above.

Treatment

- Resting decreases the demands on the heart to pump blood through it. It is important, however, to keep moving so that the blood does not become sluggish, which increases the likelihood of your developing a thrombosis. (See **Thrombosis**.) You can help the circulation in the legs by relaxing and contracting your leg muscles. Keep changing your position and sit up in an armchair rather than staying in bed.

The Doctor

- Treatment of heart failure relies on the use of a group of drugs called diuretics. These drugs make you pass more urine, and hence clear the body of the fluid that would otherwise accumulate and cause symptoms.
- Diuretics are normally given in the mornings, only because it is more convenient to pass urine during the day.
- There are many different kinds of diuretic, which vary in their strength and the way they work. Sometimes it is necessary to take them in combination with a drug that replaces some of the minerals lost in the urine. Potassium, for example, is often added.
- Heart drugs can also be given to help the heart pump more effectively.
- All these drugs must only be taken as prescribed, and blood tests may be required to check the balance of minerals in the body, particularly when they are first started.
- Heart failure may develop to such an extent that it no longer responds to any treatment. If this happens death will usually follow.

☎ British Heart Foundation, 14 Fitzhardinge Street, London W1H 4DH. (Regional offices listed in the telephone directory. Send s.a.e. for publications list.)

Heatstroke

It is common for people to suffer from a minor degree of heat exhaustion or sunstroke, which most often occurs on holiday. This is not usually serious, but if left unattended or ignored may develop into serious heatstroke which is characterised by high fever, flushed hot appearance, dry skin and rapid pulse. Only these severe symptoms normally need medical attention. A lot can be done to avoid and treat mild sunstroke.

Symptoms

Mild
* Dizzy feelings.
* Faintness.
* Headache.
* Sweating.
* Weakness and loss of appetite.
* Muscle cramps.

Severe
* Rapid pulse.
* High fever.
* Dry skin.

If severe symptoms develop consult a doctor.

Causes

☐ Prolonged exposure to sun or heat.
☐ Strenuous exercise in a hot atmosphere.
☐ Lack of adequate fluids under these conditions.
☐ Inadequate salt intake.
☐ It is the body temperature regulation system which is upset and causes the symptoms of sunstroke, which may develop into heatstroke.

Prevention

- Avoid these symptoms by limiting exposure to sun for the first few days of a holiday or change of atmo-

sphere.
- Drink plenty of non-alcoholic drinks.
- Add a little extra salt to your food.
- Wear a hat, preferably broad-brimmed.

Treatment
- Drink plenty of fluids. If you can tolerate the drinks with a small teaspoon of salt added to every two pints this can help.
- Avoid alcohol.
- Keep cool. Aids to this when symptoms develop include:
  - fanning
  - warm-water sponging
  - leaving the skin wet so the skin cools as the water evaporates
  - baths which are cool, but not cold, help to lower body temperature
- Raise the feet.
- Wear loose clothing.

The Doctor
- Should be consulted if more severe symptoms develop.
- Hospital admission is necessary to control the body temperature and balance of salt and water if heatstroke develops.

Hernia, groin

The commonest type of hernia is one which appears in the groin on either the right- or left-hand side. This is also called an inguinal hernia. A hernia is formed when there is a weakness in the outer wall of the abdomen which holds the intestines in place. Just as a weakness in an old car tyre allows the inner tube to bulge out, so the intestines may bulge through a weakness in the muscles of the abdominal wall.

An inguinal hernia is twenty times more common in men than women. It is not usually serious, but an operation is performed to repair the muscle weakness.

There are two complications of hernias which are avoided by repair. The hernia may obstruct, stopping the onward movement of intestinal contents, producing pain, nausea and vomiting. It may also strangulate when the muscles close on the hernia, limiting the blood supply to the contents of the hernia. This causes severe pain and danger of injury to the intestine in the hernia.

Symptoms
* A bulge appears in the abdominal wall in the groin. This may appear suddenly or develop slowly over months.
* There may be a sensation of heaviness or discomfort in the groin area.
* Often the bulge can be made to disappear on gentle pressure, particularly if you are lying down. It will reappear on coughing.
* Severe pain and tenderness in the area of a hernia suggests that injury to the intestine has occurred, and urgent medical attention will be needed.

Causes
- An inguinal hernia in adults occurs when there is a weakness in the muscles permitting the bulging of the intestines, which are contained in a sac, through this weakness. The muscles are designed to withstand a certain amount of pressure on the inside of the abdomen. Anything increasing the pressure makes a hernia more likely. For instance, heavy lifting, straining, even prolonged coughing and sneezing may precipitate a hernia.
- In male infants prior to birth the testicles descend from inside the abdomen into the scrotum. They drag with them a thin extension of the sac surrounding the intestines. Normally

this extension seals off, isolating the testes in the scrotum. Sometimes a patent tube remains, leading from the abdominal cavity into the scrotum. When a baby cries and increases its abdominal pressure a hernia may extend into the baby's groin and into the scrotum.

Treatment
- Surgical treatment is normally carried out to repair the deficiency in the retaining wall of the abdomen.
- While awaiting treatment avoid straining, lifting and coughing if possible.

The Doctor
- Will advise on the urgency of repair. It is usually best to operate as soon as possible. Occasionally the hernia is very large and there is less danger of the above complications. The doctor may then provide a special support, called a truss, which helps to prevent the hernia bulging out. This may also be used in the elderly if they are not fit for a general anaesthetic and cannot have the hernia repaired.
- The operation involves an incision over the abdominal wall, and the hernia is pushed back into place. The layers of muscle are then effectively darned together to create a strong barrier to prevent the hernia recurring.
- A local or general anaesthetic may be used.
- You will be up and about within one or two days of the operation. Your activities following the repair will have to be limited until healing is complete. Always take advice from your doctor over when you can resume your ordinary work. It may be necessary to avoid heavy lifting for up to twelve weeks following the operation.

Hernia, umbilical

A hernia is caused by a weakness in the abdominal wall which allows the contents to bulge out. (See also **Hernia, groin.**) A hernia in babies, appearing around the tummy button, is very common. A hernia in the area of the tummy button in adults may also occur; this is called a para-umbilical hernia. In babies there is usually no danger and repair is seldom needed (see below). In adults repair is more frequently carried out, to avoid the risks of obstruction and strangulation. (See **Hernia, groin.**)

Symptoms
Babies
* A baby is not normally troubled by an umbilical hernia.
* It may become very prominent when the baby cries.
* Usually it is easily pushed back into place.
* The opening into the hernia is wide and there is little risk of injury to the intestines.

Adults
* Adults who have a para-umbilical hernia feel symptoms of heaviness and discomfort.
* The bulge may be more noticeable on coughing or sneezing.
* If it becomes painful or tender see your doctor at once.

Causes
□ In babies there is incomplete development of the abdominal wall muscles, which allows a hernia to appear.
□ In adults a para-umbilical hernia is much more common in women than men. Repeated pregnancies may stretch and weaken the abdominal wall. Being overweight may also put you at risk of having a para-umbilical hernia.

Treatment
- In babies no treatment is usually required. The hernia usually goes by the end of the first year of life. See your doctor if it persists or becomes larger, painful or is troublesome.
- In adults, in order to prevent the complications of a hernia, repair is carried out as described for Hernia-groin. After operation, care must be taken to avoid excessive increase in abdominal pressure until healing is complete.

Hiatus hernia

A hiatus hernia occurs when part of the stomach protrudes into the chest through a weakness in the muscular division between chest and tummy. This muscle is called the diaphragm. In hiatus hernia the mechanism for closing off the stomach contents from the more delicate oesophagus, which leads into the stomach, is less effective. It may then be difficult to prevent the acid stomach contents from causing pain when they enter the oesophagus. Hiatus hernia is common in both the elderly and those who are overweight. It is not dangerous in itself but if very persistent the continuous irritation of the acid from the stomach can cause scarring at the bottom of the oesophagus and subsequent narrowing.

Symptoms
* Heartburn describes a searing or hot discomfort behind the breast bone, which is felt in hiatus hernia.
* This discomfort may be worse on lying down, or leaning forward, which causes further acid to enter the throat.
* Belching is a common feature of hiatus hernia.
* Bile or acid tastes in the mouth are common. Because the valve closing the stomach works inefficiently it is easier for stomach contents to be regurgitated.
* Many people have a hiatus hernia without symptoms, which only develop if there is a significant increase in weight or with age.

Causes
- Weakness of the diaphragm will be more marked in the elderly.
- Any slight weakness will be made worse, and a greater protrusion of stomach into the chest will occur, if there is obesity.
- Pregnancy often accentuates hiatus hernia symptoms. This is because pregnancy affects the way the stomach empties and also because the enlarging baby increases pressure on the tummy side of the diaphragm.

Treatment
- Lose weight. This is very often enough to stop hiatus hernia symptoms.
- Avoid lying down or bending shortly after meals.
- Raise the bed-head on bricks or old telephone directories to about 4–6 inches off the floor.
- Stop smoking and avoid alcohol.
- Try antacid liquids and tablets from the chemist.
- See **Indigestion** for further details of prevention and treatment of symptoms.

The Doctor
- May prescribe antacids not available from the chemist.
- There are also drugs which alter the way the stomach empties which may help hiatus hernia symptoms. These are available only on prescription.
- Your doctor will be very keen to pay great attention to any weight problem. If your weight is controlled and reasonable for your height you may

be offered surgical correction of the hiatus hernia. This can work well but is of no value if weight gain takes place subsequently.

Hips, clicky and congenital dislocation of

Many parents arrive home with their baby, having been told that the newly arrived infant has clicky hips. This puzzling description refers to the noise the hip makes when doctors are checking for dislocation of the hip, which may be present at birth (congenital dislocation of the hip). What is often not made clear is that having clicky hips does not, by any means, indicate that your child definitely has dislocation of the hip. The majority of clicky hips are normal. It is thought that the click comes from a noise made by the ligaments. Because of the possibility of dislocation of the hip you will, however, be asked to attend the hospital again for further examinations to see if the clicky hip goes on its own or if it needs further tests.

Congenital dislocation of the hip occurs when the ball-and-socket joint which comprises the hip joint is not assembled correctly. If the ball is out of the socket it is dislocated. For correct growth of the thigh bone and hip joint the ball needs to be in the correct place. The displacement of the ball at the top of the thigh bone out of the socket in the pelvis is made easier by the shallow and poorly formed nature of the socket at birth.

Females are much more commonly affected than males. There is often a family history of congenital dislocation of the hip. It is also more common in babies delivered in the breech position (bottom first instead of head first).

Symptoms
* Clicky hips are usually found on routine baby checks at birth.
* Congenital dislocation of the hip may be identified at this time; if undetected it will lead to difficulties later on.
* As the child walks, missed dislocations may reveal themselves by the child limping.
* Walking on tiptoe can indicate a hip problem.
* Discomfort on changing a nappy.
* Sitting with legs astride.
* Crawling with only one leg.
* Walking oddly.

Causes
- It is not clear why congenital dislocation of the hip occurs.
- There are some children who are born with the hip in place but, due to a problem common to their family, the socket part of the joint is poorly formed and the hip slowly dislocates.

Treatment
- Clicky hips will always be reviewed. Fortunately, most turn out to be harmless and the child develops a normal hip joint as it grows.
- It is not possible to predict which dislocated hips may correct by themselves, so all those diagnosed as having congenital dislocation of the hips are treated.
- X-rays are not helpful at birth, because the bones are not sufficiently formed. When the top of the thigh bone has developed further, at around three to six months, X-rays may be useful.
- Treatment should be carried out as early as possible as it is more difficult, and less likely to work, as the child gets older.
- The thighs are held apart using a splint. This holds the ball in the socket and allows it to develop

normally. The splint can be removed for washing. It is normally in place for six to twelve weeks, or longer. The splint makes the child look very awkward but does not cause discomfort.
- Early treatment is very successful.
- Surgery may be necessary if dislocation of the hip is diagnosed later, particularly beyond the second birthday. More than one operation may be required under general anaesthetic. The child is in hospital for several weeks and in plaster for several months following surgery, which is not always successful.
- A child who has surgery may still have problems walking in later life. A woman seen walking with a limp today is very likely to have had congenital dislocation of the hip, possibly not diagnosed at birth, which has not had successful treatment as she grew up.

Hives

This is a skin condition which is also known as urticaria and nettlerash. It is not generally serious, and although itching is often intense it usually clears quickly. Rarely, the neck and face are involved, which can lead to breathing difficulties, in which case a doctor should be consulted immediately.

Symptoms
* Red lumps appear on the skin, also known as weals.
* They appear to have a white centre on a red base.
* Itching is intense.
* The raised weals come and go over a period of hours, new ones appearing as others go.
* It often comes on within minutes of contact with triggering substance.
* Weals vary in size from pimples to several inches across.
* Face- and tongue-swelling may occur; in this instance consult a doctor immediately.

Causes
The exact cause of hives often remains unknown. Common examples of what can cause hives are:
- Skin contact with many substances, including the primula plant, which is frequently a culprit.
- Eating – many foods can bring on hives but it is commonly seen with strawberries and shellfish.
- Inhaled pollens. (See **Hayfever**.)
- Drugs, e.g. penicillin.
- Nettle stings.
- Insect bites can bring on an unpleasant form of hives called papular urticaria. Scratching of these lesions can lead to infection.

Treatment
- Must be aimed primarily at removing the cause.
- Avoid contact with the plant, food or other substances responsible.
- Calamine lotion can soothe the itching.
- Cold compresses can help.
- A warm bath may temporarily relieve itching, but it may be as intense as ever on getting out.
- Antihistamines from the chemist taken by mouth can help. Beware of antihistamines applied to the skin – prolonged use can cause skin reactions, with redness and itching.

The Doctor
- Can prescribe different antihistamines which are not for general sale at the chemist.
- Will check for infection of papular urticarial weals and prescribe antibiotics if necessary.
- May prescribe 1% hydrocortisone

cream to decrease itching.
- If there are signs of breathing difficulty the doctor will give an injection of adrenalin and steroids, which can dramatically avert otherwise fatal consequences. (See **Shock**.)

Hoarseness

The sounds produced in the larynx (or voice box) are altered when the vocal cords become swollen. Just as strings on an instrument produce a different sound when loose or damaged, so the voice box can produce a hoarse sound – usually as a result of infection. The importance of hoarseness as a symptom is that its persistence may be the only indication of a tumour affecting the vocal cords. This can nearly always be cured, so hoarseness lasting more than two to three weeks should always be reported to your doctor.

Symptoms
* Those of infection of the voice box (laryngitis).
* Often on waking the voice is hoarse.
* Two to three days later there may be loss of voice.
* It may be painful to speak.
* Flu and fever symptoms.

Causes
- Bacterial or viral infection (laryngitis).
- Irritation of the voice box due to:
  - cigarette smoking
  - alcohol
  - over-use, e.g. market traders, opera singers
- Low thyroid hormone levels. (See **Thyroid problems**.)
- A benign or malignant tumour.

Treatment
- Rest the voice.
- Inhale steamy air.
- Stop smoking and avoid alcohol.
- Control flu symptoms. (See **Flu**.)
- Usually settles in four to five days.

The Doctor
- Should be consulted if symptoms persist for more than one week.
- He may prescribe antibiotics, particularly if there is an associated sinusitis or bronchitis.
- After two or three weeks he may refer you to a throat specialist for a check-up.
- Treatment with radiotherapy can be very effective if a tumour is present.

Hyperactivity

Children are often described as being hyperactive. There may only be short periods of overactivity in children who are filled with enthusiasm; this is quite normal. For some children, however, this overactivity and difficulty in settling or concentrating to do anything is persistent, and affects all aspects of their lives. Doctors vary in opinion as to how common this problem is. In America it is very widely diagnosed and called attention deficit disorder. In the United Kingdom it is not a common diagnosis, but is increasingly recognised by child psychiatrists and other doctors working with children. It is also called the hyperkinetic syndrome.

Symptoms
* A child may have been noted to be restless from birth with feeding and sleep problems.
* When walking starts the child seems to be into everything and is prone to accidents.
* Restlessness is seen at mealtimes, and although the child may sit in front of the television for prolonged periods he will fidget continually.
* There is poor concentration on

puzzles or activities. Simple toys do not seem to hold the child's attention.
* The child is often remarkably unafraid of strangers, and behaviour is uninhibited and may even be aggressive.
* As the child grows older there may be behaviour and learning problems at school. Later there may be a persistent lack of inhibition which leads to anti-social behaviour.

Causes

No one cause has been found to explain hyperactivity; it is thought that a combination of many factors makes it more likely for a child to be hyperactive. These include:

- Hereditary (genetic) factors.
- A child's personality and temperament.
- Chemical factors in the brain; birth injury may have an effect. In America it is considered to be due to 'minimal brain dysfunction'.
- Diet is widely thought to be important, although some studies have failed to prove this. Food colourings and additives are particularly thought to cause or exacerbate hyperactivity. Dietary factors may be more important if there is:
  - a history of allergy in the child or their close relatives
  - changes in skin colour accompanying mood or behaviour changes, particularly a pale or blotchy face
  - changes in mood or behaviour in association with certain foods
- Social problems, including housing, financial and parental problems, have an influence on whether a child is hyperactive or not.
- Parental response to a child may be important; with some children hyperactivity develops as a way of seeking attention from the parent. Early separation from parents may contribute to subsequent hyperactivity.

Treatment

- Whatever the cause of hyperactivity, the parents and whole family will have to become involved in treatment if there is to be any improvement. The treatment is never instant and involves long-term help from doctors and other health workers.
- The school may have to be deeply involved. Schools can contribute by allowing some periods of free activity and others where a structure is imposed with the minimum of opportunity allowed for the child to be disruptive.
- Praise is always important when the child shows any longer periods of concentration. Bouts of hyperactivity should be ignored.
- The child should not be over-stimulated, one or two toys only being offered at any one time.
- Dietary factors can be sought by a process of elimination. If one substance does seem to worsen hyperactivity it should be excluded. It is important that major changes in diet should not be undertaken unless discussed with your doctor or a dietician. Some dietary changes if introduced too hastily or severely can affect growth. Some foods are now marked 'no additives and no artificial colourings'. The worst offenders as far as foods are concerned include:
  - processed meats and cheeses
  - pre-cooked meats or dishes
  - confectionery, including crisps, sweets, drinks, ices.
  - breakfast cereals and some breads
  - puddings and cakes bought from shops
  - margarine

The Doctor
- As well as being involved in helping with the above aspects of treatment, if the problem of hyperactivity is severe the doctor may arrange for the child and parents to be seen by a child psychiatrist.
- Medicines are sometimes given to children with this problem, but their use is always very much in conjunction with the parents' and the child's cooperation. In some children they are helpful but, partly because their side-effects can be troublesome, they are only used in very persistently hyperactive children.
- Usually the problem of hyperactivity improves by itself as the child grows older. Occasionally, poor behaviour patterns persist into adulthood and lead to anti-social behaviour and personality disorders.
- ☎ Hyperactive Children's Support Group, Sally Bunday, 71 White Lane, Chichester, West Sussex PO19 2LD.

Hyperventilation

This is the medical term for increased breathing which can lead to a variety of unpleasant symptoms. It is commonly due to emotional responses to stress or anxiety and is usually harmless. Rarely, it occurs as part of a more serious medical complaint.

Symptoms
* The rate and depth of breathing is increased; this may happen without your being aware of it.
* You may become dizzy and feel faint.
* There can be blurring of vision, numbness and tingling.
* Sweating may occur.
* You may become very aware of your heartbeat and experience palpitations. (See **Palpitations**.)
* If severe there may be spasm of the muscles (tetany), in the hands and feet particularly.

Causes
□ The increased breathing removes more carbon dioxide from the lungs. If the concentration of this gas is lowered beyond a certain point it has an effect on the balance of the chemicals and gases in the blood, which then produces symptoms.
□ Hyperventilation may occur without your being aware of any precipitating factors. Usually, however, the cause can be related to a current stress affecting you.

Treatment
- Immediate treatment is to rebreathe your own air. This can be done very adequately by breathing in and out of a bag held over the mouth. Make the neck of a paper bag or smallish plastic bag into a funnel in your hand as if you wanted to blow it up like a balloon. Hold this against your mouth and breathe in and out. As you do so the symptoms should clear within five minutes.

The Doctor
- Should always be consulted if you find you have the symptoms of hyperventilation. The doctor will be able to establish that there are no underlying medical conditions causing the symptoms and can arrange suitable help if you are having emotional or other difficulties.

Hysterectomy

Hysterectomy refers to the removal of the womb and the neck of the womb (cervix). Total hysterectomy is the medical expression used by doctors to describe what is normally understood by hysterectomy, total referring to removal of the cervix as well as the womb. It is unusual to remove only the womb, leaving the cervix, because the cervix serves no useful function and is a common cause of problems. (See **Cervical problems**.)

Periods cease after hysterectomy, but menopausal symptoms do not occur any earlier unless the ovaries are removed at the same time. The operation may be done before the menopause occurs, but is unusual during child-bearing years. In this age group it is only carried out when other treatments fail. After, or around, the menopause there are a variety of reasons for having a hysterectomy which are outlined below. Whatever the reason the ability to have children is lost, but this should not interfere with a normal sex life.

Causes

- Fibroids can be removed separately from the womb, but often this is not possible or it is more appropriate to remove the whole womb. (See **Fibroids**.)
- If the womb itself, or the cervix, is diseased hysterectomy may be performed.
- Prolapse of the womb may be treated by hysterectomy.
- Periods that are particularly troublesome and unresponsive to other treatments may have to be dealt with by hysterectomy. (See **Periods**.)
- Ovarian disease may require the removal of the ovaries. Sometimes the womb and ovaries are removed together, which is a bigger operation referred to as a Wertheim's hysterectomy.

Treatment

Before operation
- Before having a hysterectomy because of troublesome periods you should try every alternative way of controlling them. Control is preferable to hysterectomy, particularly as periods will eventually cease on their own. (See **Menopause, Periods**.)
- Whatever the reason, it is wise to make sure you are not anaemic by eating foods containing iron and having your blood checked (see **Anaemia**). Avoiding anaemia can help during recovery following the operation.

At Operation
- There are two different ways in which hysterectomy can be performed:
  - by an abdominal incision, usually along the bikini line
  - through the vagina
- The abdominal operation is more common but the vaginal method may be used, particularly if there is a prolapse or a need to tighten supportive straps around the bladder.
- On waking from the operation you will normally have a drainage tube leading from the abdomen to a container beside the bed. This helps to remove unwanted blood and fluids from the area of the operation and thereby speed healing. There may also be an intravenous drip in one arm. These appendages are very quickly removed and you will be expected to be up and about a bit within the first day or two.

Convalescence
- You will normally be allowed home after seven days.
- The operation is frequently followed by a prolonged period of marked physical tiredness, lethargy and feeling generally unwell.
- Don't expect too early a return to work, nor to be able to manage household tasks or childcare to a full extent for two to three months after the operation.

- Your doctor can advise you during this time and check for anaemia by doing a simple blood test.
- ☎ Hysterectomy Support Group, c/o Women's Health, 52 Featherstone Street, London EC1. Tel: 071 251 6580.

Impetigo

This is a common skin infection which can appear anywhere, but is usually found around the mouth and nose. Children are more often affected than adults and, because it is highly infectious, should be kept away from school until it has cleared. The same germ can affect babies and cause extensive red peeling areas of skin and general illness.

Symptoms
* Blisters appear.
* They burst, leaving red weeping areas.
* Yellowy-brown crusts appear.
* The infection spreads to affect other areas.
* The infection can be transferred to other parts of the body by touching the sores.

Causes
☐ Two particular bacteria called *staphylococcus* and *streptococcus* produce impetigo.
☐ It is resistant to certain types of penicillin.

Treatment
- You should always see your doctor as impetigo does not go on its own and will certainly spread.
- Washing the face is possible if done gently and hands are cleaned well afterwards.
- Always use only your own towel and wash things.
- Always wash hands before handling food.

The Doctor
– Will prescribe antibiotic ointment which will clear the skin in a few days. Wash thick crusts off before applying treatment.
– May prescribe antibiotic tablets if there are several lesions.

Incontinence

Incontinence occurs when either urine or stool is passed without control and against your wishes. It is an extremely common problem, affecting one person in every five over the age of sixty-five. The problem mainly affects the passage of urine; incontinence of stool is relatively rare. There is a considerable amount that can be done to help with incontinence. For problems in children see **Bedwetting**.

Symptoms
* Small amounts of urine may be lost on coughing, sneezing, laughing or exercising. (Also called stress incontinence.)
* There may be a frequent desire to urinate, but on trying to pass urine only a small quantity of urine is passed. At other times you may have to rush to the toilet as the bladder signals its sudden desire to empty. (Also called urge incontinence.)
* Some incontinence may occur due to a build-up of stool, which becomes partially blocked inside the intestine; the only stool that can pass is a liquid oozing. There may be 'overflow incontinence' of the bladder when the bladder is full but the valves and mechanism for emptying it are not working properly; it may either suddenly empty or dribbling may occur.
* Dribbling after passing urine is very common in men with prostate problems. The urine does not shut off cleanly after a quantity has been

passed. Some people find it helpful to push the base of the penis against the pubic bone to try and help clear the urine tube of the last few drops. (See **Prostate problems**.)

Causes

- ☐ Urine infection can cause incontinence. (See **Cystitis**, **Urine infection**.)
- ☐ Prostate problems. (See **Prostate**.)
- ☐ Drugs – as a side-effect of many drugs urine flow may be more difficult to control.
- ☐ Weak pelvic muscles may cause problems, e.g. following childbirth.
- ☐ Intestinal disease and lack of fibre can exacerbate, or cause, stool incontinence.
- ☐ Stroke, dementia and spinal cord injuries can all lead to incontinence. (See **Dementia**, **Stroke**.)
- ☐ Depression sometimes leads to incontinence of stool.
- ☐ Incontinence is not just an inevitable part of growing old. Although muscles forming valves, or sphincters, to close off urine and stool passages may become weaker with age, this is by no means invariable.

Treatment

- A lot can be done to help you have fewer episodes of incontinence and control the situation yourself:
  - Use the toilet regularly, setting an alarm clock or timer if necessary.
  - Keep a chamber pot or commode handy.
  - Have adjustments made to facilitate your use of the toilet, such as fitting rails round it or raising the seat. Your doctor or district nurse can help get these fitted by the local authority.
  - Wear easy clothes with zips rather than fiddly buttons.
  - Diet and drinking can greatly influence the situation. Eat a high-fibre diet and avoid excessive drinking, particularly before bedtime. If you are having trouble with stools, remember that your body's desire to pass a stool is usually around one hour after a meal.
- If you have symptoms of incontinence it is always wise to see the doctor, rather than trying to put up with the situation. There is often a readily treatable cause and, if not, other help is available.

The Doctor

- Will aim to establish the cause; this may involve tests, including checking the urine for infection.
- Examination may also reveal build-up of stool, or weak pelvic muscles. It is also possible to examine the prostate gland with a gloved finger in the back passage.
- Drugs are available to treat infections, and to stabilise partially the activity of the bladder in order to decrease urge incontinence.
- Laxatives, enemas or fibre in a convenient granule form can all be given to help stool problems (See **Constipation**.)
- The doctor, district nurse or health visitor for the elderly may be able to help with incontinence aids. These are many and varied, and it is always worth asking about them. Special pads, underwear and devices are available.
- In some cases surgery may be possible to relieve prostate problems, or tighten the muscles of a sphincter.

☎ The Association of Continence Advisors, c/o The Disabled Living Foundation, 380–384 Harrow Road, London W9 2HU. Tel: 071 289 6111.

Indigestion

Nearly everyone experiences indigestion from time to time. It is usually related to what you eat or drink. It can be very troublesome but is not serious or dangerous in itself. If the normal pattern of your indigestion changes and new symptoms develop this could indicate other illness and you should consult your doctor. Indigestion can be easily treated and avoided. Sometimes it may be quite reasonable to take a risk with eating or drinking certain substances, in the knowledge that they may precipitate indigestion, if the enjoyment of the meal or event warrants the potential discomfort.

Symptoms

* Nagging pain or discomfort in the top of the stomach or lower chest. Pain may be described as gnawing.
* General discomfort.
* Distension, with a desire to belch or break wind.
* Nausea.
* Acid or bilious taste in the mouth. There may be some regurgitation from the stomach.
* Heartburn is a general term frequently used to describe a burning or searing pain behind the breast bone. It may also be felt if there is a hiatus hernia. (See **Hiatus hernia**.)
* Vomiting, if accompanying indigestion without an obvious cause such as food poisoning or over-indulgence, may indicate more serious illness.
* Changes in symptoms to become more severe or persistent should be discussed with your doctor (see below).

Causes

▫ Indigestion is related to stomach contents, and is therefore controlled by what is eaten or drunk and the amount of acid in the stomach.
▫ Timing of what we eat is important. Hunger pain may often be felt as indigestion. If we eat snacks irregularly and then suddenly an enormous meal, it is not surprising that the stomach complains by producing indigestion symptoms.
▫ Certain foods – onions and beans, for example, and certain alcoholic drinks taken even in small quantities, may produce indigestion.
▫ Pregnancy has an effect on the way the stomach and intestine empty and digest their contents. Indigestion is extremely common in pregnancy. Early morning sickness of pregnancy can often be helped by eating a biscuit or taking antacid medicine even before getting out of bed. (See **Pregnancy problems**.)
▫ Stress over a prolonged time or being anxious about a future difficulty may cause indigestion.
▫ Indigestion symptoms may be a sign of more serious illnesses, particularly if they change as mentioned above. For example, see **Gallstones**, **Hiatus hernia**, **Ulcers**. Indigestion may very rarely indicate cancer of the stomach.

Prevention

* Eat regular meals of similar quantity.
* Avoid excesses and prolonged periods without food.
* Do not eat standing up or hurry food.
* Try and relax during a meal and for half an hour or so afterwards.
* Loosen tight clothing.

Treatment

* This is aimed at removing the cause, whether this be eating too much, too quickly or the wrong food.
* Stop smoking. Smoking is well recognised as making stomach symptoms worse. It is very important to stop if

- symptoms are severe.
- Alcohol, particularly in excess, can only make indigestion worse. Avoid completely until symptoms clear.
- Choose your diet carefully, trying to discover those substances which help most to settle your symptoms. Often milk and dry biscuits are helpful.
- Use of antacid medicines in liquid and tablet form from the chemist is often sufficient to relieve symptoms. Take your doctor's advice before using these in pregnancy.

The Doctor
- May prescribe different antacids from those available at the chemist.
- Will advise on a dietary regime to try and help, while making enquiries about social activities that may be provoking indigestion.
- If the symptoms are severe, not settling, or are part of a change from your normal pattern the doctor may arrange various tests to exclude other illnesses.
- The tests may include barium meal X-ray, gastroscopy and perhaps an ultrasound examination of the gall-bladder, for example. For more details of tests see **Ulcers, stomach**.

Infertility

Infertility refers to the inability to conceive a child. At its simplest, the failure of a woman to produce an egg, or a man to produce sperm, leads to infertility. There are many other reasons for infertility, related either to faulty egg or sperm production or mechanical difficulties preventing the two from meeting. If you are having regular intercourse once or twice a week, without using contraception, you will normally be pregnant within a year. However, despite regular unprotected intercourse, 10 per cent of couples do not achieve a pregnancy within a year. Many of the causes of infertility are simply corrected and it is always worth while seeking advice.

Causes
In couples
- Incorrect intercourse and a lack of knowledge about how sperm need to be ejaculated inside the vagina is a not infrequent cause of infertility.
- If intercourse does not take place when an egg is produced conception will not occur. Intercourse mid-way between periods is most likely to achieve a pregnancy. A woman produces an egg around the fourteenth day of her cycle, counting day one as the first day of a period. This assumes a regular cycle of about twenty-eight days. If the menstrual cycle is irregular or longer, eggs may be produced at other times, but generally a reasonable guide is mid-way between periods.

In men
- A low total number of sperm may be produced. Normally as many as 50 million sperm or more are produced at one ejaculation. In this number there will be some sperm which are abnormally formed or which move in an abnormal way. The sperm may be inadequate either in total number or there may be more abnormal sperm than usual. Abnormal sperm do not lead to a pregnancy.
- Excess alcohol, testicle abnormalities, overwork and exhaustion may all reduce the sperm count. (See **Testes problems**.)
- Rarely, there is a blockage or narrowing in the tube from the testicle to the penis which hinders ejaculation of sperm.

In women
- Hormonal problems may lead to a failure to produce an egg. This may be suggested by your having irregular

or infrequent periods. There are many factors influencing the normal pattern of periods and hence egg production. (See **Periods**.)

☐ A blockage in the tubes between the ovaries and the womb (which allow the eggs to meet the sperm) may cause infertility. This can be caused by previous infection or scarring from other gynaecological problems. (See **Pelvic infection**.)

☐ If the womb is an abnormal shape this may prevent sperm and egg from meeting and developing into a pregnancy. Sometimes the womb is an abnormal shape from birth; at other times a fibroid or other problem may be interfering with conception. (See **Fibroids**.)

Treatment

- The first part of treatment of infertility is always to discover the cause. It is often difficult to know at what stage to seek help. The following are rough guidelines:
  - Seek help after one year of unprotected intercourse if conception has not occurred (see above).
  - If you have an irregular cycle, sexual difficulties or previous gynaecological problems seek help earlier.
  - If you are a woman over thirty years of age it may be wise to seek help after only six months of unprotected intercourse as the number of eggs a woman produces diminishes as you get older.

The Doctor

- Will establish that you are having normal intercourse and that it is taking place often enough and at the time in the women's cycle most likely to achieve conception (see above).
- Simple examination of both the man and woman will be carried out to check for abnormalities and any infections.

In men

- A sperm count can be arranged, to check for the quality and quantity of the sperm. Normally at least three are done.
- Blood tests may be done to check male hormone levels and, rarely, surgery can be done to correct any blockages or testicle problems.
- Wearing boxer shorts allows the testicles to hang further from the body and hence be maintained at a lower temperature. This may be helpful.
- Abstaining from intercourse for a few days, prior to the most suitable time to have intercourse, raises the sperm count.

In women

- Blood tests will be done to check hormone levels and look for signs of egg production.
- A temperature chart may be kept daily over a period of months. This can reveal the normal change in temperature around the time of egg production, a steady temperature suggesting that no egg is being released by the ovary. Some specialists do not consider this very reliable.
- Laparoscopy may be carried out. This involves looking at the internal organs through a telescope. (A thin telescopic device is passed through a small slit in the abdominal wall.)
- X-ray tests looking at what happens to dye, which is inserted into the womb and then flows through towards the ovaries, can reveal any blockages in the tubes.
- A post-coital test is sometimes done. This involves the woman being examined within twenty-four hours of intercourse to see if sperm have

penetrated the mucus at the entrance to the womb.

- Drugs can be used to stimulate the ovary to produce eggs in some women. These 'fertility drugs' are normally taken for a few days each cycle and must only be taken as your doctor advises. Incorrect use may increase the likelihood of multiple pregnancy.
- Surgery may be helpful in women. This can sometimes unblock the tubes between the ovary and the womb. It may also be helpful if any other gynaecological problem is interfering with conception.

Techniques to aid fertility

Despite the elaborate tests and complicated surgery that are available to help achieve conception, some couples remain infertile. There are now a number of modern techniques to try and assist conception. These include:

IVF (in-vitro fertilisation)
This tries to achieve conception outside the body (or a 'test tube' baby). The sperm and egg are brought together in a laboratory and then replaced in the womb. This is one of the less successful infertility treatments and is not suitable for women who do not ovulate or have a damaged uterus. It is also less suitable for women over forty years old.

AIH (artificial insemintion by husband)
The husband's sperm is placed into the woman, but seldom more successfully than can be achieved by having intercourse.

AID (artificial insemination by donor)
If conception is not achieved because of a problem with the husband's sperm, sperm from a donor can be inserted into the woman to fertilise the egg. This should only be undertaken after lengthy consideration.

GIFT (gamete intra-fallopian transfer)
This is done by collecting eggs directly from the ovary and placing them, together with the husband's sperm, into the fallopian tube in the hope that conception will occur. It is only available in certain centres.

POST (peritoneal ovum and sperm transfer)
This works by injecting the husband's sperm and eggs collected from the ovary into a space near the ovary. It can be done in a single operation. It is only available at certain centres.

Some fertility treatments, which combine sperm and eggs together and insert several potentially successful early pregnancies into the womb, have been criticised. This is because they may lead to multiple pregnancies in which very premature babies are born, all of whom are at risk of not surviving. There are now voluntary limits which endeavour to diminish this problem. You should ask for the number of potential pregnancies to be limited if you are having this treatment.

- ☎ The Endometriosis Society, Unit F8A, Shakespeare Business Centre, 245A Coldharbour Lane, London SW9 8RR. Tel: 071 737 0380.

- ☎ National Association for the Childless, St George's Rectory, Tower Street, B19 3UY. Tel: 021 359 4887.

In-growing toenails

Commonly affecting children, but also adults, this may be a once-in-a-lifetime event or at worst recurrent and very troublesome. In short, the nail grows forward and sideways, burying itself in skin. It cuts and deforms the skin, causing injury and infection. It is never serious but certainly requires attention to treatment and prevention. Properly managed, the problem can be avoided for the future.

Symptoms
* Pain on walking.
* Pain wearing certain shoes.
* Continuous pain.
* Pain spreading up the foot.
* Red tender area on one or both sides of the nail.
* Swollen red-yellow area on nail sides.

Causes
- Incorrect cutting of nail.
- Incorrectly fitting footwear.
- Children picking the nail leads to damage to skin and nail. This is made worse as the nail regrows.

Prevention
- Correctly fitting footwear and socks.
- Cut straight across the top of the nail.
- Do not cut round or down the corners of toe nails.
- Do not cut the nails too short.

The Doctor
- See the doctor for antibiotics and advice if there are signs of infection, swelling, tenderness, pain, yellow colouration or discharge.
- Occasionally it is necessary, usually under local anaesthetic, to remove part or all of the nail to stop the problem.
- Chiropodists can give helpful advice, particularly if the problem is recurrent.

Irritable colon

This condition is also known as spastic colon or irritable bowel syndrome. Normally the intestine is continually contracting in waves along its length in order to move on the intestinal contents. These contractions occur regularly without your being aware of them. If you have an irritable colon the normal pattern of contractions is disorganised and irregular. This leads to a number of unpleasant and painful symptoms. Irritable colon tends to be a life-long condition but you may go for long periods, of a year or more, without any symptoms. It is not dangerous.

Symptoms
* Cramp-like pains felt generally on one side of the lower part of the stomach.
* Pains are intermittent and may be worse at certain times of the day or in association with passing stools.
* Stools may be frequent, and can be either soft and runny or hard pellets. Sometimes diarrhoea and constipation occur alternately.
* Nausea, bloating and flatulence are common.

Causes
- It is not known what causes irritable colon; many factors, including diet, are probably involved.
- Many people who have irritable colon find it is worse at times of stress or emotional upheaval.

Treatment
- Many people learn to live with the symptoms, only rarely having severe symptoms.
- It is worth avoiding any foods that exacerbate symptoms. Stopping coffee and tea and cutting down on smoking may be helpful. Avoid alcohol excesses and very spicy foods.
- Increasing the fibre in your diet may help, particularly if you tend to be constipated. If you are already on what you consider a high-fibre diet it may be necessary to double your fibre intake to help the problem.
- When symptoms of irritable colon first appear it is important to see the doctor.

The Doctor

- Before a diagnosis of irritable colon can be made, other intestinal problems have to be excluded. The doctor may arrange tests, including examination of the back passage and X-ray examinations of the intestines (barium meal and/or barium enema). If tests fail to reveal any other cause of the symptoms, and the pattern of symptoms remains the same, a diagnosis of irritable colon may be made.
- Some people find increasing their fibre intake helpful. If dietary measures have not produced improvement, sachets of the husk of a plant called ispaghula can be taken. This increases the bulk of the stool and may help to relieve symptoms. It can be purchased at chemists or prescribed.
- Other drugs affecting the intestine may be given, as used in the treatment of constipation. (See **Constipation**.)
- Drugs which decrease the spasms and contractions in the intestine may be used, e.g. merbentyl. These are usually only useful for severe abdominal pain and are best taken for brief periods. There may be unpleasant side-effects and they are not suitable for everyone.
- All drug treatments will only provide temporary relief of symptoms. There is no cure and symptoms tend to fluctuate on and off over many years.

Itching

This is one of the commonest problems brought to the doctor. The variety of causes below illustrates the enormous range of possibilities when itching starts. Fortunately, almost all causes of itching are easily treated and not at all serious.

Symptoms

Itching may be associated with:
* Redness.
* Local swelling.
* Flaky skin.
* Discharge from the skin, sometimes staining clothing.

Causes

Generalised itching

- Allergy: exposure to plants, foods, animals, dyes, cleaning materials or other products can produce a rash or urticaria. Urticaria is characterised by weals that come and go as raised patches on the skin. (See **Hayfever**, **Hives**.)
- Sensitisation to certain products can occur, e.g. disinfectants in the bath, washing powders (rinsing is important), drugs, or nickel in jewellery leading to dermatitis.
- Skin problems: a wide variety of skin problems cause itching, the commonest being eczema. (See **Eczema**.)
- Infection, for example: scabies, ringworm, insect bites, chicken pox or thrush.
- Illness elsewhere in the body can cause generalised itching.

Limited itching

- Anal itching, common in men, can be caused by threadworms, thrush, piles, anal fissures and also occurs with no specific cause being found.
- Vulval itching: women may get itching of the genital area due to thrush, allergic reaction, dryness or soreness (common around the menopause).
- Skin folds: for example, at the elbows and back of knees in eczema, below breasts or in the groin due to thrush or other fungi such as ringworm.
- Feet: for example, athlete's foot, sweat rash.

- Hands: contact with chemicals, cleaning products or even rolling tobacco in the palm can cause a contact dermatitis which is a kind of eczema
  - scabies infection commonly affects the hands
  - thrush can affect fingertips
  - herpes can appear on fingers
- Hair: itching of the scalp can be caused by headlice, psoriasis, seborrhoeic eczema, dandruff, fungal infection. (See **Hair problems**.)
- Armpits: can develop a sweat rash, a sensitisation reaction to deodorants, or be infected with fungi.
- Anywhere an antihistamine or local anaesthetic cream is used over a prolonged time, a local sensitisation reaction can occur.

Treatment
- This must aim to find the cause, whether it be a clasp on a piece of jewellery, a jean-stud causing a sensitivity reaction or an infestation with headlice.
- Specific treatments are listed in various sections of the book covering those problems mentioned above.
- General aids to decrease itching include:
  - cooling with compresses or ice
  - calamine lotion
  - keeping the area clean helps to prevent itching and avoid infection of the area
  - fanning
  - loose clothing; cotton is preferable to nylon and acrylics (see **Thrush**)
  - antihistamine tablets from chemists, e.g. promethazine; these can cause drowsiness and must not be taken if driving or involved in delicate manual work

The Doctor
- Will examine and ask about the cause.
- May look for lice, take skin scrapings to look for fungi, blood tests to check on the body's response to any parasite or general disorder causing itching.
- Will provide a wider range of tablets and lotions to decrease and relieve itching.
- Will review the condition after an interval during which you may be asked to eliminate dietary factors, cosmetics, cleansing agents, etc. that may appear to be the cause.
- May refer you to a skin specialist for more detailed skin examination and testing.

Jaundice

Jaundice is a symptom of disease. The commonest cause of jaundice is a viral infection of the liver called hepatitis. However anything that damages the liver can lead to jaundice. The liver is essential in processing a pigment called bilirubin, which is made up of old and damaged blood cells. If the amount of bilirubin builds up, either because there are too many old and damaged blood cells or because the liver cannot work as normal, the typical yellow colour of jaundice appears in skin and eyes.

Symptoms
* May appear in days or slowly come on over weeks, the skin gradually becoming a darker shade of yellow.
* The whites of the eyes may be the first part to show the typical yellow discoloration.
* First symptoms may be dark urine and pale cream-coloured stools.
* Itching may be noticed.

Causes

- Liver damage due to viral infection may lead to hepatitis. One type of hepatitis is called 'infective' or type A hepatitis. This is passed from person to person by finger and mouth contact, and can also be caught from contaminated food or water (shellfish abroad are common culprits). Another type of hepatitis is called 'Serum' or type B hepatitis. This is caught either through sexual intercourse, injections, tattoos or transfusions.
- Infections such as malaria and glandular fever can also cause liver damage and subsequent jaundice.
- Liver damage can also occur following excess alcohol or certain chemicals, including drugs; e.g. some people become jaundiced following the use of a gas called halothane in anaesthetics.
- If too many blood cells are destroyed a process called haemolysis is said to be taking place. This haemolytic jaundice is seen in blood disorders such as sickle cell anaemia, and thalassaemia. (See **Anaemia**.)
- Jaundice may also follow a blockage in tubes, thus obstructing the drainage of bilirubin into the intestine from the liver. This is called obstructive jaundice and may be caused by gallstones or a cancer near the liver, e.g. cancer of the intestine or pancreas.
- In babies jaundice may occur due to normal immaturity of the liver. This jaundice may last for about two weeks after the birth. In premature babies it may last longer.
- Other causes of jaundice in babies include excess bruising, inherited blood defects, inherited liver defects, and a reaction between the mother's blood cells and those of the baby, called rhesus incompatibility.

Prevention

- Hepatitis A can be prevented by taking simple precautions with washing hands and food carefully, e.g. avoid shellfish in an area where hygiene standards are low.
- Hepatitis B can be prevented through the use of a vaccine. This is used to protect those at risk either through their work, e.g. nurses, or through their sexual contacts, e.g. some homosexuals. Babies of mothers with hepatitis B can be given the vaccine at birth.
- Other causes of liver damage can be avoided where possible, such as excess alcohol or exposure to certain chemicals. (See **Alcoholism**.)

Treatment

- Treatment of hepatitis A is usually unnecessary, the illness clearing on its own over a few weeks.
- Blood tests can give an indication of the possible causes of jaundice and can identify the type of hepatitis (A or B).
- Rest, a good diet and alcohol avoidance for six months are usually all that is required.
- Severe liver problems will need hospital treatment. Tests, which may be used to establish how severe the effects on the liver are, include using ultrasound to build up a picture on a screen of the internal structure of the liver, and liver biopsy, when a small piece of liver is removed by needle for examination under the microscope.
- Often the management of severe or prolonged liver problems involves frequent analysis of blood and other tests to monitor the progress of the disease. Little in the way of specific treatment may be possible.
- Jaundice in the newborn can be monitored by examination of blood from small heel pricks. If the level of

bilirubin causing jaundice is not settling, exposure of the baby to special lights for a short time each day (with the eyes covered) quickly helps to reduce the jaundice. Failure to control the level of bilirubin can have effects on the baby's hearing and brain.

Knock knees

Knock knees are very common in toddlers. Because the knees press together there is a gap between the ankles. Most children will grow out of this by the age of seven.

Symptoms
* On lying down the gap between the ankles should be less than two inches.
* You should see your doctor if the gap is more than four inches.
* There may be generally loose ligaments.
* There may be associated flat feet.
* Symptoms of bone disease are as for bowlegs.
* Children over seven, with knock knees should see the doctor.

Causes
☐ These are usually normal.
☐ Rickets may cause a toddler to have severe knock knees.
☐ Damage to the inner knee by infection or injury.

Treatment
● You do not normally need to worry or see a doctor.
● If you are worried your doctor can usually reassure you.
● If there are signs of bone disease, X-rays and blood tests are done.
● Rickets is treated with special vitamin drops.
● Very rarely, a corrective operation is needed.
● See also **Bowlegs** for more information about rickets.

Limp

There is usually a time in everyone's lives when we have to limp for one reason or another. Limping implies that we are not able fully to use a leg or part of a leg because of pain or weakness. This leads to reluctance or inability to put our full weight on the affected side when walking.

Symptoms
* Walking in such a way as to avoid using one leg to the full.
* A child may refuse to walk.
* Use of a stick may disguise a limp which would be more pronounced without it.

Causes
☐ Polio as an infant can lead to weakened muscles and a permanent limp.
☐ Congenital dislocation of the hip. (See **Hips**.)
☐ Arthritis of the hip. (See **Arthritis**.)
☐ Infection of the skin on the foot from a splinter or injury. (See **Splinter**.)
☐ Infection of the bone may present as a limp. This may occur with or without a tender spot over one of the leg or foot bones. It is serious and always needs treatment by a doctor. This is called osteomyelitis.
☐ One condition that may cause a limp to appear suddenly in children usually less than six or seven years old is called irritable hip. It is common, occurring more often in boys than girls, and is thought to be caused by an inflammation of the hip

joint which may occur after an injury or viral infection. The limp, and difficulty with moving the hip, recovers after a few days' rest. X-rays of the hip are important to exclude other causes of limp, both when this occurs and afterwards. Irritable hip rarely causes long-term problems.
- Perthes' disease may appear in a similar way to irritable hip. X-rays are important to see what is happening to the upper part of the thighbone. In Perthes' disease this part of the thigh bone breaks down before growing back together again. Recovery is usually good, but severe cases may require surgical correction. This disease is much rarer than irritable hip and affects children between four and ten years old. One or both hips may be affected.
- Slipped femoral epiphysis is another cause of limping in children around early teenage years. The top part of the thigh bone, which forms the hip joint, can become displaced away from the rest of the bone forming the thigh bone. Limping occurs suddenly, with pain which may be felt in the knee. Surgical correction with pins is necessary; the long-term outlook is very good.
- Injury: any muscle sprain from foot to hip may cause a limp.
- Ill-fitting shoes and/or discomfort in the foot from a verruca are further causes of limp.

Treatment
- This is aimed at settling the underlying cause.
- It is important, in children particularly, to have careful follow-up of all causes of limping. This is to exclude the serious bone and joint causes mentioned above.
- The pain of a hip problem may commonly be felt in the knee. The absence of signs of infection or injury around the knee should not deter you from seeking a doctor's advice and X-ray examination of the hip if necessary.
- Using a stick can provide enormous relief for a temporary or a long-term limp. To people's surprise it should be held and used on the opposite side to the affected limb.

The Doctor
- You should always consult a doctor for any unexplained limp, particularly if it does not quickly settle on resting for a day or two.
- He will order X-ray examinations and possibly blood tests. The blood tests can help in the diagnosis of certain types of arthritis. (See **Gout, Arthritis**.) They may also help to reveal an underlying infection such as osteomyelitis, which may not appear at first on X-ray examination.
- If the limp is unexplained or due to a serious cause your doctor may refer a child to a children's doctor (paediatrician) or bone specialist (orthopaedic surgeon). Adults may be referred to a joint specialist (rheumatologist).

Lipomas

These are lumps of soft tissue which appear on various parts of the body. Lipomas are one of the commonest growths. They are very slow-growing and generally harmless. Women have a greater tendency to develop lipomas than men.

Symptoms
* They usually appear as a soft fatty lump just below the skin surface.
* They are not usually painful unless interfering with other structures in the body.

* The size varies from that of a pea to a small tangerine and, rarely, even larger.
* Growth is very slow. Any sudden change in size of a lipoma should be reported to your doctor.
* They may occur singly or in clusters.

Causes
□ A lipoma is made up of fat cells. Why the fatty tissue should increase in size, causing a lipoma, is not known.

Treatment
- As with any unexplained lump on the skin, when it first appears you should consult your doctor. If the doctor is not able to confirm that the lump is a lipoma it will usually be necessary to remove the lump for examination under a microscope.
- Usually lipomas are best left alone.
- If the lipoma is causing problems, or changes in any way, it can be removed at operation. Sometimes they are removed because they are unsightly, but removal will usually leave a scar.

Manic-depression

This condition is characterised by mood swings from mania to depression. The interval between these phases of the illness may be very variable, from months to years. Often there is a family history of others who have had similar problems. Women appear to be more commonly affected than men, being particularly at risk following childbirth and at the menopause. With modern treatment, which may have to be continued for life, the outlook is good, particularly if you have friends and relatives around who can ensure that you have early treatment if you enter a phase of illness. Uncontrolled illness may lead to job loss and possible bankruptcy.

Symptoms
These are often felt and noticed by those around you before you are aware there is anything wrong.

Early mania (hypomania)
* Early-morning waking.
* Extreme restlessness and inability to settle.
* Being unproductively busy; nothing ever gets completed.
* Likely to go on a dramatic spending spree or start elaborate projects which are never finished.
* Irritability, with frequent violent outbursts and rages.

Full mania
* Rapid and wild speech.
* Illogical thinking and speech.
* Elaborate rhyming, joking, word-matching.
* Showing off, singing, dancing, making speeches.
* Occasional quiet or sad moments.
* Poor concentration.
* Exhaustion and loss of weight.
* Frustration and anger at uncompleted grand schemes.

Depressive phase
* Gradual onset.
* Increasingly introverted and withdrawn.
* Late rising and poor sleep pattern.
* Slowness of movement and speech.
* May hide away in shut rooms.
* Talk of suicide, but not frequently carried out.
* Increased risk of suicide as depression lifts.

Causes
□ Exactly why some people have manic-depressive illness is poorly understood. It may have something to do with the chemistry of the brain.

- ☐ Episodes of mania or depression may be provoked by severe stress, such as impending job loss or relationship difficulties.
- ☐ Occasionally, severe illness or injury can precipitate either mania or depression.
- ☐ Often there is no obvious cause.

Treatment
- If you think someone around you may have manic-depressive illness, seek help early. Early treatment is much more likely to shorten the illness.
- A family doctor or someone who knows the ill person well is usually much better equipped to help than a stranger. It is much easier to persuade someone who is becoming either manic or depressive to make contact with a friendly doctor known to them.

The Doctor
- May initiate treatment at home with tranquillisers for the early manic phase, or anti-depressant medication for the depressive phase.
- May involve a psychotherapist to explore ideas and feelings with the ill person to try and help the situation.
- It is often necessary to involve a hospital psychiatry department in planning management of the illness.
- Treatment with a drug called lithium has transformed the lives of manic-depressive people. Before treatment is started blood tests will be done to check how the body is functioning, so any later side-effects of the drug, on thyroid hormone, for example, can be quickly detected.
- Lithium treatment is usually continued long term. There will be occasional blood tests to check the drug is at the most suitable dose and is having no adverse effects.
- If hospital admission is necessary, be sure of obtaining adequate instructions from the hospital to enable you to detect early signs of a further manic or depressive episode, should this occur at home in the future.

Measles

Measles is highly infectious. It is caused by a virus and spread from person to person. After a few days of a cold, the typical rash develops, and lasts for about five days. In poor countries, it is a common killer, but in this country it is usually less serious. Serious complications, including brain inflammation, do occur and although they are rare make vaccinating toddlers very worthwhile.

Symptoms
* Symptoms start between one and two weeks after contact.
* They are those of a cold – fever, runny nose, cough, sore throat.
* Red eyes, earache, diarrhoea and vomiting are common.
* Temperature reaches a peak after four days.
* Temperature should be controlled, or it may lead to a convulsion.
* The typical rash then starts behind the ears.
* Red blotches spread from the face on to the body.
* The rash fades in the same order.
* The skin may peel, or leave brown marks which fade.
* Croup is quite common. (See Croup.)
* Mild bronchitis is common, pneumonia less so.
* Middle ear infection is common.
* Return of fever or drowsiness a week later may signal a rare but serious

complication. This is brain inflammation with fits, leading to coma. Rapid improvement may occur with treatment in hospital, but a few children die.
* Absence of cough makes measles an unlikely diagnosis.

Prevention
- Keep an infected child at home and inform the school.
- The child is infectious from five days before the rash appears until a week afterwards.
- Keep away from any children whose bodies' defences are diminished by serious illness such as cancer or its treatment.
- If you have had measles, your baby is usually protected for up to nine months.
- Life-long immunity follows a single attack of measles.
- Immunisation of children at around fifteen months is very effective.
- It may be given within two days of contact to prevent illness developing.
- Widespread immunisation, as in America, could wipe out the disease.
- All children should be immunised if possible; it is one of the safest immunisations.
- Immunisation should be delayed if the child is unwell with fever.
- Children who are at risk from fits may be immunised with a separate protective injection given at the same time as measles immunisation.
- An allergy to eggs used to be a reason for not immunising, but it is only extremely rarely that egg allergy leads to such a severe reaction that this would be a reason for not immunising.
- Asthma is not a reason for not immunising against measles. Children with asthma should definitely be immunised to protect their chests.

Treatment
- Contact your doctor if you suspect measles.
- He will look for signs of complications.
- Most people can be treated at home.
- Paracetamol, sponging with a lukewarm cloth, or giving the child a bath of normal temperature will reduce the temperature.
- Do not dress up the child; one layer of clothing is usually enough.
- Extra drinks are needed.
- Diarrhoea may need careful adjustment of diet. (See **Diarrhoea**.)
- Croup can usually be managed at home (See **Croup**.)
- Fits due to temperature are mostly short-lived, but to be safe your child will often be sent to hospital. (See **Convulsions, febrile**.)
- Your child should be in hospital if there are signs of brain inflammation: i.e. repeated or prolonged fits, excessive drowsiness or irritability.
- Your doctor may prescribe antibiotics if there are signs of ear infection or pneumonia.

Meningitis

Meningitis is an infection of the brain linings, called the meninges. It is not strictly infection of the brain, which is called encephalitis. The symptoms of meningitis can be confused with those of many other infections. The disease is suspected in any person who is very unwell with a fever. It occurs at any age but most commonly affects babies and young children. It is caused by many different bacteria and viruses. There are outbreaks of the most serious form every few years. Diagnosis depends on a test called a lumbar puncture. Untreated bacterial meningitis will usually lead to serious handicap or death. Treated early with the right antibiotics there will usually be a full recovery. Viral meningitis is less serious, in that although there is no specific treatment there will usually be a good recovery.

Symptoms

* Starts with a fever, and being generally unwell.
* May follow an ear or chest infection.
* There is a severe headache made worse by light and head movement.
* There is repeated vomiting and increasing drowsiness.
* In the most serious form a rash like bruising develops.
* The symptoms can be confused with those of flu, ear or throat infection, sinusitis or migraine. The important difference is that the person appears more unwell and drowsy.
* If nothing is done, a bacterial meningitis will progress rapidly to fits and coma.

In babies

* An infant is irritable and may make a high-pitched cry and look vacant.
* Feeds are refused or vomited.
* The fontanelle is tense and bulging. (See **Soft spot**.)

Causes

☐ These vary depending on the age of the person infected.
☐ Newborn babies may catch particular bacteria from the birth canal.
☐ A skull fracture may allow bacteria to enter the spaces around the brain, causing meningitis. Bacteria may also affect the meninges following an ear, nose, sinus or chest infection.
* Outbreaks of the most serious form, caused by the bacteria *meningococcus*, can occur in institutions.
* TB can cause meningitis, particularly in old or weakened people.
* Many viruses, including mumps, cause meningitus.

Prevention

● The close contacts of people with meningococcal infection (i.e. people who live with them at home or in an institution) are given antibiotics. Contacts at day school do not normally need treatment. Swabs are taken from the nose to check if anyone is carrying the germ.
● A vaccine is available against some particular bacteria causing meningitis. It is not yet available against the type which causes the most serious form.

Treatment

● If you or your child become suddenly or very unwell see a doctor straight away. Most cases of feverish illness are not meningitis.
● You will do no harm by giving a dose of paracetamol to control the fever.
● One sign of meningitis, not always present early on, is a stiff neck. Bending the neck is painful because it stretches the meninges. This also happens when the legs are bent upwards from the hips. Your doctor will balance these signs against those of other illnesses. For example, swollen glands will also cause pain on bending the head.
● If meningitis is suspected you will need to go to hospital.
● In hospital a lumbar puncture may be done. A needle is inserted into the back to obtain a sample of the

fluid which bathes the brain and surrounds the spinal cord.
- Examination of the fluid under a microscope will often give the diagnosis. If it suggests bacterial meningitis, antibiotic treatment is started. The fluid is kept to see which germs grow, and which drugs are effective in treating them.
- Antibiotic treatment usually continues for about ten days.
- Bacterial meningitis carries risks of permanent defects in hearing, vision, understanding and movement. Prompt, correct treatment will, however, lead to full recovery in most cases.

Menopause

This is the expression used to cover a wide range of events surrounding the last menstrual period. It is a natural and healthy moment in a woman's life. Although a quarter of all women have distressing symptoms, it should not be seen as an illness or a disease. Another quarter of all women have no symptoms other than noting their periods stop. Half of all women have some symptoms which they can adjust to and treat themselves. Although symptoms may go on for several years, there is no need for the menopause to stop you leading a normal life. The onset is unpredictable, anytime between forty and fifty-eight, but the average is around forty-eight to fifty. Smokers tend to experience the menopause earlier, and daughters often have the same pattern of events at the menopause as their mothers.

Symptoms
* Periods may:
  - suddenly stop
  - gradually decrease in amount
  - become more widely spaced apart
  - become irregular
  - be sometimes heavier, sometimes lighter
* The overall pattern is for periods to generally decrease until stopping.
* Other physical symptoms include:
  - fluid retention
  - palpitations
  - sweating and feeling hot (hot flushes); this can come on suddenly and be either severe or mild
  - breast discomfort
  - headaches
  - joint pains
* Non-physical symptoms include feeling:
  - nervous
  - edgy and upset
  - depressed
  - anxious and lacking in confidence
  - unable to concentrate as well as before
  - tired
* Some of these symptoms may be made worse by other events not related to the menopause.

Causes
□ There is a normal hormone pattern in the body, which leads to egg production from the ovaries, and to periods. In the months before the menopause this regular pattern is upset, eventually leading to the last period and no further egg production. This is a normal process, just as breast development happens as a result of hormonal changes in puberty.

Treatment
- None of the symptoms of the menopause present a risk to health. The treatment is therefore aimed at making life more comfortable.
- Some measures that may help include:
  - watching weight
  - making time to rest adequately

- decreasing fluid intake if you are feeling bloated
- wearing comfortable, good, supporting bras
- wearing layers of light cotton clothing so you can peel off to cool off
- keeping a spare nightdress by the bed to change into if sweating is a problem
- avoiding alcohol or coffee if they make symptoms worse
- using a vaginal lubricant to make intercourse comfortable
• Contraception is necessary for around eighteeen months after the last period, though there is no fixed rule about it. Sex can certainly be continued and enjoyed as before, or more so when it is no longer necessary to take precautions against pregnancy.

The Doctor
• If bleeding returns more than six months after it has stopped, or if spotting of blood appears between periods, or if bleeding is prolonged, a doctor should be seen immediately. These could be signs of abnormal, possibly cancerous, growth in the womb.
• The ways in which a doctor can help severe menopausal symptoms involve a variety of treatments, including:
  - water tablets to ease fluid retention
  - sleeping tablets, only for a very brief period of difficulty and preferably not at all (see **Sleep problems**)
  - oestrogen creams for the vagina can ease dryness and irritation
  - rarely, anti-depressants can help
  - above all, discussing symptoms and being examined to confirm the normal changes of a healthy menopause, is much more important than using drugs

Hormone replacement therapy
This is often misunderstood, and many people do not realise that it means you go on having artificially induced periods, although ovulation is not induced. Many women prefer to cope with the symptoms than go on having periods. It is not effective as contraception.

The advantage is that it does alleviate the totally incapacitating symptoms of those so severely affected that they cannot lead normal lives. It is normally continued for anything from six months to two years, but may have to be continued much longer.

There are different types of hormone replacement therapy. You should ask for a combined oestrogen and progestogen therapy, which is given cyclically. There is now thought to be no increased risk of developing cancer of the lining of the womb from this type of therapy, and some people can benefit.

☎ Women's Health Concern. Helpline: 071 938 3932 (London); 0222 549888 (Cardiff).

Migraine

This is a particularly severe kind of headache, usually on one side of the head. It affects all age groups, but most frequently adolescents and young adults. In children it may cause severe stomach pain, called abdominal migraine. The severity varies from only one or two attacks in a lifetime to as many as one a week. They can vary in length from a few hours to several days. People can sometimes learn to control or even stop an attack, or may be very disabled by it over many years. Often other members of the family are migraine sufferers.

Symptoms
* One of the features of migraine is the variety of symptoms found.

* The aura refers to sensations felt before or at the onset of a headache, including:
  - flashing lights or zig-zags
  - peculiar smells
  - strange noises
  - numbness or tingling, sometimes quite obvious and affecting the whole of one side of body
  - desire to pass urine
* Nausea and vomiting are sometimes part of the aura, or follow it. They may also accompany the headache, and be severe and very difficult to cope with, or a mild sensation only.
* A headache may be the only feature, or accompanied by the above symptoms. It:
  - is usually one-sided, but sometimes spreads to affect the whole head
  - is often piercing and excruciating, making it difficult to concentrate or do anything but lie down
  - does not usually prevent sleeping

Causes

- The sensations of migraine are thought to be caused by changes in blood vessels in the scalp and brain which trigger nerves to send pain messages.
- Many substances have been described as possible causes. There is no doubt that some people can have a migraine started by eating a particular substance, such as: cheese, chocolate, fruit, spices, medicines, wine, fish, pickles, cocktails, milk, meat extracts, tea or wheat.
- Hormonal changes can bring on migraine before periods or while taking the contraceptive pill.
- Changes in the surroundings can be a factor, e.g.: noise, heat, light, travelling, high winds or smells.
- Exhaustion, stress and anxiety all play a part, and may make migraine worse.

Treatment

- This aims to prevent or shorten an attack at best, or to help cope with an attack at worst.
- Resting, lying down or sleeping can all shorten an attack. Struggling on can lead to a longer attack.
- Some sufferers find a quiet, darkened room very helpful.
- Icepacks and showers can sometimes help.

Simple painkillers

- It is better to take these by the clock than waiting 'to see if I can manage'.
- Try paracetamol as first choice (less likely to aggravate sickness than aspirin).
- Soluble forms of painkillers may be better absorbed.

Stronger painkillers

- These help, but may require a doctor's prescription and can be associated with nausea or sickness as a side-effect.

Anti-vomiting pills

- Taken early, these can help to keep the painkillers down and clear the symptoms.
- They are sometimes combined in one drug with a painkiller, e.g. Paramax (prescription required).

Ergotamine

- This is a special drug affecting blood vessels which must be used very carefully. Too much of it can actually cause headaches.

The Doctor

- There is a family of drugs called betablockers which can prevent or very much reduce the number of attacks. Your doctor can advise you. Not all sufferers can be helped in this way.
- Special migraine clinics can help

when all else fails. They can advise on the usefulness of stronger drugs or may advise other remedies, such as the leaves of the feverfew plant.

☎ The Migraine Trust, 45 Great Ormond Street, London WC1N 3AY. Tel: 071 278 2676.

☎ The British Migraine Association, 178a High Road, Byfleet, West Byfleet, Surrey KT14 7ED. Tel: 09323 52468.

Miscarriage

A miscarriage occurs when a pregnancy is lost naturally during the first twenty-eight weeks of pregnancy. It is much commoner than most people realise, happening in as many as one in eight pregnancies. You may miscarry without realising it has happened. A late period may be heavier than normal and actually contain a failed pregnancy in the menstrual loss.

More commonly, a wanted pregnancy is threatened by the appearance of bleeding from your vagina. This may settle down and the pregnancy continue, or pain may develop and the pregnancy is expelled by the womb. Some of the womb contents which made up the early pregnancy may not be completely expelled, giving rise to further bleeding or infection; this is called an incomplete miscarriage. It is also possible for the pregnancy to cease without symptoms and without expulsion from the womb. This may only be revealed by failure of the womb to grow and is called a 'missed' miscarriage. An operation is then usually required to empty the womb.

Whichever way the miscarriage occurs, although very distressing, it is not usually dangerous to the mother. Often it may not be necessary, if the miscarriage occurs very early, to see the doctor, but if bleeding or discharge persist medical advice must be sought. The outlook is usually good, with a subsequent pregnancy continuing normally. Some people, however, have difficulty in maintaining a pregnancy and may require special treatment, such as the insertion of stitches in the neck of the womb.

Symptoms

* Fresh bleeding in pregnancy before twenty-eight weeks. (If bleeding occurs after this time it is called an ante-partum haemorrhage; the baby may still be born alive – seek medical help immediately.)
* Brownish discharge. This may also be caused by a problem on the neck of the womb, such as an erosion, which may lead to slight bleeding or discharge. Brown discharge may precede the bleeding of a miscarriage.
* Bleeding may range from a few days to flow which is much heavier than a normal period.
* Pain, if it occurs, usually follows the bleeding and may indicate that miscarriage has become inevitable. Expulsion of the womb contents usually follows.
* You may be aware of passing the pregnancy through the vagina. Sometimes it is possible to save the foetal remains for the doctor to examine subsequently. In late or recurrent miscarriages full labour may occur, with delivery of an undeveloped foetus.
* In late miscarriages bleeding can be very heavy and is called a haemorrhage. You should lie down with the legs raised and summon emergency help to take you to hospital immediately.
* Pregnancy symptoms such as fullness of the breasts or morning sickness may disappear, making you suspect that the foetus has stopped growing. This will be reflected in failure of the

womb to increase in size and be picked up on your next ante-natal visit. It can be confirmed by an ultrasound examination.

Causes

- Miscarriage most often occurs because there is a problem with the developing foetus. By a little-understood mechanism this is identified by your body and the pregnancy is expelled.
- There may be a problem with the womb or neck of the womb which makes it difficult for you to retain a pregnancy. This will often lead to recurrent miscarriages and the help of a gynaecologist will be required.
- Hormonal imbalance in the mother may lead to miscarriages. This can occasionally be detected and corrected.

Prevention

- Usually there is little that can be done to prevent a foetus miscarrying. If the foetus is not growing correctly it will miscarry. Intercourse in pregnancy does not normally lead to miscarriages.
- If you have recurrent miscarriages your doctor will refer you to a gynaecologist, who may be able to identify a structural problem with the womb, correctable by surgery. It is also possible to sew the neck of the womb shut in later pregnancy to hold the foetus in and prevent a miscarriage. This is only done in later pregnancy so that a wrongly developing foetus may be expelled early on if necessary. (The neck of the womb in this situation is called an incompetent cervix.)

Treatment

- When bleeding occurs in early pregnancy the only way of trying to treat or prevent progression to a miscarriage is by resting. Some doctors feel that resting makes little difference, and that if the pregnancy is going to miscarry it will do so.
- You should refrain from intercourse if bleeding occurs. It may be necessary to avoid intercourse throughout pregnancy.

The Doctor

- You should inform your doctor if bleeding occurs in pregnancy. Initially he may only advise you to rest at home.
- If pain occurs you may become very uncomfortable and the bleeding heavier. If this occurs after the sixth to seventh week of pregnancy it is likely that you will have to go to hospital.
- In hospital you may have an ultrasound examination, which reveals the contents of the womb and can indicate if the pregnancy is continuing.
- It will usually be necessary for you to have a general anaesthetic and a simple operation to ensure that no remains of the pregnancy are left in the womb. This is referred to as a scrape or D and C operation.
- After a miscarriage it is quite normal to feel very depressed and upset. It may be some time before you wish to plan another pregnancy, but it is possible to do so whenever you wish.

☎ The Miscarriage Association, c/o Clayton Hospital, Northgate, Wakefield, Yorkshire. Tel: 0924 200799.

Mouth ulcers

These are small painful ulcers appearing in the mouth (also called apthous ulcers). They can affect all ages, and are common in children and young adults. They are not serious but can be very uncomfortable and interfere with eating. Some people have a tendency to have them more often than others. After about one week they will almost always go away by themselves. They are not infectious.

Symptoms
* Usually single painful ulcers; a large crop of ulcers generally indicates a viral infection and has a different origin such as the cold sore virus. (See **Cold sores**.)
* Red angry area inside cheek or lips, on the tongue or gums.
* Yellowish-white centre to the red area which appears as a hollow.
* Severe pain if rubbing against teeth when eating.
* Stinging and discomfort with certain drinks and food, particularly fruit juices.
* Continual pain and discomfort if in a 'busy' place in the mouth, e.g. tip of tongue.

Causes
- It is not clear exactly what causes these ulcers.
- They are sometimes more common when you are run down or ill.
- Large ulcers can be caused by injury from a rough tooth or biting; check for this.

Treatment
- Tricks to try are:
  - choosing food carefully to avoid adding to the discomfort; milky and non-spicy foods are good, as are liquid or runny foods which don't need chewing
  - ice cubes to suck can amuse children and numb the painful area; unfortunately, ice-lollies usually contain stinging fruit juices
- Teething gels such as Dentinox can help, or try Ambesol; both are available from the chemist.
- Rubbing a child's lip or inner cheek with vaseline can sometimes help, and reassure the child.
- The doctor can prescribe small pellets of hydrocortisone to leave against the sore area in the mouth (corlan pellets). While giving some relief, this does not provide a cure.
- These ulcers will go on their own in seven to ten days.

Mumps

Mumps is an infection caused by a virus. It is not as infectious as other childhood illnesses and many people pass through childhood without catching it. They are still at risk as adults. Mumps is most common between the ages of five and fifteen. It is spread by close contact. The infection may be very mild, causing only a fever. It typically causes swelling of the glands around the angle of the jaw. Cheeks may look swollen like a hamster.

Symptoms
* Symptoms may be very mild.
* Rarely, you can have mumps without knowing it.
* Symptoms start two to three weeks after contact.
* There may be one or two days of fever, headache and reduced appetite.
* It is the glands which produce saliva which swell in mumps.
* One or both sides may be swollen; swelling may appear at different times, one side following the other, or at the same time.
* The swelling lasts up to ten days.
* The glands may be very painful and tender.
* The pain is made worse by eating and it hurts to swallow.
* Fever, which may be high, lasts up to a week.
* Mumps is easily confused with

swelling of the lymph glands in the neck, which happens in many throat infections.
* Many of the body's other organs may be inflamed and swollen, causing:
  – severe headache made worse by light, stiff neck, excessive drowsiness; this could indicate mumps meningitis which is rare but serious, though usually recovery is good
  – tummy pain, usually mild
  – pain in the testicles, which may be severe; one-fifth of boys who develop mumps after puberty may have their testes affected; sterility is very rare after mumps

Prevention
- Vaccine has not been widely used because the illness is mild.
- There is a combined vaccine for mumps, measles and German measles. This will be introduced at around fifteen months of age.
- Life-long immunity follows a single attack.
- It is usual to keep infected children away from school, but some doctors would not advise this, saying it is better to catch mumps as a child.
- Your child is infectious from a few days before the swelling until it has settled.

Treatment
- You can usually treat all the symptoms by yourself.
- Paracetamol will lower temperature and ease pain.
- Warmth applied to the gland will ease the pain.
- Give plenty of drinks.
- Your child may find it easier to swallow soup, mashed food and ice cream.
- You do not have to call your doctor if the infection is mild.
- Call your doctor if there are signs of increasing illness or complications such as the testicles being affected.

Nail problems

Infected nails

It is very common for nails to become infected, particularly if hands are often immersed in water. The infection often comes up quickly, is never serious, but can be extremely painful.

Symptoms
* Pain and throbbing, made worse by the solid nail preventing the infection from finding its way to the surface.
* A red bulge of pus may develop alongside the nail (a whitlow).
* Symptoms often appear very quickly.
* If severe, infection may spread up the hand.

Causes
☐ Germs get into the space around the nail, particularly if the skin is damaged or there is repeated soaking of the skin. These germs (bacteria) cause sudden infections, usually around one nail only.
☐ More slowly developing and longer lasting infections are caused by fungi. Again, wet hands are more vulnerable. It is often the same yeast type of fungus as causes thrush. Several nails may be affected at the same time.

Prevention
- Use rubber gloves with a cloth inner lining.

Treatment
- Germs or bacteria usually respond quickly to antibiotics given by your doctor. It may be necessary to make a small cut to one side of the nail to

allow the infection out. This generally heals quickly.
- Fungi are more difficult to treat; you will be given creams or paints to apply to all the nails. Treatment has to be continued for several months to be sure to clear the infection. If the problem is severe anti-fungal tablets are occasionally given and may have to be continued for six months or longer.

Painful nails

* May be due to infection (see above).
* A sharp blow to the nail, such as when hammering, can lead to a black nail or a black area under part of the nail. This is painful at the time but usually ceases within a few minutes.
* Continuous and increasing pain below the nail can be because a blood blister has formed below the nail following a blow. It will be visible as a black patch, often in the middle of the nail (see above). The blood has nowhere to escape to, being limited by the nail. The intense pain is due to pressure. Pain can be instantly relieved by piercing the nail with a sharp needle previously sterilised in a flame. See a doctor if your first attempt does not work or if you don't feel confident about doing it!
* (See also **In-growing toe nails**.)

Unsightly nails

Symptoms

* Lines or ridges across the nails, which are a sign of where nail growth has temporarily ceased, perhaps during a period of illness. They will grow out with time.
* Cracked, damaged-looking nails, sometimes seen in association with skin problems. (See **Psoriasis**.)

* Creamy-white, thickened nails, often with the end of the nail separated from the skin, can be a sign of fungal infection (see above).
* Thickening of the whole nail may take place (particularly on feet) due to pressure on the nail-growing area. Tight-fitting shoes can cause this.
* White patches that move forward as the nail grows are often caused by knocks to the nail.

Nappy rash

This is a red rash appearing around the napkin area which varies from a widespread, vivid, painless pink to weeping red sores causing great distress. (It can last for a matter of hours or persist for several days.) All babies have at least a touch of a red rash at some stage, but some are undoubtedly more prone to it than others.

Symptoms

* Symptoms are as described above. Very often it is only discovered when the nappy is undone, not having produced specific symptoms.
* Can cause distress, presenting as crying and irritability.
* Greater distress after urine or faeces comes in contact with the skin.
* Distressed mothers; it is often worse to see than for the baby to have.

Causes

- Prolonged wet nappies.
- Urine and/or faeces left in contact with the skin sets off a burn-like reaction.
- Changes of diet, leading to 'stronger' urine or faeces, can quite suddenly affect the skin. (Hence the awful rash after the baby has been left with someone else for the weekend.)
- Fever often produces strong urine and runny faeces, hence nappy rash.

☐ Infection: nappy rash can become infected with (1) (most commonly) the yeast candida which causes thrush (see **Thrush**); (2) other skin germs which take advantage of the rash to make it worse.

Treatment
- Frequent nappy changes at least six times daily.
- Frequent cleansing of the area with simple soap and water, good rinsing, good drying. No talc.
- Avoid chemical cleansers, or rinse well after using.
- A barrier cream such as zinc and castor oil, which can be bought from a chemist, should be applied thickly like icing on a cake.

The Doctor
- May give a cream to treat yeast (e.g. clotrimazole or other anti-fungal cream) or other skin infection if yeast is not the cause.
- A swab test may be necessary if the rash has become infected.

Note
Thrush can occur in babies' mouths. It is worth checking the tongue and sides of mouth for white patches which do not come away easily on touching. (Milk does.) When there is mouth thrush this needs to be treated at the same time as any thrush in the nappy area. Different preparations are necessary from those used in the nappy area:
- a clear gel, easy to use inside each cheek, e.g. miconazole oral gel; no prescription needed
- anti-fungal drops, e.g. nystatin; prescription needed

Neck problems

Neck problems considered here are:
Stiff and painful neck (including cervical spondylosis)
Wry neck (torticollis)

Stiff and painful neck

In the middle-aged and elderly a stiff and painful neck frequently develops with no apparent cause. This is usually due to a condition called cervical spondylosis. This problem is due to wear-and-tear changes in the neck bones which are described below. Cervical spondylosis tends to be a long-term neck difficulty which may intermittently become very troublesome. If care is taken and treatment is followed most of the severe symptoms can be avoided.

The neck may also be uncomfortable after an injury or if you develop wry neck. In this case the symptoms may point to an obvious cause. (See **Wry neck** below.)

Symptoms
* Pain:
  - this may be felt in the neck itself
  - it may be felt in the arm or shoulder (see **Shoulder pain**)
  - one or both sides of the body may be affected
* Stiffness of the neck is common:
  - there may be considerable limitation of movement (turning round in the car to see behind may be difficult)
  - stiffness may gradually increase over a period of years
  - it may be more severe after increased activity
* Bending the neck can lead to:
  - dizziness
  - severe pain
  - tingling, numbness or pain felt in arms or hands
  - headaches, double vision or sickness
  drop attacks (see below)
* Rarely, there may be symptoms in the legs or urinary problems.

Causes

- Exactly why cervical spondylosis should affect some people and not others is not known.
- The symptoms of cervical spondylosis are caused by the changes in the neck bones and the joints between them.
- The bones of the neck become worn and torn, losing their regular shape. Small growths on the edges of the bones, called osteophytes, may appear. The normally smooth discs which lie between the neck bones, instead of acting as a flexible cushion, became hardened and misshapen.
- Nerves are trapped or pinched, causing pain.
- Stiffness occurs because of the damaged bones and discs limiting movement.
- Because everything below the neck has to be connected with the head in order to work properly it is not surprising that there are so many different structures packed tightly into the neck. This tight packing of nerves, blood vessels, muscles and bones means that if the bones are not well aligned or become irregular there may be serious consequences for structures around them.
- It is due to this that drop attacks in the elderly may occur. The main blood vessel carrying oxygen to the brain passes very close to the bones. An elderly person with cervical spondylosis may bend the neck and temporarily cut off the blood supply to the brain, causing sudden collapse. A typical story is a simple action such as stooping to turn off an electric plug causing a nasty fall. Consciousness returns quickly, but there may be injuries caused by the fall.
- Similarly, severe deformity of the bones, or the discs between them, may press on the spinal cord itself, producing symptoms in the legs or affecting the bladder. These symptoms should be reported to your doctor at once.

Treatment

- It is not possible to reverse the changes of cervical spondylosis, but it is possible to limit their effects and to some extent prevent exacerbations.
- Avoid movements or activities which produce symptoms or which could lead to a flare-up of symptoms later on.
- Adjusting your pillows can be surprisingly helpful, although it may be difficult to find what is best for you, since both too low or too high a position may aggravate symptoms.
- Simple painkillers such as aspirin or paracetamol can be helpful. These may have to be taken over a long period due to the long-term nature of the condition. Increase the dose and take them regularly during bad spells.
- It is possible to make a temporary collar out of folded newspapers pushed into a stock or wrapped in a cloth, which may provide temporary relief.

The Doctor

- Can arrange for you to have a special collar. Wearing a stiff plastic collar during the day supports the head, limiting movements which might otherwise cause pain and may prevent more serious symptoms. A soft collar at night may be helpful. It may be necessary to wear a collar for three months until symptoms settle.
- The doctor may prescribe different painkillers or a trial of an anti-inflammatory drug. The effect of this group of drugs, (NSAIs, see **Gout**) is

not always helpful in cervical spondylosis.
- Muscle relaxants are sometimes prescribed, but long-term use may prevent them from being so effective. They may also be difficult to discontinue.
- X-rays may be taken but, other than confirming wear-and-tear changes, will not usually alter treatment significantly. The position of the most visible changes on the X-ray may bear little relation to the position where most problems are occurring in the neck.
- Referral to a physiotherapist can provide great relief from a variety of treatments. These may include:
  - traction to help separate the neck bones, taking pressure off other structures in the neck
  - mobilisation of the neck through a variety of movements and exercises
- Referral to a specialist for more intensive physiotherapy or investigation of nerve pain in more detail may be necessary.
- Very rarely, surgery may be required to relieve serious symptoms. This may, however, reduce mobility further.

Wry neck

Typically, you wake up and have difficulty in straightening up your neck. It can be painful and distressing, made worse by the surprise when it happens. It is not serious and will usually pass off within one or two days. It is common in children and young adults. This is also called torticollis.

Symptoms
* Head held to one side.
* Pain and discomfort on moving.

Causes
□ It is not known why it happens, but it is caused by the muscle that pulls the head down towards one shoulder going into spasm.

Treatment
- This is aimed at relieving the muscle spasm.
- Heat from a towel wrapped round a hot-water bottle may help.
- An icepack may also help. Frozen peas make good ones, but don't eat them after re-freezing.
- A newspaper folded into a long thin sausage, wrapped in a towel, can be wrapped around the neck. This supports the head and helps the muscle to relax.
- A physiotherapist can help, and may use a cold spray on the skin called ethylchloride.
- Regular painkillers such as paracetamol are worth taking, and may be the only treatment possible or suitable in young children.

Non-specific urethritis (NSU)

Non-specific urethritis is a common infection caught through sexual intercourse. It affects sexually active men, usually after a change in sexual partner. It is an infection of the urine passage and was named when the cause was not known. Although painful, it is not dangerous to the infected man, who usually does not feel unwell. The main danger is to his female partner, who may have no symptoms at first but is at risk of pelvic infection (see **Pelvic infection**) and of passing the infection on to her newborn baby during childbirth.

Symptoms
* The symptoms usually start about two to three weeks after infection, although the gap may range from a few days to six weeks.
* There is pain on passing urine and sometimes a clear discharge from the urethra.
* The infection sometimes spreads to the testicles and prostate gland, causing pain.
* The back passage may also be infected during anal intercourse, causing discomfort and discharge.
* A rare complication is called Reiter's disease – arthritis affecting particularly the knees, ankles and feet; red eyes may also be a feature.

Causes
☐ All the above conditions are caused by a small germ called chlamydia.

Prevention
● As with all venereal diseases (those transmitted through sexual intercourse), some protection is offered by barrier methods of contraception, such as the sheath and cap.
● An infected man or woman should inform any recent sexual partners, who may also need treatment.

The Doctor
● It is important that you should see the doctor or visit a special clinic, listed as a VD clinic in the phone book.
● Samples of any discharge may be taken, and a urine sample may be asked for.
● You will be given a two-to-three week course of antibiotics: usually tetracycline or erythromycin.
● This will usually cure the infection, although a second course is sometimes needed.
● It is important to avoid intercourse, and sensible to avoid alcohol during treatment.
● Painkillers are also important.
● Pain in the testes will be helped by wearing a support, which can be obtained from chemists.
● Anti-arthritis drugs and bed rest will help Reiter's disease.
● An infected woman will have swabs taken from the vagina and be given a similar course of antibiotics.

Nosebleeds

Very frightening, usually sudden and sometimes recurring, nosebleeds are not a sign of any serious illness. It is a myth that they are nature's way of relieving high blood pressure. If occurring as part of another illness there will be signs of that illness elsewhere. People often think their blood won't clot. If this were the case, as happens in unusual circumstances, there would be bleeding gums and bruising to be seen. Nosebleeds can almost always be stopped quickly and easily. They are more common in children.

Symptoms
* One nostril suddenly bleeds. Although the amount of blood can appear dramatic, it is extremely rare for it to cause any significant anaemia.

Causes
☐ Often it just happens. The lining of the nose is very thin over the blood vessels and breaks easily.
☐ It is more likely to happen if you have a cold.
☐ Nose-picking and over-vigorous nose-blowing can be causes.
☐ Infection, either in the nose or sinuses on either side, makes the nose lining even more fragile and liable to break, leading to bleeding.
☐ Injury to the nose. Even if this causes

frequent bleeding, it is very unusual to require surgery to the nose other than for cosmetic reasons.

Treatment
- Sit forward.
- Breathe through mouth.
- Hold nose, pressing with thumb on affected side.
- Continue holding nose, applying pressure for more than five minutes, preferably ten.
- Release your grip slowly.
- Do not blow, pick or touch your nose during the next day.

The Doctor
- If bleeding persists it may be necessary to attend your local casualty department or surgery.
- Your nose will be packed with a long, thin gauze strip left in place for about four hours.
- If bleeding still persists or is recurrent the blood vessels in the nose may be cauterised; this seals the ends of the blood vessels.
- Sometimes your doctor may prescribe an ointment to use gently in the end of the affected nostril for a few days to clear any germs that might be in the nose causing recurrent bleeding, e.g. chlorhexidine with neomycin (naseptin).

Obesity

Obesity occurs because you eat more food than you need to, and any surplus intake gets turned to fat. This may be very hard to accept but is almost always the case. Obesity often runs in families, obese children being more common in families where the parents are overweight. This may not only be due to family eating habits, but particular rates at which the body burns up energy may run in families. The body's requirement for food varies enormously between individuals; what makes one person overweight may keep someone else slim.

Symptoms
- Increase in weight due to build-up of fat.
- Feeling of heaviness, and being short of breath.
- Easily becoming overheated and sweaty.
- Other illnesses or problems are more likely to occur, including: diabetes, strokes, heart disease, kidney or gallbladder trouble, raised blood pressure and arthritis.

Causes
Adults
- Food intake exceeds energy requirements.
- Very rarely, you may suffer a problem affecting your metabolism, the rate at which your body uses up energy. This can be checked by your doctor, but is very uncommon.

Children
- Children gain weight for the same reasons as adults, i.e. their food intake is greater than their requirements.
- It is normal for children to pass through phases of chubbiness, especially babies and adolescents. This affects girls, particularly, at puberty. The excess fat seen in boys and girls during adolescence goes as growth occurs and muscles develop.

Prevention
- Prevention starts in childhood. Throughout life prevention is much easier than cure.
- Regular weighing of babies and infants can allow you to record clearly the pattern of weight gain. In this way, if a child is steadily becoming heavier than average for their age it

can be detected at an early stage. Your doctor or health visitor can advise you on the extent to which your child is above average weight.
- Regular weighing can also help adults. You are more likely to be successful in lowering weight if you are aware of excessive weight gain when it first occurs.
- Don't put a child on a special diet to lose weight. Often a change of diet to include fibre-rich foods such as wholemeal flour, brown rice, fresh fruit and vegetables is enough. Cut down on sugar and refined flours in cooking. Avoid sweets, cakes, biscuits and sweetened drinks. If a snack is necessary give apple pieces, celery or carrots.
- What you eat, and when you eat, will have an enormous influence on your child's eating habits and pattern of weight gain.
- Regular exercise can be very helpful in avoiding obesity.

Treatment

If you are overweight the following suggestions may be of some help in reducing your weight.

- Concentrate on yourself and your intake of food, not on comparisons with what others eat. Others may eat the same as you and stay slim while you gain weight. It is important to find the intake that allows you to lose weight comfortably.
- A combination of diet and exercise is helpful. Start gently doing something you enjoy and are likely to be able to continue over several months.
- Be realistic when choosing a diet. Aim your total daily intake at around 1,500–2,000 calories. Choosing food you like is more likely to enable you to continue the diet. Crash diets – fasting for several days – are usually a waste of time. While crash-dieting you only lose body water; the quantity of body fat remains the same. On stopping a crash diet you quickly regain any weight lost as fluid is rapidly replaced.
- A loss of 1 lb a week is a good target. This may not seem much, but added up over three months makes you nearly a stone slimmer.
- Avoid high-calorie, low-bulk foods such as fatty, sugary foods. Choose watery, fibrous, low-fat, low-carbohydrate foods. Potatoes should be boiled not fried. Bread should be wholemeal and used to mop up sauces rather than eaten with butter. Cut fat off meat before cooking; grill or steam instead of frying. Drink water, not sweetened drinks or alcohol.
- Choosing a fixed timetable for meals can be helpful. Stick rigidly to eating only at the time you have selected. Never eat between the fixed times. When eating – eat slowly, always use a knife and fork, pause between items.
- Joining a group such as Weight Watchers benefits many people. The knowledge that you have set a reasonable target can be a great spur to losing weight, particularly if you can share your hopes and successes with others.

The Doctor

- If, despite all your efforts, you make no progress it may be helpful to see your doctor.
- The doctor will be able to check your weight and height on charts to calculate your ideal weight. Together, it is usually possible to draw up a plan of diet and exercise.
- The doctor or a dietician may be able to go over a diary you have kept of everything you have eaten and make suggestions.

- Blood tests can be done to check some of your body chemicals and hormones to ensure you are using energy at the normal rate. Hormonal problems causing obesity are very rare.
- Blood pressure and other checks may be made to monitor the extent to which your obesity has affected you.
- There is no place for the use of drugs in the treatment of obesity. Drugs affecting appetite have potentially dangerous side-effects. There is little evidence to suggest they are useful in the long-term treatment of obesity problems.
- Drastic forms of treatment such as jaw-wiring or surgery are not recommended. Not only are such procedures sometimes dangerous, but the underlying pattern of eating is rarely addressed and subsequent weight gain is therefore very likely to occur.

☎ Weight Watchers Enquiries. Tel: 0628 777077 or 071 491 1929.

Palpitations

Different people understand different sensations to be palpitations. Usually it is an awareness of the heartbeat being more noticeable and more rapid than normal. There are lots of factors that may produce palpitations; fortunately the commonest ones are not at all serious. Occasionally the symptoms are persistent and only tests can reveal exactly what is happening. The outlook for most people with an attack of palpitations is good. They are usually short-lived and do not necessarily mean you have heart trouble. If you do have heart trouble there are treatments available.

Symptoms
* Feeling of loud, obvious heartbeat, the heart thumping in the chest.
* Rapid heartbeat.
* Feeling of breathlessness, especially when excited.
* Sweating, headaches.
* Feeling of fear.
* There may be some pain in the chest.
* Often an abrupt onset and end to the sensation.

Causes
- Cigarette-smoking and drinking too much tea or coffee are among the commonest reasons for palpitations.
- Lack of physical fitness. Most people have had the sensation of palpitations when running upstairs and finding themselves breathless at the top. If you are unfit the fast heartbeat needed to get you up there may continue for some moments after you stop, giving a feeling of palpitations.
- A lion jumping out of the jungle will give us a fright and make us feel stressed. In more usual circumstances an event such as nearly having a car accident or sneaking past the boss late in to work may be enough to give us palpitations. This is due to adrenalin having an effect on the heart. Stress in general can make you more prone to palpitations.
- Palpitations may be felt at the menopause. (See **Menopause**.)
- Thyroid disease affects the heart, causing palpitations. (See **Thyroid problems**.)
- Fever can often cause palpitations.
- Anaemia, if severe, can cause palpitations.
- Drugs may cause palpitations. They may also change the balance of minerals and chemicals in the body, making palpitations more likely.
- Some heart problems do cause palpitations. Just as a pump in a central-heating system may work less efficiently and do odd things when

undue demands are made on it, so the heart may give us palpitations in certain circumstances. These are all usually diagnosed and treated.

Treatment
- Stop cigarette-smoking and tea/coffee-drinking straight away.
- Having looked at the likely causes above, you may find you have a fever or other simple explanation.

The Doctor
- Will, if symptoms persist, take a blood test to look for thyroid disease or confirm the menopause. Blood tests can also reveal upsets in body chemicals, sometimes brought on by drugs, that cause palpitations.
- Will do a heart tracing. Although this may be normal it can reveal how large the heart is and, to some extent, how well it is working.
- If the explanation of your symptoms is still a mystery the doctor will arrange for you to have a small recording machine attached to you to record the heart rhythm over twenty-four hours. You can still walk about normally. This machine has a button on it for you to indicate when you feel the palpitations. The doctor can then look at the recording and advise on treatment.
- A number of drugs are available to stop palpitations, but much of the treatment is aimed at removing the underlying cause. Beta-blocker drugs are particularly useful, but there are many other different types of drug available which may be suitable.

Pelvic infection (or PID)

Pelvic infection usually affects sexually active women. PID stands for Pelvic Inflammatory Disease, which is caused by infection in the tubes which lead from the womb to the ovaries. The infection usually spreads up from the vagina into the womb and then along the tubes. It is most commonly caught after sexual intercourse, or may follow childbirth, miscarriage or abortion when the area is raw and bloody. It may also follow fitting of a coil, and is more common if a woman has a coil fitted. It is a serious disease because of its long-term complications, including blockage of the tubes which can cause infertility.

Symptoms
Acute infection
* May follow a few days after one of the above causes.
* You feel unwell with a high fever and severe pain across the lower part of the abdomen and into the back.
* The pain is worse on movement.
* There is pain also on intercourse.
* There is usually a vaginal discharge.

Chronic infection
* The pain is not as severe but may be almost continuous, making you feel unwell.
* The periods are often heavy and painful and may be irregular.
* There may be a discharge which is heavier than normal.

Causes
- Different germs cause the infection, depending on how it was caught.
- Sexually transmitted infections include gonorrhoea and chlamydia. (See NSU.)
- Several types of germ cause infection after childbirth, coil insertion etc.

Prevention
- This is afforded by barrier methods of contraception such as the sheath and cap.
- Do not have intercourse if you or

your partner have an untreated genital infection, or one that is being treated.
- Tell any recent partners if you are found to have an infection.
- Do not have a 'back street' abortion but go to your doctor or a local clinic.
- Report any feverish symptoms after childbirth to your midwife or doctor.

The Doctor
- It is important to see your doctor with these symptoms in order to prevent the long-term complications.
- The pain in acute infection may be so bad that your doctor may refer you to a specialist.
- The doctor will do an abdominal and internal examination and take samples of any discharge.
- Sometimes doctors cannot be sure that it isn't appendicitis or an ectopic pregnancy, and the specialist may need to look into your stomach with a small telescope under anaesthetic.
- The pain in appendicitis is different because it is mainly in the lower right abdomen. (See **Appendicitis**.)
- After examining you, the doctor may be sure that you have pelvic infection and may start a course of several antibiotics.
- It is important that you say if you are allergic to penicillin.
- One of the antibiotics may be metronidazole, and it is important not to drink alcohol at the same time because it may bring on sickness and headaches.
- If the doctor is not sure about the diagnosis he may wait for the results before starting treatment.
- If you have a coil in place this will be removed once treatment has started, and you will be advised not to use a coil again.
- Bed rest and warmth to the lower abdomen both help the pain, as do simple painkillers such as aspirin or paracetamol.

Periods

The monthly bleeding that occurs in women is often upset and disturbed. There are numerous factors that influence the amount and frequency of the bleeding (see below). Most of the problems causing changes in the periods are simple and easily sorted out. A normal cycle is a regular pattern of bleeding occurring over two to seven days, about every twenty-eight days.

During the month the inner lining of the womb becomes thicker in order to receive an egg from the ovary. If a sperm fetilises the egg it will normally remain in the womb and a pregnancy commences. If the egg is not fertilised by a sperm it will not remain in the womb, but is shed with the womb lining in normal menstrual flow.

Both the release of the egg from the ovary and the changes in the lining of the womb are controlled by a delicate 'chain-reaction' of chemicals and hormones. These controlling substances are released by the brain and by the ovaries themselves. The factors that upset periods may do so by affecting the womb and ovaries, or they can act directly on the brain.

The following subjects are discussed here:
Periods, infrequent
Periods, irregular and unexpected
Periods, no
Periods, painful
Periods, too heavy

Periods, infrequent

In some women periods are infrequent throughout their adult life. This reflects the pattern of their particular hormone cycle, being perhaps much longer than the usual four to five weeks.

Causes
- This is common in the first few years of adolescence, when periods start. It is not generally serious, and indicates a failure of egg production.
- As you approach the menopause, periods may decrease in frequency, similarly reflecting a failure of egg production.

Treatment
- There is normally no need for treatment if periods are infrequent.
- It may be necessary to trigger egg production, using hormones, in order to achieve a pregnancy. This is not only because few eggs are produced, but also because it is difficult to predict when they will be released. (See **Infertility**.)

Periods, irregular and unexpected

Apart from when periods commence, and towards the menopause when periods may be infrequent, many women experience an upset to their menstrual pattern.

Symptoms
* Bleeding between periods.
* Bleeding after an interval when no periods have occurred.
* Bleeding more frequently, or in an irregular pattern.
* Bleeding after intercourse.
* Bleeding while taking the Pill.

Causes
Any factors influencing the hormonal cycle may cause irregular or unexpected bleeding.
- Stress.
- Confusion in taking the Pill, missed Pills or starting a packet incorrectly.
- The Pill may also cause bleeding between periods. This can often be stopped by changing the Pill for a different one containing different levels or types of hormones.
- Other drugs or illness upsetting the hormone balance can also interfere with the normal pattern of bleeding.
- Breast-feeding.
- Thyroid problems.

Other factors:
- Polyps at the neck of the womb may bleed irregularly or after intercourse.
- The neck of the womb (cervix) may bleed after intercourse if it is inflamed or infected. (See **Cervical problems**.)
- Infection in the womb may cause irregular bleeding. (See **Pelvic infection**.)
- Bleeding after the menopause can be the only symptom to indicate the presence of cancer. In this instance consult your doctor at once.

Treatment
- This is aimed at treating underlying causes listed above.

The Doctor
- May prescribe a different Pill.
- May take a blood test to check hormone levels and platelets.
- May carry out an examination and smear test.
- May refer you to a gynaecologist, particularly if you are past the menopause or if the bleeding is not explained.
- Details of tests and examinations which may be carried out are listed under **Periods, painful**, and **Periods, too heavy**.

Periods, no

This is called amenorrhoea and does not normally indicate any risk to health or to the womb. It is not essential to have a period every month in order to remain healthy.

It may be difficult to conceive while there is amenorrhoea, but this does not mean that contraceptive precautions can be avoided, as an egg may be produced at any time.

Symptoms
* Periods never start.
* Periods suddenly cease after being normal and regular.
* Patches of amenorrhoea occur, with the odd period now and then. (See **Periods, irregular and unexpected**.)
* Periods eventually cease altogether, usually after gradually diminishing. (See **Menopause**.)

Causes
- Being late starting to have periods:
  - girls often experience the same pattern as their mothers
  - childhood illness can delay periods starting
  - emotional factors can be responsible
  - rarely, a hormonal problem prevents periods from starting
- Periods may cease after previously being normal. Anything that upsets the balance of hormones and chemicals controlling egg production may cause periods to disappear:
  - pregnancy
  - breast-feeding
  - severe stress, bereavement, job problems
  - anorexia
  - drugs
  - following use of the contraceptive Pill
  - during continuous use of the contraceptive Pill without a break between packets; used by some to prevent periods on holiday (take your doctor's advice on this)
  - menopause
  - hysterectomy
  - rarely, hormonal problems which may produce other symptoms, such as hairiness, spottiness and change of voice (see also **Thyroid problems**)

Treatment
- If you are over sixteen years old, and your periods have not started, see the doctor. Usually no cause is found and periods start naturally.
- If periods are delayed after having been normal, this may indicate pregnancy – see the doctor as soon as possible.

The Doctor
- If there is no pregnancy the doctor may advise waiting for periods to start naturally, or may proceed to do simple blood tests and examinations. These frequently reveal no underlying problem and periods return in due course.
- If you wish to conceive, drugs can be given to stimulate ovaries to produce eggs.
- It is still necessary to use contraceptive precautions during amenorrhoea, as an egg may be released at any time.

Periods, painful

More than half of all women complain of severely painful periods. There is no risk involved in having painful periods unless they are caused by some underlying disorder.

Symptoms
* Typically, the pain is at the beginning of the period.
* Dull pain in the back and lower stomach.
* Cramping stomach pain, which can be severe.
* Headache.
* Vomiting and diarrhoea.
* Irritability and lethargy.

Causes
- Usually the pain of periods is caused by muscle contractions of the womb and cervix. The pain may or may not be caused by pelvic disease.
- Pain may start when periods first begin, and sometimes continues throughout life until the menopause. Pain of this kind is often due to hormonal imbalance and is less likely to be due to underlying pelvic disease. This type of period pain is commonly at its worst around 17 to 24 years of age.
- Pain following previously less painful periods can be due to:
  - fibroids: the womb may contract on a fibroid, which is attached by a stalk, trying to expel it with the menstrual flow and causing severe pain (see **Fibroids**.)
  - endometriosis: this is when fragments of tissue, which behave exactly as the lining of the womb, are found in the wrong place outside the womb; as they swell and bleed each month they can cause severe pain and may impair fertility
  - pelvic infection (see **Pelvic infection**)
  - coils, which may make period pain more severe
  - hormonal imbalance

Treatment
- Initial treatment should be with a simple painkiller such as paracetamol in regular doses, taken from the onset of period pain.
- If the pattern has changed from normal, or the pain is not tolerable, see the doctor.

The Doctor
- Will prescribe stronger painkillers and may prescribe a drug called mefenamic acid, which can be particularly useful for period pain.
- For the 17–24-year-old age group it is possible for the contraceptive Pill to be used to control period pain. By imposing an artificial hormonal cycle, period pain can be greatly reduced.
- If period pain is a new feature, or very persistent, examination and tests to look for the causes listed above will be carried out. This may include:
  - blood tests to check on hormonal balance
  - ultrasound examination (as used in pregnancy), which reveals the shape of internal organs by using soundwaves to create a pattern on a television screen
  - laparoscopy examination, when a thin telescope is passed through the tummy wall under anaesthetic; this may be necessary to reveal other diseases, such as endometriosis
- If all these prove normal, a variety of hormone preparations can be used to try and decrease period pains. The Pill, which is a combination of oestrogen and progestogen, or progestogen alone, may be given. It is certainly worth persevering in the search for a suitable preparation, because although one may not suit you another may be of great benefit.

Periods, too heavy

This is also called menorrhagia. More than one in ten women experience distressingly heavy periods at some stage.

The commonest problem is the development of anaemia as a consequence. As there are important causes of menorrhagia which can affect your health and future fertility, the doctor should be consulted.

Symptoms
* Heavy loss.
* Prolonged loss over a greater number of days than normal.
* Blood clots, often quite large, may be passed after lying down.

Causes
- Usually a hormonal imbalance causes menorrhagia.
- Fibroids.
- Pelvic infection.
- Coils, also called intra-uterine contraceptive devices (IUCDs).
- Miscarriage: a delayed period may be heavier because a pregnancy has been started and lost. If this is suspected, consult your doctor.
- Rarely, disturbance of blood-clotting, e.g. a low platelet count.

Treatment
- If your cycle returns to normal the next month it is not usually necessary to see your doctor for one heavier period than normal.
- Eating foods rich in iron will help prevent anaemia, e.g. beef, liver and other meats, green-leaf vegetables, dried fruit. Iron may be prescribed if you are found to be anaemic.

The Doctor
- It is important to see the doctor if heavier loss occurs after a delayed period, as this may indicate miscarriage. If the delay is for more than two weeks, and a pregnancy is suspected, admission to hospital may be necessary in order to ensure that nothing remains of the early pregnancy in the womb. An incomplete miscarriage can cause further problems with bleeding or infection. This may require a scrape operation under anaesthetic, also called D and C.
- The doctor will normally examine you, e.g. to check for fibroids.
- He will take blood tests to check for anaemia, hormonal abnormalities (see **Thyroid problems**), and the number of platelets in the blood (responsible for clotting).
- If no abnormality in other tests is found, referral to a gynaecologist may lead to a D and C operation to check for disease of the lining of the womb.
- While this procedure may reveal the cause of bleeding, often the scraping of the womb in itself helps menorrhagia.
- If menorrhagia is very persistent and uncontrolled, as a last resort hysterectomy may be offered, but this should not be undertaken lightly. (See **Hysterectomy**.)
- It is important to eat foods rich in iron, or to take iron supplements.

Piles

These are varicose veins around the back passage. They are also called haemorrhoids and are common particularly in pregnancy. They do not usually require surgical treatment, but it is important to see a doctor if you have any bleeding when passing a stool. Piles are not serious, but the other causes of rectal bleeding can be.

Symptoms
* Often the only symptom is blood seen on the paper, stool, or in the loo.
* A painful grape-size lump may appear at the back passage, sometimes a whole bunch of grapes.
* There can be a slimy mucus discharge with the piles.

Causes

- The bleeding is because varicose veins have thin walls and can easily rupture.
- The pain is often because the blood in the vein clots (thrombosed pile) and sets up an angry reaction in the vein.
- Anything that causes an increase in pressure on the veins around the back passage may cause piles. This happens during pregnancy and in constipation. When there is an inadequate diet to provide a large soft stool, piles may occur (see below). Straining particularly increases pressure and causes piles. Piles in pregnancy are worse after the straining and pressure effects of childbirth.
- Pain may also be from an anal fissure which is a slit in the muscles closing off the back passage. This can cause severe pain. Many of the treatments for piles help anal fissures.

Treatment

- A significant change of diet, to include more fruit and vegetables, whole-grain cereals and bran, is important. If you already have a diet such as this, you should double the amount of bran above your usual intake.
- Suppositories can be bought, which cause some shrinkage of the piles and can relieve pain.
- Use of frozen peas as an ice pack can give great relief. Many new mothers find sitting on such an ice pack provides relief for the few days it takes for piles to settle after childbirth. (Note: once peas are unfrozen they can be refrozen as often as you like but never eaten.)
- Simple painkillers such as aspirin or paracetamol taken regularly may help.
- Salt baths may help.

The Doctor

- Will examine you to make sure that piles are the cause of the problem. If he is not sure, examination with a special metal tube to look inside the back passage will be necessary and perhaps a barium enema X-ray examination
- For piles he may prescribe
  - ointments and suppositories containing steroids and sometimes local anaesthetic; note that local anaesthetic preparations can cause a skin reaction if used repeatedly for more than seven days
  - powders to make up with water; these are usually derived from the husk of a plant called ispaghula, which helps to give a soft, easily passed stool and makes very effective treatment; some people find it easier to continue the powders than trying to eat bowlfuls of unappetising bran
- Rarely, surgery is necessary if bleeding and pain are very troublesome and do not respond to the above measures. Surgical treatment is usually carried out on you as an outpatient, with local treatment applied to the piles to make the veins seal off, thus preventing, hopefully, further bleeding or pain. Banding, injection or operation are some of the techniques used.

Pins and needles

The sensation when you bang your 'funny bone' at the elbow is caused by pressure on a nerve that is near the skin's surface. The sensation is of pins and needles and normally passes off quickly. Pins and needles can be felt in many different parts of the body, due to pressure on nerves. The symptom itself is not serious, but the cause of the pins and needles, although usually minor, can reflect a more troublesome cause of pressure.

Symptoms
* The description 'pins and needles' is applied because the sensation is like many gentle pricks from sharp points.
* Often there is associated numbness.
* There may be pain in the area of the pins and needles or some distance away.
* It usually passes off quickly but may recur frequently.
* Tingling is another word sometimes used to describe a similar sensation due to the same causes.

Causes
- The feeling of pins and needles at the elbow, which is mentioned above, occurs frequently because the nerve concerned is near the surface. In other parts of the body nerves are deeper inside and less vulnerable to pressure.
- Unusual posture is a common cause of pins and needles. Prolonged squatting, sleeping in an awkward position and sitting on an uncomfortable chair may all cause nerve pressure and pins and needles.
- Wear-and-tear arthritis in the spine can lead to irregularly shaped bones and the discs between them. This causes pressure on the nerves, causing pain, numbness and pins and needles. (See **Neck problems, Backache**.)
- Wherever nerves pass through narrow passages in the body they are liable to pressure effects, particularly if the body retains fluid. For example, in pregnancy wrist discomfort and pins and needles in the hands are common, because of carpal tunnel syndrome. (See **Wrist pain and tingling fingers**.)
- Pins and needles may also occur when the brain is affected. For example, in migraines this sensation may occur in the arm, although it is the brain, connected to the arm by nerves, which is affected.

Treatment
- This is aimed at relieving the cause. Usually this will be obvious and the symptoms of pins and needles will ease as pressure effects on the nerve wear off.
- Shaking the affected limb or raising it in the air may help to relieve symptoms.
- If symptoms are persistent, recurrent or without any obvious cause you should see the doctor.

The Doctor
- May mark out on your skin the exact area affected. This often reveals that the pins and needles sensation is limited to the skin affected by one particular nerve.
- The doctor may advise no treatment if he considers the sensation will go on its own.
- If the pins and needles sensation persists, or it is not clear what the cause might be, further tests may be arranged. These will include X-rays of any bones which may be pressing on the nerve. Electrical tests on the nerve supplying the area may be carried out to try and identify what is happening to the nerve and at what point along its pathway.

Pleurisy

The word pleurisy is often incorrectly used to describe a general chest infection. In fact, true pleurisy refers to a problem in the pleural space between the lungs and the ribs, which may be due to several different causes. The use of antibiotics has fortunately led to pleurisy becoming much less common. The presence of pleurisy symptoms should always lead to your seeking a doctor's advice. (See also **Bronchitis, Pneumonia.**)

Symptoms
* Pain on deep breathing.
* Pain on coughing.
* Pain usually confined to one side and often severe.
* Sometimes fluid accumulates in an area where there is pleurisy. The presence of fluid will stop the pain but the illness may still be present. This fluid is called a pleural effusion.
* There may be a fever.

Causes
The lungs inside the rib cage expand and contract as we breathe. Between the lungs and the ribs is an area called the pleural space. This space is almost imperceptible and allows the lungs to glide smoothly against the ribs. Pleurisy occurs when the space becomes either inflamed or made larger by the lung pulling away from the rib cage (as in pneumothorax, see below). Causes include:

- Infection, such as pneumonia or tuberculosis, leading to irritation of the pleural space. (See **Pneumonia.**)
- Injury, such as a damaged rib, can irritate the pleural space and cause inflammation.
- Underlying lung disease such as cancer can also affect the lung edges, causing pleurisy.
- Pneumothorax is relatively rare but causes pleurisy symptoms when the lung pulls away from the ribs and air enters the pleural space. The severity of symptoms depends on your fitness and the size of the area affected. Pain is usually sudden, and there may be breathing difficulties.

Treatment
- A doctor should be consulted for treatment of the cause of pleurisy symptoms.
- By listening to the chest the doctor may be able to identify exactly the area of pleurisy. If fluid has entered the pleural space, causing a pleural effusion, this can sometimes be identified by examination.
- An X-ray of the chest will be arranged, and can often clearly show the reason for pleurisy. Appropriate treatment can then be commenced.
- Infections will normally respond well to antibiotics. Painkillers may be required until the infection is treated.
- Pneumothorax may heal by itself, or a special tube may need to be inserted into the pleural space to remove the air.
- Other lung problems, such as cancer, will require specialist treatment.
- If fluid builds up, forming a pleural effusion (see above), this can cause breathing problems. It may become necessary to remove some of the fluid. This can be done easily by the insertion under local anaesthetic of a syringe needle between the ribs.

Pneumonia

Pneumonia is an infection of lung tissue. It varies from a fairly mild infection to one which threatens life. Babies, young children and the elderly are most at risk. People with diseases of nerve, muscle, chest or immune system are more at risk. Pneumonia is more common in the winter months. Many different bacteria, viruses and moulds can cause it; bacterial infections are treated with antibiotics. There is usually a full recovery, though permanent scarring of lung tissue may occur.

Symptoms

* There is a chesty cough with phlegm; this may be coloured yellow or green or be streaked wth blood. (A dry, irritating cough may keep you awake but is unlikely to be pneumonia.)
* The cough, catarrh and runny nose of a cold will usually get better.
* There is fever and sweating.
* Breathing is noisy and more rapid than normal.
* There may be a sharp pain on breathing in. (See **Pleurisy**.)
* Babies may vomit or refuse feeds. Their breathing is rapid, and they may appear to be working very hard to breathe. The nostrils flare, the stomach and ribs are sucked in.
* Older people may become confused.
* Blue lips caused by pneumonia suggest a severe lack of oxygen.

Causes

- Many bacteria cause pneumonia. Most are spread by coughs and sneezes.
- Many viruses cause pneumonia. These include measles and chicken pox viruses.
- Tuberculosis also causes pneumonia.
- People with weakened immune systems are most likely to have fungal pneumonia. This may be because of AIDS, leukaemia, malnutrition, or high doses of steroids.
- Cystic fibrosis is an inherited disease which causes frequent pneumonia.
- Muscular or nervous weakness makes infection likely.
- Influenza leaves the lungs more prone to infection.

Prevention

- Do not smoke. Cigarette smoke paralyses the action of hairs which keep the airways clean; this reduces the ability of cells to fight off infection.
- Vaccination is available against whooping cough and measles. These infections can cause pneumonia and may damage the lungs.
- A vaccine is available against the *pneumococcus*, one of the commonest germs causing pneumonia. This may be given to people who are vulnerable to infection because their defence systems are weakened in some way (see above).

Treatment

- Paracetamol will help with fever and sore throat.
- Cough mixtures from the chemist are soothing, but may have little more effect than honey-and-lemon drinks. (See **Cough**.)
- Signs that indicate you should see a doctor are:
  - a chesty or persistent cough productive of coloured phlegm
  - breathing which is rapid, difficult or painful

The Doctor

- Your doctor will examine your chest with a stethoscope.
- Antibiotics will be prescribed if there are signs of pneumonia. Painkillers and cough mixtures may be recommended.
- A chest X-ray may be required.
- Some people will need hospital treatment, particularly most infants with pneumonia and the elderly.
- Blood tests and tests on the phlegm may be arranged.
- Antibiotics can be given by injection if necessary.
- A physiotherapist will help with your breathing and coughing. This can often be as effective, or more so, than the antibiotic treatment.
- Oxygen can be given through a mask.
- Very rarely, ventilation via a res-

pirator (breathing machine) is needed.

Poisoning and over-dosage

Accidental ingestion of drugs and poisons is common. It is usually not fatal, but urgent medical attention must always be sought immediately. Drugs are the commonest substance taken, but household products and berries also cause problems. Poisoning usually affects children, but adults may also take a dangerous substance accidentally or deliberately. The immediate actions required after poisoning are the same, whether the ingestion of the substance was deliberate or accidental. In deliberate overdoses there will obviously be a need for further psychiatric help and intervention. This is not considered further here.

Symptoms
* These may be immediate: burns from caustic substances, or stomach pains, for example.
* They can often appear some time after the poison has been taken.
* Bizarre symptoms such as awkward or strange movements may occur.
* Confusion may be seen.
* Loss of consciousness may occur.
* Breathing difficulties may occur.

Causes
- Common drugs which cause problems when they are taken incorrectly include:
  - anti-depressant drugs; some of these, particularly the tricyclic group, cause heart problems (abnormal heart rhythms) and overdosage may be fatal
  - diarrhoea medicines, e.g. Lomotil, may cause loss of consciousness and breathing problems, sometimes occurring after an interval
  - aspirin can be dangerous, causing breathing and bleeding problems and upsetting the body chemistry
  - iron, which is often thought to be harmless, can be very dangerous in overdose, causing diarrhoea, vomiting, bleeding and nervous problems.
  - distalgesics may lead to coma and fatal breathing problems
  - paracetamol, if taken in overdosage, leads to dangerous liver changes; early action may be able to halt some of the changes
- Household products commonly causing problems include:
  - bleach
  - lavatory cleaners
  - detergents
  - paint thinners and cleaners
  - weed killers and garden products
  - paraffin
- Many berries cause problems. Interestingly, the laburnum plant, which is often a cause for alarm, caused no deaths over a recent twenty-year period.
- Glue-sniffing may lead to a variety of symptoms, and is effectively a form of poisoning common in children and adolescents. (See **Drug abuse, Glue-sniffing**.)
- There are examples of an unusual form of child abuse where poisoning occurs due to the deliberate administration of substances to children by their carers.

Prevention
* Most instances of poisoning in children could be avoided by the adequate storing of dangerous products or drugs in the home.
* All medicines should be kept in a locked cupboard out of reach of children. After giving a dose of even a simple medicine to a child, the

bottle should be kept out of reach of the child even if another dose is due in a few hours' time.
- Choose household products with childproof tops and store away from children.
- Never store any substances in old lemonade bottles; this is a common cause of poisoning from weed-killers.

Treatment
- Immediate action on suspecting or witnessing poisoning or over-dosage should be to seek medical help.
- Do not try to induce vomiting by sticking fingers down the throat or giving salty drinks. If the poisoning is due to a caustic substance this could worsen the situation.
- Wash any chemicals away from round the mouth with water, but do not give water to drink.

The Doctor
- Will be able to ascertain quickly if the substance is safe or dangerous by contacting a special national poisons unit that handles such enquiries. Always show the doctor any containers or bottles that might indicate what has been taken.
- If the substance is not safe, vomiting may be brought on by giving a medicine called Ipecacuanha. The dose may need to be repeated. If vomiting does not occur it may be necessary to pump out the stomach contents by inserting a tube down the gullet. (Ipecacuanha will not normally be used if corrosive poisons or paraffins have been taken, nor will it be used in semi- or unconscious people.)
- Blood and urine samples may be taken to estimate the amount of the substance in the body.
- Specific antidotes will be given if available. Unfortunately, there is rarely a specific antidote to counteract a poison.
- Careful monitoring after the initial treatment is completed may be required. For example, continuous heart recording may be required following tricyclic antidepressant drug ingestion.
- Unless there is a need for a further period of observation in hospital, or attention from a psychiatrist, discharge from hospital will take place very quickly. When at home, plenty of fluids and a gradual return to a normal diet is all that is required.

Pregnancy problems

Pregnancy is a normal condition. There are many problems that may occur, making the supervision of the pregnancy by your doctor, midwife and health visitor of considerable importance. The problems considered here are:

Anaemia in pregnancy
Raised blood pressure in pregnancy
Sickness in pregnancy

Anaemia in pregnancy

Anaemia commonly occurs in pregnancy. It is detected by taking blood tests which measure the ability of the blood to carry oxygen. Doctors watch for a fall in the haemoglobin (the red pigment in the blood that carries oxygen) count in pregnancy.

The importance of anaemia in pregnancy lies in the fact that if you are anaemic your body will be able to cope less well with infection or bleeding around the time of birth. The baby may also be affected if you have severe anaemia.

Symptoms
* Minimal anaemia may not cause any symptoms, only being detected on routine blood tests.
* Pallor.
* Tiredness and weakness.
* Breathlessness and palpitations if severe.

Causes
☐ In later pregnancy the growing baby makes increasing demands for iron and folic acid. These are vital ingredients for production of haemoglobin and prevention of anaemia.
☐ In pregnancy there are changes in the body which lead to the blood being diluted. Because the blood is diluted the same quantity of haemoglobin does not go so far. Insufficient haemoglobin to match the previous concentration leads to anaemia.

Prevention
- Eating foods rich in iron (see **Anaemia**) helps to prevent anaemia. The absorption of the iron in these foods can be helped by eating other foods rich in vitamin C, such as citrus fruits and fresh vegetables.
- Fresh green vegetables contain folic acid. It is important to avoid folic acid deficiency to avoid anaemia in pregnancy (see **Anaemia**).
- Despite adequate dietary iron and folic acid, anaemia may develop, so it is important to attend for regular blood tests and check-ups. This ensures early detection of anaemia, so you have time to correct it before the baby arrives.

Treatment
- Iron and folic acid tablets are commonly given in pregnancy. These may be provided even if your blood test does not yet reveal anaemia. They are safe if taken correctly and can prevent anaemia, as well as restoring a reduced haemoglobin level. Problems with indigestion have been greatly helped by newer formulations of iron and folic acid.

The Doctor
- As well as monitoring your blood for anaemia, the doctor may prescribe a different type of iron and folic acid if the one you have tried doesn't suit you.
- The doctor can advise on measures to combat constipation, which may be aggravated by iron therapy. (See **Constipation**.)
- Constipation can add to the problems of piles in pregnancy. The doctor can provide advice and assistance with treatment for piles (see **Piles**). (Also see **Varicose veins**.)
- If anaemia is persistent, further measures may be taken to correct your haemoglobin, as described under **Anaemia**.

Raised blood pressure in pregnancy

Raised blood pressure may be present before you become pregnant, only being detected for the first time during routine check-ups. It can also develop during pregnancy, and possibly become dangerous towards the end of pregnancy. Because the effects of raised blood pressure are so important to both the baby and the mother, it is very important that blood pressure is monitored throughout pregnancy. Raised blood pressure can interfere with the function of the placenta and hence the baby's development.

Symptoms
* Usually none, especially if blood pressure was raised before pregnancy.
* Urine may be found to contain pro-

tein, which could be a sign of pre-eclampsia developing (see below).
* Swelling of ankles and fingers may occur, indicating pre-eclampsia if the blood pressure is raised.
* Symptoms of severe pre-eclampsia or eclampsia (see below).

Causes

☐ Pre-existing high blood pressure. (See **Blood pressure, high**.)

☐ Pre-eclampsia, which is a condition of pregnancy where the blood pressure is raised and there is excessive body fluid. It is not understood why this should happen. It occurs more commonly in first pregnancies. If, in addition to swelling and raised blood pressure, the urine is found to contain protein you are at risk of developing:

Eclampsia, which may be preceded by a period of headaches, visual difficulties and vomiting, which are symptoms of severe pre-eclampsia. If the blood pressure is not controlled there is a risk of fits, loss of consciousness and even maternal death.

Prevention

- Resting in pregnancy can avoid and treat raised blood pressure.
- Regular check-ups must be attended. This enables any changes in blood pressure to be detected early so treatment can be started.

Treatment

- Often rest is adequate. Once the diagnosis of raised blood pressure is made, and the consequences explained, it is usually easier for mothers to rest, as any necessary help is more likely to be forthcoming.
- Frequent measurement, even daily at home, may be carried out by the midwife or doctor.

The Doctor

- Drug treatment will be started if the blood pressure is persistently above a certain level. Only drugs considered safe in pregnancy will be used. The risk to mother and baby of continuing with a dangerous level of blood pressure is usually much greater than any potential risk to the foetus from the drug.
- Hospital admission is often necessary if blood pressure remains high. If symptoms of severe pre-eclampsia or eclampsia develop it will be essential. Drugs will be given to prevent fits, and an early delivery of the baby either by induction or caesarean section may be necessary.
- Following delivery of the baby the blood pressure will continue to be monitored, but the symptoms of pre-eclampsia normally cease shortly after birth.

Sickness in pregnancy

In early pregnancy most women have at least a feeling of nausea, if not actual vomiting. This varies enormously in severity. Some people have only a few days' trouble, and feel 'off' certain foods; others have such severe vomiting that their body chemicals get out of balance and treatment in hospital is necessary. Fortunately, very few people indeed have very severe vomiting. Normally, sickness in pregnancy is quite harmless and, despite the unpleasantness of symptoms, most people can tolerate them until they wear off.

Symptoms

* Feeling of nausea and/or being sick, starting from around four weeks of pregnancy and lasting until fourteen to sixteen weeks of pregnancy.

* Nausea and vomiting may be worse in the morning but can occur all day long.
* Acid tastes in the mouth may be caused by heartburn, a searing discomfort behind the breastbone which may occur in pregnancy. This adds to feelings of nausea and vomiting. It is caused by lax muscles that normally close off the stomach. This laxity allows stomach acids to irritate the more sensitive gullet. (See **Hiatus Hernia**).
* Heartburn usually occurs in late pregnancy and is aggravated by the pressure of the growing baby on the stomach.

Causes

- In very early pregnancy symptoms of nausea and vomiting may be caused by many different factors. It is thought that hormonal changes, diet and emotional factors all play a part.
- The way the stomach empties is altered in pregnancy. The intestines do not work as efficiently as before pregnancy. This may lead to the build-up of acid in the stomach and subsequent symptoms.
- The chemicals that are found in the liver are also present in different quantities in pregnancy. Some of these changes may produce sickness symptoms.
- In later pregnancy hiatus hernia symptoms may occur, with heartburn and bilious taste in the mouth (see above and **Hiatus hernia**).

Prevention

- Avoid becoming overtired; this exacerbates symptoms.
- Eat frequent small meals, avoiding long periods without eating.
- Greasy foods are best avoided. If there are particular foods that upset you, put everything connected with them out of sight.

Treatment

- Food taken before you get up in the morning can help symptoms. Some people find a milky drink and dry biscuit taken first thing in the morning can decrease the severity of nausea.
- Eating frequently ensures that acid in the stomach is absorbed. Carbohydrate foods, such as bread and potatoes or dry crackers, may be particularly helpful.
- Some people find antacid medicine helpful, though unfortunately this is by no means always the case. It is wise to discuss with your doctor what kind of antacid to try. Antacids may be helpful in later pregnancy, when heartburn and hiatus hernia symptoms occur (see above).

The Doctor

- Will test the urine for traces of body chemicals, which are increased if vomiting is severe. These are called ketones and can indicate that you are not taking enough fluids to counterbalance the vomiting.
- A blood test may also be done to check that you are not in danger of upsetting the balance of minerals and chemicals in the body.
- The urine may also be tested for infection, although this is a relatively rare cause of vomiting in pregnancy.
- It is unusual for drugs to be prescribed, as nausea and vomiting are usually not sufficiently severe to justify their use. The vast majority of women prefer to put up with the symptoms, knowing they will cease at around fourteen weeks.
- If symptoms occur later in pregnancy, or are very severe, the doctor may prescribe antacid medicine or, less commonly, a drug such as promethazine.

- The persistance of severe symptoms is called hyperemesis. This may require hospital treatment. If blood tests show that the balance of mineral and chemicals is upset, hospital treatment will certainly be necessary. This involves replacing fluid into a vein, using an intravenous drip. This special replacement fluid can give directly to the body all the necessary minerals and chemicals required. This allows the stomach to remain empty, while also providing an important means of giving any drugs that may be necessary. Usually symptoms settle over five to seven days, but occasionally a longer stay in hospital may be required.

Pregnancy, unwanted

If you find yourself unexpectedly pregnant, making the difficult decision to seek an abortion or continue the pregnancy can be extremely distressing. Unfortunately, you do not have long to make up your mind because the ease and safety with which you can have an abortion are related to how early you have the operation. It is increasingly difficult to have an abortion beyond twelve to thirteen weeks. This is because doctors do not like doing them later than this, because of the nature of the operation involved, and because of the risk to your health.

An early termination of pregnancy is not dangerous, nor should it have implications for your future fertility. The psychological consequences of having an abortion are, however, impossible to estimate. Some people appear to cope well with the upset, while others may have considerable emotional difficulties, either immediately or well into the future.

In Britain it is legal to have an abortion. Two doctors must agree to your request under specific legal conditions. The pregnancy must represent sufficient risk to your well-being, or your existing children's well-being, to satisfy the legal requirements. The pregnancy may also be terminated if there is evidence that the baby would be at substantial risk of serious handicap if it were born.

Prevention

- Obviously, correct use of contraceptive measures is paramount in avoiding an unwanted pregnancy.
- There are now many methods available. These include:
  - the combined contraceptive Pill (containing oestrogen and progestogen), taken for twenty-one out of every twenty-eight days
  - the progestogen-only Pill, taken every day of the year and working in a different way from the combined Pill
  - the coil or intra-uterine contraceptive device (IUCD)
  - the cap or diaphragm
  - condoms or sheaths, e.g. Durex
  - injections of a contraceptive drug lasting three months
- Other methods which are much less reliable include:
  - withdrawal technique
  - rhythm method
  - contraceptive sponges
- It is always wise to discuss these methods with your doctor or local family planning clinic before you start having intercourse. Even if you are under sixteen your doctor is able to discuss contraception in confidence with you.
- The morning-after pill is not a method of contraception and should only be used in emergency situations when unprotected intercourse has exposed you to the risk of an unwanted pregnancy. You should always see your doctor if considering using this.

- It is not guaranteed to stop a pregnancy developing but usually does so.
- To take the morning-after pill involves taking a total of four special-dosage type pills. Two are taken as soon as possible after intercourse, followed by two twelve hours later. All the pills should be taken within seventy-two hours of intercourse. If previous unprotected intercourse has occurred, as well as the occasion for which you need help, the morning-after pill should not be taken, as you may already be pregnant.
- Ordinary contraceptive pills you may have at home should not be taken in this way.
- You must always see your doctor for follow-up checks after taking the morning-after pill, so any necessary checks to ensure that pregnancy has not occurred may be carried out. Three weeks after taking the pills is a good time to see your doctor again.
- Some people experience feelings of sickness after taking these pills. Contact your doctor if you actually vomit within three hours of taking the pills.
- Fitting a coil following unprotected intercourse is a possibility. Your doctor may consider fitting an IUCD up to one week after unprotected intercourse. Not everyone is suitable to have a coil fitted, and this is not a reliable form of contraception following unprotected intercourse. Such a measure will only be considered by the doctor if it is felt likely to be safe and successful.
- If a coil is fitted it can remain in place and can continue as your method of contraception.

Treatment
- Once you have decided you would like to consider an abortion, contact your doctor, family planning clinic or one of the addresses listed below.
- Don't delay – the sooner you are seen the better. You can change your mind right up to the last moment before you have the operation.

The Doctor
- Your doctor cannot refuse to help you. He or she is duty bound to refer you to a local family planning clinic or another doctor if, for one reason or another, they do not wish to help you or do not agree to your needing a termination.
- You will have counselling from either your doctor or another worker trained to answer your questions. During the counselling you should not be influenced one way or the other by the opinions of the counsellor. Counselling is very important to ensure that you are confident of your feelings and are sure of your need for an abortion. Your needs must always be sufficient to meet the legal requirements.
- Normally your doctor signs part of a special form called a Schedule A and contacts a local gynaecologist with details of your situation. The gynaecologist may then agree to do the operation and must sign the same form.
- You will be asked to sign a consent form for the operation. If you are under sixteen a parent normally signs the form.

The operation
- This may be carried out without your having to stay in hospital. There may be a local hospital offering what is called day-patient facilities.
- If the operation is done in this way it may be carried out using a suction method which uses a straw-like structure inserted through the neck of

the womb to withdraw the pregnancy. This leaves the womb empty. A general anaesthetic may not be necessary.
- Staying overnight will usually be necessary if you are more than a few weeks' pregnant. In this instance the operation will be done using either the suction method described above or an instrument inserted through the cervix which scrapes the lining of the womb clear, (also called a D and C or scrape operation).
- In the much more unusual situation where an abortion is required after around fourteen weeks, termination of the pregnancy is more difficult and more unpleasant. This is usually required when tests done during the pregnancy show there is substantial risk that if the child were born it would be seriously handicapped. Unfortunately, these extremely important tests have not yet been widely developed to be able to give answers about the baby's abnormalities before the eighteenth week of pregnancy.
- If a later termination is required it will normally be done by inducing labour using a drug called prostaglandin. This is injected into the womb and/or inserted into the vagina. As the full process of labour will take place, with an undeveloped foetus being expelled, the distress for everyone concerned can be considerable.
- The risks of abortion are small if it is done early in pregnancy by a doctor recommended by your own doctor or reputable clinic (see list below). At the time of operation there is a small risk of perforation of the uterus, damage to the cervix and heavy bleeding. After the operation, there is some risk of infection or further heavy bleeding, both of which will require urgent medical attention.

After the operation
- Follow-up from your doctor, not just to discuss contraception (see above), but to check for complications is important. Your doctor will also be keen to help you through any psychological difficulties you may have. If difficulties arise in the future, do not hesitate to discuss your feelings as a lot can be done to help.

☎ Pregnancy Advisory Service, 11–13 Charlotte Street, London W1. Tel: 071 637 8962.

☎ British Pregnancy Advisory Service, Austy Manor, Wootten Wowen, Solihull, West Midlands. Tel: 0564 793225. (Ring for details of local branches.) London: 071 828 2484 (Victoria), 071 602 3804 (Hammersmith).

☎ Brook Advisory Centre, 153A East Street, London SE17. Tel: 071 708 1234. (Ring this number for details of local services.)

☎ (Family Planning Clinics are listed in the telephone directory.)

Premenstrual tension

This refers to a variety of symptoms that occur prior to menstruation. A combination of both physical and emotional symptoms may occur. For some women this is very mild, while for others several days are lost each month due to the severity of their symptoms. Treatment is poorly understood and controversial. There is no doubt that a number of different preparations can give considerable benefit. Premenstrual symptoms are less common in women under thirty years old. It may only appear after having your first child. Being on the contraceptive pill seems to make you less likely to suffer premenstrual tension.

Symptoms
* Some authors have suggested more than a hundred different symptoms as part of premenstrual tension. It is also called premenstrual syndrome.
* The most common symptoms include:
  - tension
  - irritability
  - depression
  - feeling bloated
  - fatigue
  - breast tenderness
  - swelling, particularly of ankles and fingers

Causes
☐ Hormonal changes occur throughout the menstrual cycle (see **Periods**). It seems likely that variations in the levels of these hormones account for the symptoms. Some specialists consider that psychological factors may also play a part.

Treatment
- Various forms of treatment have been suggested.
- Very often symptoms of premenstrual tension fluctuate, being severe for several months before improving by themselves. If you are troubled, it is worth persisting in finding a treatment that suits you. Your doctor may be able to advise you on one of the following treatments.

The Doctor
- Use of a hormone called progesterone has proved very successful in many women. This can be taken either as tablets, injections or suppositories. Norethisterone, taken as tablets three times daily from the 19th to the 26th day of the cycle, may for example, be useful. (Available on prescription only.)
- Vitamin B6, or pyridoxine, has been claimed by some people to be helpful. Excess dosage can lead to toxic symptoms.
- Evening primrose oil is another common treatment. (Not available on prescription.)
- Sometimes use of a contraceptive Pill can relieve symptoms. This may be worth trying for a few months. On discontinuing the Pill symptoms of premenstrual tension may be less severe.

☎ Women's Health Concern. Helpline: 071 938 3932 (London); 0222 549888 (Cardiff).

☎ The Premenstrual Society (PremSoc), PO Box 102, London SE1 7ES.

Prostate problems

The prostate is a small gland about one inch across, which encircles the urine passage as it leaves the bladder. It is only found in men. Its exact function is not clear, but it is known to secrete substances into the urine passage to add to the fluid at ejaculation. Its position around the urine passage means that changes in the prostate may have an effect on the free flow of urine.

Problems considered here are:
Cancer of the prostate
Enlargement of the prostate
Inflammation of the prostate

Cancer of the prostate

After about eighty years of age, nearly every male has cancer of the prostate gland. It is different from other cancers in that it lies dormant in the gland for many years, seldom causing any problems. In most cases the cancer does not spread elsewhere; when it does the first sign may be of cancer in the bones. Often the fact that the growth of the prostate is malignant is only discovered at the time of operation for enlargement of the prostate (see below). It is not a very dangerous cancer, death usually occurring due to some other unrelated condition rather than the cancer of the prostate.

Symptoms

* Usually none. It there are symptoms they are usually those of enlargement of the prostate (see below).
* Occasionally, symptoms related to the prostate itself do not occur and the presence of bone pain is the first sign of cancer of the prostate, indicating spread to the bones.

Treatment

- If suspicion of cancer of the prostate is raised after examination of the prostate by a gloved finger in the back passage, your doctor will refer you immediately to a specialist called a urologist.
- Blood tests will be done to measure a body chemical called acid phosphatase, which is sometimes raised if you have cancer of the prostate.
- A piece of the prostate gland will be removed for examination under a microscope. This is called a prostate biopsy.
- Pieces of tissue removed at an operation for normal enlargement of the prostate are sent for microscopic examination, as this may be the only indication of the presence of cancer in the prostate.
- If you have cancer of the prostate a special X-ray examination called a bone scan will be done to reveal the spread of any cancer to the bones.
- Treatment for cancer of the prostate may involve radiotherapy and drug treatment, both of which can be very effective.
- The prostate gland is not necessarily removed if cancerous, because the cancer normally remains limited to the prostate and causes no problems. Removal of the entire prostate is a major operation, not without its problems, and does not guarantee cure of the cancer.
- You will have regular check-ups to ensure the cancer has not spread. As mentioned above, other conditions are much more likely to cause death than the cancer of the prostate, particularly if this is discovered after about fifty years of age.

Enlargement of the Prostate

The commonest problem affecting the prostate is for it to become enlarged. As a natural part of the ageing process, particularly beyond the mid-forties, some prostate enlargement is usually found. The changes in the prostate are not just increases in size, but small areas of gristle-like substance may appear, which may make the prostate harder. In order for the urine to flow freely through the middle of the prostate it must relax. Hard gristle in the prostate and its enlargement make it less able to relax, and may cause it to press on the urine pipe, causing a variety of symptoms.

Fortunately, most prostate enlargement is harmless and troublesome symptoms, if they do occur, can be treated by surgery to the prostate. There is little danger from prostate enlargement, although if severe it can obstruct the urine passage completely, causing urine to be retained. If this happens acutely it is very painful and must be immediately relieved by passing a thin tube into the bladder through the penis. If it happens over a longer period of time, with the bladder not fully emptying, there is a danger of infection. See your doctor if these situations arise.

Symptoms

* The stream of urine becomes weaker.
* There is a desire to pass urine more frequently, but only small quantities may be passed each time.
* At the beginning and end of passing urine there are difficulties. It is sometimes difficult to start passing urine, and after doing so the urine may dribble to a stop rather than ceasing abruptly.
* Starting to pass urine may be particularly difficult first thing in the morning.
* There is no pain associated with enlargement of the prostate.
* Rarely, there can be some blood in the urine. If this happens you should see your doctor.

Causes

☐ It is not clear why the prostate enlarges, but it is known to be extremely common, affecting most men.
☐ The enlargement is usually not malignant. Cancer of the prostate does, however, occur and may have the same symptoms as benign enlargement of the prostate. (See above for **Cancer of the prostate**.)

Treatment

● When symptoms first appear, many men find ways of passing urine effectively to overcome the symptoms.
● Sitting down to pass urine can help.
● Using the tummy muscles to help expel the urine by contracting the muscles helps. In the long term, if the bladder is having to work harder to expel urine the muscles in its wall become thickened and stronger.
● You should see your doctor when prostate symptoms occur. No action may be taken in mild cases, symptoms often clearing up without treatment.

The Doctor

● Will examine the prostate, easily done by inserting a gloved finger into the back passage. This gives information about the size and consistency of the prostate.
● A blood test to check for changes in a body chemical which may be present in increased amounts in cancer of the prostate is sometimes done (see above).
● You may need to be seen by a doctor called a urologist who specialises in the way the kidneys, bladder and urine passages work. The urologist will organise further tests and any treatment required.
● He will arrange for an X-ray examination which reveals how the urine passages are working and gives information about the size of the prostate (intravenous pyelogram or IVP).
● If treatment is required there are two ways of having surgery to the prostate. Firstly, transurethral resection or TUR. This is done by inserting a tube containing a telescope and a cutting device up through the penis to the prostate. Using this, it is possible to core out the prostate from the inside of the urine passage, in much the same way as you would an apple. The hardened and enlarged shavings from the operation are flushed out, using liquid, at the time of operation. There is usually some bleeding after this operation, seen in the bag beside your bed when you wake up. The bag is attached to a catheter, which is left in the penis for

a short time after the operation. You are normally home from hospital after about four days. The urine stream may be remarkably improved after this operation. Secondly, the prostate can also be removed to prevent problems via an incision in the tummy. This is a much bigger operation with more dangers associated with it. It is technically difficult and can damage the nerves to the penis, leading to subsequent impotence. This way of dealing with prostate problems is sometimes necessary because transurethral resection is not feasible due to other problems with the penis. The hospital stay following this operation is longer than after transurethral resection. You may be in hospital for ten to fourteen days.

- After prostate surgery the semen at ejaculation may enter the bladder instead of coming out of the penis. This is harmless, the semen eventually coming out with urine, but sterility is a consequence. Due to the age at which most prostate operations are done sterility does not normally present a problem.

Inflammation of the prostate

This is not common, but may occur particularly in those with an enlarged prostate.

Symptoms

* Feeling unwell.
* Fever.
* Pain at the base of the penis and inside the back passage.
* Difficulty or discomfort passing urine.
* Symptoms may be recurrent.

Causes

□ Infection in the urine is uncommon in men. If it does occur it may spread to affect the prostate.
□ Rarely, a chronic infection may affect the prostate, with the accumulation of pus in the gland causing little in the way of symptoms until the pus discharges.

Treatment

- The doctor, by examining the back passage with a gloved finger, may feel a swollen and painful prostate gland.
- A urine sample will be taken to look for infection before treatment is started.
- Antibiotics usually clear the infection and the symptoms settle down. Occasionally, the inflammation of the prostate is not affected by antibiotics, and if the symptoms do not settle on their own a chronic inflammation may occur, causing more problems. This is rare.

Psoriasis

This is a common skin condition which may occur at any time from infancy to old age. There are various forms, but the commonest type is a long-lasting condition. It is often seen between ten and thirty years of age and its severity is very variable, from a few patches to many larger ones. There is often a family history of others with psoriasis. It is not infectious and is not dangerous except in a very rare severe form. A few people have an associated arthritis, which may resemble rheumatoid arthritis. (See **Arthritis**.) Although the tendency to develop psoriasis may remain for life, most people can control their outbreaks well with a variety of creams and ointments. Psoriasis may also quite spontaneously clear from the skin.

Symptoms

* There are reddish raised patches on the skin.

* These patches have white or silvery scales.
* There may be one small patch half an inch across or many large patches up to several inches or more across.
* Itching is slight, but the lesions may be very uncomfortable. On the hands and feet in particular fissures may appear in thick lesions, causing considerable discomfort.
* Knees, elbows and scalp are most commonly affected, but it may appear almost anywhere.
* The nails may become thickened, indented with little pits, and may sometimes lift away from the skin beneath.

Causes

□ In psoriasis there is a problem with the normal skin turnover, which is designed to replace our skin as we shed scales daily. There is a lack of a substance called keratin which should give the skin its firm surface and helps to hold the skin together.

□ Infection may precipitate psoriasis; it commonly follows a sore throat.

□ It is a myth that psoriasis is primarily a stress disorder. Some people may find stress worsens the psoriasis but it is not a general rule and may occur without any specific upsets or emotional problems.

Treatment

- There is no permanent cure, but much that can be done to help control and diminish skin patches. The illness may also clear of its own accord. For some people, however, it remains throughout life as severe, angry-looking lesions widespread on the skin, which are extremely difficult to control, although there may be occasional remissions.
- Sunbathing with care helps, although actual sunburn can make it worse. Use sun lamps with great care, always remembering to protect the eyes.

The Doctor

- It is usually necessary to seek a doctor's advice to obtain one or more of a variety of treatments.
- For each cream or ointment available there are many different strengths. Treatment should always be started with the mildest, gradually increasing the strength. Avoid applying to normal skin as this may be adversely affected by psoriasis treatments.
- Salicylic acid is useful for scalp and scaling lesions; often used with soft paraffin. Many preparations containing tar exist. As the tar content increases, so does the amount of mess involved in using them. Some people use these while at home over weekends, using other 'cleaner' preparations during the week.
- Dithranol can be used. It is important to start with very weak preparations as this can have a 'burning' effect.
- There is a limited place for the use of steroid cream preparations in psoriasis. Their use should always be under a doctor's supervision. Great care must be taken as the psoriasis is likely to be a prolonged problem and all steroids used over a long time on the skin, except very mild preparations, can have an adverse affect. Resistance to steroids may develop in some cases and the condition return, or even worsen, after their use.
- Ultraviolet light can be administered by a hospital clinic.
- PUVA is a special light treatment, also available in hospital skin clinics.
- Rarely, hospital admission and drug treatment by mouth may be used. Usually, intensive application of

local skin treatments during a period in hospital can achieve good results.

☎ The Psoriasis Association, 7 Milton Street, Northampton, NN2 7JG. Tel: 0604 711129

Rashes

Children particularly may often suddenly develop skin rashes. The vast majority of rashes are harmless and part of a transient infection. Other rashes may be serious and the sign of a severe infection. Some types of rash occur more frequently in people with certain skin characteristics or a tendency to have allergies.

Symptoms

* Areas of rash affected may vary, e.g. local rashes in one area – maybe just the arms and legs – or all over the body.
* Itching (common in allergies).
* Blisters may appear, which may later scab over (chicken pox or coxsackie infection).
* Fine pinpricks may be seen which may later become purple blotches (possible meningitis).
* Fine red spots or red blotches may appear (possible viral infection).
* Weals may appear (possible urticaria).

Causes

□ Viruses are one of the commonest causes of rashes. Some are well recognised, such as measles, german measles and chickenpox. Others may be very difficult to distinguish from these since they produce very similar rashes. The coxsackie virus, for instance, produces blisters which can be confused with chickenpox. The fact that different viruses cause similar rashes frequently accounts for why people think they or their children have had a specific illness twice.
□ Rashes may also be caused by allergies and drugs. (See **Allergies**, **Hives**.)
□ Bacteria may cause rashes, e.g. those of scarlet fever and meningococcal meningitis.
□ Skin problems may cause rashes, e.g. certain types of psoriasis and fungal infections.
□ There are a few other rare causes of rash, including bleeding problems and tropical diseases.

Treatment

● An unexplained rash in a well person is not usually a cause for alarm, but it is advisable to see the doctor to try and identify the type of rash.
● Occasionally the cause will be obvious and no action need be taken, the rash clearing on its own.
● The advice given for itching can be applied to most rashes if required. (See **Itching**.)

The Doctor

● Will check for the source of the rash and often be able to identify a likely cause. If a drug is found to be responsible a note of the reaction will be made on your medical file.
● Treatment will be aimed at the underlying cause, and any necessary tests can be done by taking blood tests, skin swabs or scrapings, or throat swabs to look for particular bacteria. (See **Scarlet fever**.)
● Often the cause of a rash only becomes clear as the rash develops or changes over the course of a few days.

Ring stuck on finger

There are occasions when a ring has to be removed after several years' wear and it is either difficult or impossible to do so. To avoid cutting a ring, which most casualty departments will do for you if necessary, it is worth trying the method of removal described below.

Causes
* Pregnancy may cause finger swelling, which makes removal of the ring both desirable and necessary. As finger swelling is likely to become more marked as pregnancy progresses, remove the rings sooner rather than later.
* Arthritis can lead to swollen joints. It may be impossible to remove rings if the neighbouring joints become swollen; however, at a later date, swelling may subside sufficiently to enable rings to be removed.
* Growth and weight gain can both account for a ring which fitted loosely in the past becoming firmly fixed.

Treatment
- Vigorous pulling and tugging can cause swelling and make eventual removal more difficult.
- An effective method of removal is as follows:
  - insert a string or thread through the ring from the nail end of the finger towards the hand
  - in close circles, starting at the nail end of the finger, gradually encircle the finger with the thread, working towards the ring; this will squeeze swelling out of the finger, thinning it down
  - apply soap all over the thread-encircled finger
  - it is now possible to release the ring by a combination of pulling and unwinding the thread; start with the end which has been passed below the ring and is on the hand side
- Failure of these attempts may require the ring to be removed by cutting. If this is not done the ring may seriously impair both the circulation to the finger and your ability to use the finger.

Scabies

This is an infestation caused by a tiny parasite called an itch mite, normally only occurring below the head and face. It can affect anyone but is more common where there is poor hygiene and overcrowding.

Symptoms
* Intense irritation.
* Red lumps on the skin.
* Sores and scabs caused by scratching.
* White or red lines on the skin.
* Commonly on the hands but also wrists, armpits, buttocks and genitals.
* Overall rash on trunk often occurs.

Causes
☐ The mite burrows into the skin to lay its eggs; this causes the 'lines' seen in scabies.
☐ The eggs hatch mites, which cause the itching.
☐ It is caught from personal contact or infested clothing or bedding.

Treatment
- Insecticide based on malathion is available either on prescription or over the counter. This can be in either a lotion form or a cream-based shampoo. Both types may be useful.
- Apply all over the body from below the neck.
- Leave on for twenty-four hours before washing.

- Repeat treatment after one week if necessary.
- Treat clothes and bedding. (Mites will not survive more than four or five days if removed from skin; so any items not treated should be free of infestation after this time.)

Scarlet fever

Nowadays scarlet fever is a much less serious illness than it used to be, largely because of the development of antibiotics. The particular germ causing it, the *streptococcus*, is a common cause of sore throats. Children are most commonly affected by scarlet fever, which is seen particularly between the ages of two and ten. It is infectious to others. Recovery is usually complete, although very rarely after an interval of about five weeks the kidneys or heart may be affected.

Symptoms
* These are as in tonsillitis. (See **Tonsillitis**.)
* Fever, headache and vomiting, which may start quite suddenly.
* A bright red rash starts in the armpits and groin after about twenty-four hours of fever. It looks like fine red pimples, which may join together into scarlet patches.
* The rash spreads all over the body, legs and arms. It may leave a pale patch around the mouth.
* Doctors describe the tongue as 'strawberry tongue', red and swollen.
* The rash fades after a few days.
* After about a week the skin, particularly on the hands and feet, may peel off.
* Rarely, as mentioned above, the kidneys and heart may be affected.

Treatment
- Keep your child away from others. Scarlet fever is infectious until at least one day after treatment has commenced.
- Treatment is with penicillin or erythromycin (if there is a penicillin allergy).
- Sometimes the close contacts of someone who is infected will also be given antibiotics to prevent them developing scarlet fever.
- It is important to control symptoms of fever in children to avoid convulsions. (See **Convulsions, febrile**.)

Schizophrenia

In schizophrenia normal thoughts and feelings become disorganised. The illness tends to be lifelong but, with treatment, someone with schizophrenia can be helped to lead a normal or near-normal life. Occasional alterations to treatment or admissions to hospital may be necessary. Schizophrenia tends to occur first in late adolescence or young adulthood. There is a family tendency towards having schizophrenia. Children of parents who both have schizophrenia have about a 50 per cent chance of contracting the illness.

Symptoms
* Symptoms may gradually come on over months, or may develop quite suddenly.
* Speech becomes vague and conversation increasingly difficult.
* Thoughts are disorganised and may suddenly dry up in midflow, leaving the mind empty, or they may suddenly appear out of the blue, as though the sufferer were under someone else's control.
* People with schizophrenia may feel that other people are affecting them or their body. The radio or television may be felt to be giving them instructions or making them ill.
* A fantasy world may develop in

which someone with schizophrenia can live happily but is not in touch with reality.
* Feelings and emotions may be absent or exaggerated.
* There may be strong feelings of paranoia (being over-sensitive and distrustful).
* Symptoms may return after being absent for months or years. Sometimes such a relapse is precipitated by stress.

Causes
☐ It is thought that there is an actual malfunction of the brain's cells in schizophrenia. The difficulties created by disordered thoughts may at times be so severe that the sufferer is a danger to themselves or others.

Treatment
- Anyone with symptoms of schizophrenia will need to see a doctor. It may be very difficult to persuade someone with schizophrenia or a relapse of schizophrenia to seek help. Advice to see a doctor may lead to fears of being locked away, even if the affected person realises that something is very wrong.
- A familiar relative or friend can be of enormous help in persuading someone to seek medical help and reassuring them until treatment has started to work.

The Doctor
- Admission to hospital will usually be necessary when schizophrenia symptoms first appear. Tests may be carried out to ensure that there are no other medical problems upsetting the brain or body chemistry, such as a brain tumour or severe hormone disturbance.
- In hospital special tranquillisers will be used which have an effect on the brain's functioning. These do not necessarily cause sedation, so other drugs may need to be given to help restore a normal sleep pattern. Often a combination of drugs is necessary, and several adjustments of the dose will be made before symptoms are controlled.
- In the acute and severely disturbed stage psychotherapy techniques are usually of no help, though they may become more helpful as symptoms improve. Group work and activities can later be introduced to help a return to normal living.
- In the long term, medication often needs to be continued to prevent relapses. This can be given either as tablets or injections. Injections may only need to be given at weekly or two-weekly intervals. Some of the medication does have side-effects which can fortunately be cleared, or greatly reduced, by taking a small dose of another medication.
- With the help of modern drugs it is no longer necessary for people with schizophrenia to spend very long periods in hospital. They can live in the community with the support of family, friends, social workers, psychiatric nurses and doctors. This may be either in their own homes or a hostel. Regular help and advice from the family doctor or out-patient clinic is often enough contact to ensure that medication is helping appropriately.

☎ The National Schizophrenia Fellowship, 28 Castle Street, Kingston, Surrey, KT1 1SS. Tel: 081 547 3937

☎ MIND (National Association for Mental Health), 22 Harley Street, London W1N 2ED. Tel: 071 637 0741.

☎ Schizophrenia Association of Ireland,
4 Fitzwilliam Place, Dublin 2, Eire.
Tel: Dublin 761988.

School refusal

This is a common problem which occurs most frequently in adolescence. It can be summarised as an irrational fear of attending school. It is not the same as truancy, which is a deliberate and concealed absence from school. Children who play truant from school have different reasons for staying away than those involved in school refusal. This does occur among small children, around five years old particularly, but it is most common around fourteen to fifteen years old and at school change around eleven years old. Most mild and acute episodes of school refusal resolve quickly. Even children severely affected, where there may be considerable emotional difficulties, usually grow into adults without serious mental health problems.

Symptoms

* It may first occur after a change of school or brief absence through illness.
* There are often symptoms such as headache, tummy pain, limb pains, tiredness.
* The child may simply refuse to go to school.
* Symptoms are often absent during evenings and weekends, when the child may be quite happy to go out.
* Once school refusal has started there is often a gradual increase in the frequency of absences.
* Often it is children who have previously been very good and quiet who develop school refusal.

Causes

□ The child is usually nervous or frightened of separation from parents.
□ There are often family problems and the child may feel he has to stay at home to make sure his mother is all right.
□ The child may be depressed and anxious.
□ A school problem such as bullying is less likely to be the cause than stress at home. If related to a difficulty at school, school phobia is a more appropriate description of the problem.

Treatment

● The distress of the child may be matched by your distress that he is not attending school.
● Do not encourage the child to avoid school.
● Seek help early in getting the child back to school. The longer the problem continues the more difficult it is to treat, the child's isolation from school becoming greater and increasing even more his dependence on the family.
● Most cases are dealt with by educational psychologists or school welfare officers, without health professionals being involved.
● If there are marked physical symptoms, or if the problem persists, see the doctor.

The Doctor

● Can usually quickly establish whether the symptoms – e.g. of tummy or limb pain need treatment, or are part of the child's distress.
● Will almost certainly want to involve all the family and establish the whole picture of what is happening at home. Liaison with the school is important.
● The aim will be to support and encourage the child towards an early return to school. To do this it may be necessary for a child psychiatrist to

meet the family and the child. As nearly 15 per cent of adolescents need some psychiatric help the family should not be put off by this suggestion from the doctor. A lot can be done to help.

Sexual problems

Many people experience sexual problems at some point in their lives. Those considered here are:
Absence of orgasm
Impotence
Painful intercourse
Premature ejaculation

Absence of orgasm

This may have a psychological basis but can develop following illness, or after impotence has developed. There is much that can be done to help.

Symptoms
* Many women are unable to reach orgasm while having intercourse. Additional stimulation of the clitoris may be necessary and is normal.
* Some people never reach orgasm even during masturbation.
* Men can also have difficulty reaching orgasm.

Causes
□ This is often related to inadequate sexual technique between partners.
□ Hasty intercourse or intercourse spoilt by anxiety over becoming pregnant are common causes.
□ It can be psychological in origin.

Treatment
• Talk frankly with your partner. Often taking longer to enjoy being together before actually having intercourse, or having intercourse more slowly, can help you reach an orgasm.

• Changing position, using fingers or having oral sex can all help. Some people benefit by using a vibrator.
• It is very helpful if the problem persists to seek help. Psychosexual counselling is available from a number of clinics and can be arranged through your family planning clinic. It is not necessary to see your doctor in order to obtain this help. For further details see **Impotence**.

Impotence

This refers to the failure of a man to have or maintain an erection. All men are impotent at some stage in their lives; this may be after too much alcohol or in a stressful situation. The influence of anxiety on the ability to maintain an erection is complex and poorly understood. If impotence is a recurrent or persistent problem much can be done to help, although treatment may have to be carried on over a long period.

Symptoms
* It may not be possible to have an erection at all.
* An erection of the penis may be poorly sustained and disappear after a few minutes.
* It may be possible to have an erection while alone, but not possible when with your partner.
* Waking from sleep, it is normal to have an erection. This may not be sustained if you attempt then to have intercourse, despite your desire to do so.

Causes
□ There are both physical and psychological causes.
□ Temporary impotence is more likely to be due to a psychological difficulty. This may be related to a new partner

191

or a difficult life situation.
- Impotence may be due to chronic illness, tiredness, stress or excessive alcohol.
- Surgery, for example to the prostate gland, may cause impotence. This is less common with the more modern trans-urethral prostatectomy operations. (See **Prostate problems**.)
- Drugs may cause impotence, e.g., methyl-dopa, a drug used for high blood pressure. A drug which causes impotence in one person may not have any noticeable effect on another.

Prevention
- Do not drink excessive alcohol.
- Have intercourse in the most relaxed and pleasurable surroundings. Use comfortable positions and a lubricant if necessary. Allow your partner to participate as much as possible in your arousal.
- Talk about any difficulties or embarrassments you may have. If impotence develops, often being frank with each other and sharing the problem can be helpful. As most men are impotent from time to time this is not a reason for giving up and never trying again.
- If impotence develops and you are not able to have satisfactory intercourse, seek treatment.

Treatment
- Treatment can only start when a physical cause for the impotence has been excluded. Some physical causes, such as disease of the spinal cord affecting the nerves to the genitals, may not be treatable.

The Doctor
- May be able to establish quickly whether there is a physical or psychological difficulty.
- Tests may be carried out to look for physical causes, e.g. a simple blood test can indicate if your alcohol level over a long period of time has been persistently raised above what the body can normally cope with.
- Sometimes it is necessary to be admitted to hospital for 'tumescence studies', which monitor what happens to the penis while asleep.
- If no physical causes are found, often discussing the situation with the doctor, either alone or with your partner, can help. It may become clear that your partner is not aware of what stimulation you need.
- Your doctor may suggest the use of hormones or a drug to decrease anxiety, but these are often not successful. Why they should help some people is not clear, though it may be that the knowledge of taking a treatment gives you enough confidence to be able to have satisfactory intercourse.
- Counselling from a trained professional is of the most benefit. There are now many different centres offering sex therapy or psycho-sexual counselling. Many of these are available on the NHS. Usually, both you and your partner will be asked to attend the sessions, which may continue weekly over a period of several months. Often there are other benefits from attending such sessions, and different areas of your relationship improve.
- Surgery to the penis and use of a prosthesis (artificial device to assist in maintainance of an erection) is rarely used as a method of treatment. This may help the physical problem of impotence, but any psychological difficulties may remain or be increased by the need to rely on such measures.

- ☎ Family Planning Association, National Office, 27 Mortimer Street, London W1. Tel: 071 636 7866. (Family planning clinics are listed in the phone book. Your local clinic can put you in touch with a centre offering psycho-sexual counselling.)
- ☎ The Association of Sexual and Marital Therapists, PO Box 62, Sheffield S10.

Painful intercourse

This affects both men and women. There are both physical and psychological causes. It is important that the pain is not attributed to psychological causes before a full exploration of the possible physical causes has been carried out.

Symptoms
Men
* Pain on having an erection.
* Pain on intercourse.
* Pain in certain positions.

Women
* Pain felt at the entrance to the vagina.
* Pain on penetration and during the movements of intercourse.
* Pain on deep penetration.
* Pain made worse by certain positions or felt more severely at different times during the menstrual cycle.

Causes
Men
- A tight foreskin. (See **Foreskin problems**.)
- Inflammation of the penis in balanitis. (See **Foreskin problems**.)
- Local infections such as thrush or genital herpes. (See **Genital herpes**, **Thrush**.)
- Small tears on the skin at the end of the penis, following vigorous intercourse or made worse by you or your partner not having sufficient secretions to provide lubrication.
- Coil strings can make intercourse uncomfortable.
- An allergic reaction can develop to spermicidal creams or jellies. Rarely, condoms irritate the skin.
- An infection in the prostate or urethra (see NSU, **Prostate problems**) can cause pain. A urethral stricture may cause pain (this is when there is a narrowing in the tube of the penis which carries urine and sperm. It is usually caused by previous infection.)
- In homosexuals pain can be due to piles, anal fissure or inadequate lubrication. (See **Piles**.)

Women
Pain at entrance to the vagina
- Vaginismus is when the muscles at the entrance to the vagina go into spasm and intercourse becomes difficult or impossible. It is often very distressing. Treatment can help.
- A tight hymen may cause discomfort, but can be easily dealt with.
- Following childbirth there may be temporary discomfort in any area of scarring due to a tear or episiotomy. (See **Episiotomy**.)
- Infections around the vaginal entrance or on the skin can cause discomfort, e.g. infected cysts or glands, herpes infections. (See **Genital herpes**.) A Bartholin's cyst forms when glands at the entrance to the vagina, which normally help lubricate the area during intercourse, become swollen and infected. Antibiotics are normally required to settle the infection, or surgery to drain the abcess may be required.
- Piles or other varicosities, found particularly in pregnancy, can cause discomfort.

Pain in the vagina or on deep penetration
- ☐ Commonly caused by infection. (See **Genital herpes**, **Pelvic infection**, **Thrush**.)
- ☐ Allergic reactions to spermicides or douches.
- ☐ Endometriosis. (See **Periods, painful**.)
- ☐ Ovarian problems.
- ☐ Constipation.
- ☐ Dry vagina. (See **Vaginal problems**.)
- ☐ Anxiety may also cause intercourse to be painful or uncomfortable, usually due to muscle tension. There may be fear of the penis causing damage or of pregnancy.

Treatment
- Simple measures can often help, e.g. use of a different method of contraception or different spermicide.
- Use of a lubricant such as KY jelly, available from chemists, can often ease discomfort.
- If you cannot discover why there is pain on intercourse, or if you think you may have an infection, see your doctor.

The Doctor
- Will often be able to discover the cause by examining you. Antibiotics may be prescribed for infection.
- Referral to a gynaecologist may be necessary for further tests, including a laparoscopy (see **Periods, painful** for further details of tests that may be carried out).
- If the pain is due to vaginismus or a tight hymen a doctor can help you by teaching you to use a series of what are called vaginal dilators. The doctor shows you how to use these and you practise at home. Your partner may be able to help you. This treatment is often very successful.
- Psycho-sexual counselling or sex therapy is available from your local family planning clinic. These clinics are listed in the phone book, and you do not necessarily have to see your family doctor to seek help. You and your partner may attend weekly sessions over several months, if necessary. Often there are other benefits for your relationship and a much greater understanding of each other is achieved. This counselling is available as part of the NHS.

Premature ejaculation

This is the commonest male sexual problem. It is normal at the beginning of a relationship. As the relationship develops, better control of when orgasm occurs is usually possible. You and your partner can greatly influence the timing of ejaculation.

Symptoms
* Ejaculation may occur before the penis has entered the vagina.
* Ejaculation may occur very shortly after intercourse has begun; this can lead to impotence in men and your partner may lose interest in sex.
* It occurs frequently, and can be considered normal, at the start of a relationship.

Causes
- ☐ Usually there is a psychological basis to premature ejaculation; rarely, diseases of the nervous system or an inflammation of the prostate or urethritis can cause the problem.
- ☐ If sexual experiences are rushed or anxious it is more likely to occur.
- ☐ Control over ejaculation can be learnt with the aid of counselling.

Treatment
- No treatment is necessary if this occurs at the start of a relationship.

The problem usually goes on its own as your sexual relationship and knowledge of each other increases.
- Avoiding intercourse for a time and only having other body contact can help. Either you or your partner can squeeze just below the glans, on the shaft of the penis, when you are on the verge of having an orgasm. This can be repeated regularly over a period of weeks if necessary, and control usually increases dramatically.
- Sex therapy or psycho-sexual counselling can provide excellent results. Further details are listed under **Impotence**.

Shingles

This appears as an ugly crop of blisters on the skin, often in a 'stripe' around the chest. This is because blisters appear along the line of the nerve infected by the virus. It is most common in the elderly but can be seen in younger people or those with serious illness such as cancer. It is possible to catch chicken pox from shingles; a child visiting a grandparent with shingles may develop chicken pox eleven to twenty-one days later. Shingles can be a very distressing illness, making you unwell over several months.

Symptoms
Before the blisters appear
* Feeling generally unwell and run-down.
* Pain along the line of the infected nerve.

When the blisters appear
* Pain.
* Fever.
* Blisters are confined to one side of the body along the line of the nerve.

When blisters clear
* Unpleasant pain may persist for weeks, months or even, rarely, years.

* Depression. It is not uncommon to feel very pulled down after shingles, particularly in the elderly. Treatment may be necessary.

Causes
□ Shingles is causes by a virus called *herpes zoster* or *varicella zoster*, the same virus that causes chicken pox.
□ Rarely, shingles can develop after contact with chicken pox.
□ It is thought that in most cases of shingles the chicken pox virus has been lying dormant in the nerve for years.
□ Being very run down or exhausted may bring on an attack.
□ Illness elsewhere in the body can lead to an attack of shingles.

Treatment
- It is usually necessary and best to see the doctor early.

Anti-viral drugs
- Treatment has been greatly helped by the introduction of an anti-viral drug called acyclovir (Zovirax). This is available as cream, paint or tablets on prescription only.
- Your doctor may advise acyclovir tablet treatment to shorten the severity and length of attack.
- Paint or cream acyclovir applied locally may stop blisters developing and reduce the severity of attack.
- It is important that anti-viral drugs are used correctly.

Painkillers
- These are often necessary.
- Start with a mild one, taken regularly, such as paracetamol or paracetamol and codeine combined.
- Stronger ones such as dihydrocodeine may be prescribed if pain is not being relieved.
- Take them regularly, by the clock, as by doing so you often need less. If you try and 'be brave' you may need

a higher dose to stop the pain.

Anti-depressant medicines

- Doctors do sometimes prescribe this in the elderly. As they take some time to work, they may be started early. They can help depression, and any drowsiness felt at first can help with pain relief.

Skin treatments

- Calamine lotion, although messy, can give some relief and help stop itching.
- Wear loose clothing.
- Lightly applied dressings, such as melolin squares (available to buy or on prescription), absorb fluid from the blisters and keep the sore area clean. They also protect the blisters from clothing and from being rubbed.

Shock

To many people 'shock' means the feeling of intense upset when a sudden event has a dramatic effect on them, such as after a road accident, when you are not injured but may be overwhelmed by the experience. This emotional reaction may lead to overwhelming sadness or severe stress symptoms, including loss of memory.

'Shock' considered here, however, means something quite different. If you are next to someone who collapses, you may witness the medical effects of shock. The body ceases to function, and if left untreated death usually occurs.

Symptoms

* Loss of body colour, especially pale face, hands and feet.
* Sweating.
* Rapid pulse.
* Faintness.
* Rapid breathing.
* Cold wet skin.
* Low blood pressure.
* Confusion and drowsiness.
* Loss of consciousness and death.

Causes

☐ Anything which prevents adequate supply of oxygen to the body's vital organs causes medical shock. For example:
 – if the heart stops pumping (see **Heart attack**)
 – if there is a severe injury or burn, leading to a loss of blood or body fluid (see **Burns**)
 – if there is a severe allergic reaction (this is called anaphylactic shock; see **Allergies**)
 – if there is serious infection
 – the lack of oxygen in shock only makes the condition worse, as the brain is unable to respond and correct the situation; medical treatment must be given urgently

Treatment

- Summon medical help immediately.
- Arrange transfer to hospital.
- While awaiting help:
 – lie the shocked person down with head low and feet up
 – if unconscious, lie on the side with upper leg and arm bent and in front of the body
 – cover with a blanket and give no food or drink; do not give alcohol
- Hospital treatment will be aimed at watching the blood pressure and heart record carefully.
- The blood pressure will be restored to ensure that oxygen returns to the vital organs before they are damaged. This is done by adding fluid to the body directly into a blood vessel. A small tube is inserted into a vein and more blood or a special fluid is given. This restores the necessary volume of blood, and with it the blood pressure.
- The cause of the shock will be treated: e.g. blood loss stopped, heart stimulated to work again, allergic

reaction counteracted, infection treated.
- During this time a record will be kept of how the kidneys are functioning by watching the outflow of urine. It may be necessary to use drugs called diuretics to help the kidneys until blood pressure and oxygen supply can be restored.

Shoulder pain

Pain in the shoulder is often put down as being 'a touch of arthritis'. This is usually incorrect. The shoulder is a complex joint and numerous different problems may cause pain. The commonest of these are called tendonitis and frozen shoulder, which are both considered in detail separately. For all shoulder problems, the sooner treatment is started the sooner the problem is likely to clear.

Symptoms
* Shoulder pain may occur on its own, or other joints may be painful at the same time.
* Pain may be continuous and limit movement severely. (See **Shoulder pain – frozen shoulder**.)
* Pain may be present only on certain movements and absent at rest. (See **Shoulder pain – tendonitis**).
* Injury to the shoulder joint may cause pain through muscle strain or damage to muscles or ligaments around the joint. (See also **Dislocation**.)
* There may be pain in nearby joints which is felt as pain in the shoulder joint.
* Moving the neck may cause shoulder pain.

Causes
☐ Tendonitis (see separate entry).
☐ Frozen shoulder (see separate entry).
☐ Rupture of a tendon surrounding and supporting the joint can cause pain.
☐ Over-use of the shoulder joint can lead to shoulder pain.
☐ There is a part of the shoulder blade near the shoulder joint, which is called the acromion. It is linked in a joint to the collarbone or clavicle, and this acromio-clavicular joint may give rise to pain felt in the shoulder.
☐ Below this joint there is a soft cushioning pad called a bursa. Bursas are found throughout the body near joints. They help to minimise friction between moving parts. If there is injury to the bursa it becomes red, inflamed and fills with fluid, causing a bursitis.
☐ If the neck bones are arthritic they may nip a nerve as it leaves the spine. Although the nerve is pinched in the neck it is not unusual to feel pain in the shoulder. There may be associated numbness or tingling in the arm. (See also **Neck problems, cervical spondylosis**.)
☐ If other joints are involved a diagnosis of arthritis is more likely. (See **Neck, stiff and painful**.)

Treatment
- When shoulder pain occurs, rest the joint without allowing it to become totally immobile.
- Simple painkillers such as aspirin or paracetamol taken regularly may provide good relief.
- The pain of many conditions settles quickly over a few days. Avoid repeating any activities that brought on the pain.

The Doctor
- If the pain persists or becomes more severe you should see the doctor.
- He may well diagnose tendonitis or frozen shoulder and arrange appropriate treatment (see separate entries).

- If other joints are involved, suggesting an arthritis, he may arrange blood tests and X-rays of the joint. (See **Arthritis**.)
- Other conditions may settle down on the use of a special NSAI drug (See **Gout** for further details of this kind of drug.)
- Referral to a joint doctor (rheumatologist) may be required.
- Some conditions settle with an injection of a steroid into the affected area. This does not have the side-effects of steroids taken by mouth. (See **tendonitis** below.)
- Physiotherapy may also help to relieve shoulder pain. (See **frozen shoulder**, **tendonitis** below.)

Shoulder pain – frozen shoulder

This is a painful condition of the shoulder joint which is not cold, but stiff. Frozen shoulder occurs most commonly in people between forty and sixty years old. Pain is often severe but treatment can be very effective.

Symptoms
* Usually comes on gradually, with the shoulder becoming increasingly stiff.
* There is limitation of nearly all joint movements.
* Pain may be continuous and is sometimes worse at night.
* Pain gradually settles, but may persist for several months.
* Movement gradually improves, but may be limited for up to a year or longer.
* The hand can be affected, becoming swollen and painful; this is largely due to lack of movement.

Causes
☐ Frozen shoulder may follow an injury which has restricted movements of the joint.
☐ More often, it comes on with no obvious cause.
☐ The capsule surrounding the shoulder joint is similar to the capsule surrounding other joints in the body (see **Gout**). In frozen shoulder this becomes inflamed and severely limits movement. The surfaces of the capsule, instead of being smooth and lubricated, are angry, tender and swollen.

Treatment
- Unlike when tendonitis causes shoulder pain, the treatment for frozen shoulder is not rest, but movement.
- Unless the pain is very severe it is important to keep the joint moving to prevent it stiffening up further. Swinging the arm and exercising as much as possible is helpful.
- Using painkillers regularly can help with pain relief, start with simple ones such as aspirin or paracetamol.
- Pain can also be relieved by using ice packs or hot-water bottles. These should be left on the joint for about fifteen minutes three times a day. (Frozen peas make a good icepack; they can be refrozen and used again but not eaten.)

The Doctor
- If frozen shoulder continues to be troublesome the doctor may prescribe stronger painkillers and/or anti-inflammatory drugs. (See **Shoulder pain – tendonitis**).
- A steroid injection may also be of great benefit. This may need to be repeated.
- Physiotherapy is very useful. You may be shown simple exercises to

keep the joint mobile while at home, as well as having a variety of treatments.

Shoulder pain – tendonitis

This is the commonest problem affecting the shoulder joint.

Symptoms
* The joint is not stiff.
* Keeping the arm at rest allows the pain to settle.
* Symptoms generally only last a few weeks.
* If the joint is not rested adequately the pain may persist for months.
* As you move the shoulder through certain movements there may be only a limited range of movement that is painful. Typically, raising your arm away from your side is painful, but the pain goes as you continue to raise the arm.

Causes
- Over-use of the joint, perhaps due to repeated activity which the shoulder is not accustomed to, may bring on tendonitis.
- The symptoms are caused by an inflammation of a tendon around the joint. The tendon becomes swollen and is painful if moved.
- Surrounding the shoulder are numerous tendons. The symptoms will vary depending on which tendon is involved.

Treatment
- Stop the movement causing the pain. If you continue moving the affected tendon it will aggravate the tendonitis.
- Use of simple painkillers such as aspirin or paracetamol, taken regularly, can often provide relief.
- The tendonitis may settle without further treatment.

The doctor
- If the pain persists your doctor may recommend a steroid injection to the affected area. This does not have the side-effects of steroids taken in tablet form.
- Following the injection there will often be more severe pain for the first twenty-four to thirty-six hours, but this should clear, leaving the joint more mobile. If pain does not settle you should inform your doctor. The injection may have to be repeated.
- Avoid movements which aggravate the pain for six weeks or so after the injection, but do not immobilise the arm to such an extent that it stiffens up.
- Steroid injections can be repeated if tendonitis does not clear completely, or if it recurs.
- Ultrasound treatment is used by physiotherapists and may be helpful in tendonitis.
- Anti-inflammatory (NSAI) drugs may be used. These generally take much longer to help and may cause unpleasant side-effects such as indigestion. (See **Gout** for further details of this kind of drug.)
- Very rarely, surgery is required to try and relieve problems of tendonitis or repair a ruptured tendon.

Sinusitis

This is a common, painful condition which affects the air spaces behind the cheeks and the lower forehead. These air spaces are called sinuses; they have the same kind of lining as the nose and air reaches them from the nose. An infection in the nose can easily spread to the sinuses, causing inflammation and discomfort. Sinusitis is not usually serious and tends to follow a cold. It may happen just once, which is acute sinusitis, or may linger on and become chronic sinusitis.

Symptoms
* Often follows a cold.
* Greeny-yellow nasal discharge.
* Nasal speech and general congestion.
* Generally feeling ill.
* Pain over cheeks and above and between the eyes.
* Tenderness over central forehead and cheeks.
* Headache.
* Pain worse on leaning forward.
* See also **Foreign body in the nose**.

Causes
- The inflammation in the sinuses is caused by infection.
- This usually follows a cold, when the congested symptoms are due to blockage of the passages between the sinuses and the nose. This blockage prevents the sinuses clearing properly and helps trapped bacteria to produce an infection.
- It occasionally follows dental treatment when germs enter the sinus from a dental abcess around the root of a tooth.

Treatment
- Mild sinusitis symptoms often clear of their own accord.
- Steam inhalations, taken with care to avoid burns and scalds, can decongest and alleviate symptoms. This is made more pleasant by the addition of menthol, either as crystals or in a solution such as 'Menthol and Eucalyptus for Inhalation', available from chemists. It is, however, the steam and warm moist air that helps most.
- Keeping air in the room humid can also help; this can be done by drying washing on radiators.
- Decongestant medicines, some available without prescription, may help. Many cause drowsiness (avoid driving and operating machinery if taking antihistamines, for example).
- Simple painkillers such as aspirin or paracetamol can relieve discomfort.

The Doctor
- Will prescribe antibiotics, which can be very effective. The use of antibiotics has made what used to be a potentially serious illness much less worrying.
- If sinusitis is persistent or chronic a longer course of antibiotics may be required.
- X-rays of the sinuses may reveal fluid trapped in the cavities, promoting infection.
- Referral to an ear, nose and throat specialist may lead to a simple operation. This involves washing out the sinuses, via the nose, and ensuring that good drainage passages exist between the sinuses and the nose.

Sleep problems

This section covers the following subjects:

Insomia and sleep problems in adults
Night terrors in children
Nightmares
Sleepwalking in children
Wakefulness in children

Insomnia and sleep problems in adults

Although the average sleep required by an adult is around seven to eight hours, individual variations on this may be considerable. If you feel awake and refreshed after five hours that is fine. Often what you consider to be a very restless night does provide you with adequate sleep. Several days in succession of poor sleep will do you little harm. Staying up the whole night may even help to break an episode of insomnia. Occasionally, sleep problems are part of an underlying difficulty such as anxiety or depression. (See **Anxiety**, **Depression**.)

Symptoms
* Difficulty in getting to sleep.
* Waking in the night.
* Early-morning waking.
* Restless sleep.
* Uneven sleep pattern.
* Nightmares. (See **Nightmares**.)

Causes
- Sleep requirements decrease with age. It is not unusual for someone over sixty, living quietly, to require much less sleep than the busy family with whom they may be living.
- Pregnancy often leads to sleep problems, particularly towards the end as discomfort increases.
- Tea and coffee commonly keep people awake, or cause them to wake later in the night. If you have already tried not having these in the evening, try stopping them completely.
* Overeating can lead to sleep difficulties. Eat large meals at least three hours before bedtime.
- Lack of exercise can lead to or exacerbate sleep problems.
- Illness can cause sleep problems, e.g. breathlessness in asthma, or heart failure.
- Stopping tranquillisers or sleeping pills often leads to a prolonged period of sleep problems. It is best to discontinue these slowly, gradually cutting down the number and strength of tablets under your doctor's supervision.
- (See also **Anxiety**, **Depression**.)

Treatment
- Avoid the above causes as far as possible.
- Drinking a hot milky drink or having a whisky at night can be helpful.
- Read a book at bedtime on a subject totally unrelated to your work; this helps you to relax.
- Exercise during the day or going for a walk shortly before bedtime can be helpful.
- A warm bath or long hot shower can help.
- Sexual intercourse may have a relaxing, if not actually sedative effect.
- Room temperature, ventilation and comfort are important. A hot-water bottle may help.
- Try practising a relaxation technique such as breathing exercises, muscle relaxation or meditation. There are now many books available on these techniques.
- If necessary, stay up rather than fighting to get to sleep. Often a short read or snack may help you to go back to bed and sleep. Listening to the radio can be very helpful and allow you to drop off to sleep.

The Doctor
- It is only normally necessary to consult your doctor when disturbed sleep is upsetting your daily life.
- The doctor will make enquiries about your routine, and may arrange simple tests to check for any underlying problems or illnesses.
- If there is a recent event that has upset you, it may be possible to use a sleeping medication for a very short period to help you continue with normal living. Used sensibly, sleeping medication can be of great help at very difficult moments.
- Ask your doctor for a medicine which

will leave you fresh for work the next day. Only accept a small supply and try and see your doctor for any more. This is preferable to obtaining a repeat prescription without seeing your doctor.
- Never use sleeping medication over a prolonged period, because not only does it usually cease to have any benefit after two or three weeks, but discontinuing it may be very difficult.

Night terrors in children

These occur in a different part of the normal sleep pattern from nightmares and have different features. The response of a parent to a child with night terrors should also differ from that made to a nightmare (see **Nightmares**). The child does not fully awaken during a night terror, and they may be very frightening for a parent to witness.

Symptoms
* The child suddenly cries out, usually very loudly, in his sleep – often about two hours after going to sleep.
* The child sits bolt upright, staring in a glazed way in one direction.
* There is no response to your presence. Indeed, you may become incorporated into the terror and be pushed away. The child is still asleep.
* The child does not remember the events of a night terror.
* The child may appear hallucinated and even try to get out of bed.
* The terror settles over a few minutes, the child never fully awakening.

Causes
□ It seems to be a single moment or feeling from an event that has influenced a child that triggers a night terror.

□ This may include:
  - frightening moments seen on television or experienced while playing with friends
  - bad moments when the child has had an injection or hospital procedure against their will
  - an unpleasant event recalled by the child happening to a close family member

Treatment
- The child does not waken during a night terror and should not be woken up.
- The terror usually passes on its own, the child settling back on the bed.
- If the child tries to get out of bed, supervise and gently guide back to the bed. (See **Sleepwalking**.)
- It is not generally helpful to talk about what happened next morning. This can be very frightening to the child, who has no recollection of events.
- Night terrors generally cease well before adolescence, very rarely persisting into adult life.

The Doctor
- It is generally not necessary to consult the doctor. If the problem is severe a mild sedative may be prescribed.

Nightmares

Everyone dreams at night while asleep, but we do not normally recall our dreams unless awakened during or immediately following them. As well as good dreams everyone also suffers bad ones, some sufficiently unpleasant to be described as nightmares. If a nightmare occurs it usually has nothing to do with your being any more mentally unwell than anyone else. Nightmares occur both commonly and naturally.

Symptoms
* Unpleasant or frightening dreaming.
* Waking in the same state as occurred during the dream, e.g. in tears, struggling or shouting.
* The heart may be pounding when you waken; you may be shaking or sweating.

Causes
- Nightmares occur as part of normal dreaming.
- Certain factors may make them more likely to occur:
  - anxiety
  - previous unpleasant experience such as a car crash
  - fever accompanying an illness
  - stopping sleeping medication; often on coming home from hospital sleeping tablets are discontinued and nightmares may occur as part of a general sleep disturbance
  - alcohol, or decreasing amounts of alcohol if your intake has been heavy
  - television or films containing unpleasant or frightening images
  - medicines, including those given for sleep; in particular, medicines given to children, often as part of a cold remedy, may cause them to have sleep disturbance and hallucinations; this may include seeing spiders, e.g. Actifed

Treatment
- Adults usually adopt their own mechanism for dealing with nightmares. This may include getting up and having something to eat or reading for a short time. Listening to the radio may also help and allow you to drop off to sleep.
- In children a number of things can help to diminish the impact of a nightmare:
  - go quickly to the child
  - reassure as much as possible
  - if not fully awake, allow the child to go back to sleep
  - if awake, put the light on to reassure the child that it was only a dream
  - avoid asking about the nightmare
  - distract by talking about something else, or reading a book if necessary
  - talk the next day about the nightmare to try and reveal any underlying fears or anxieties
  - tell the child that everyone has bad dreams and nightmares from time to time and that it is quite normal

Sleepwalking in children

This usually occurs in the same part of a normal sleep pattern as night terrors; the child never fully awakens. There is a myth that a child should not be woken during sleepwalking. This in fact does no harm, but it is not usually necessary. Normally, sleepwalking ceases well before adolescence and is only rarely part of an emotional disturbance. The tendency to sleepwalk does run in families, though sleepwalking is unusual in adults.

Symptoms
* The child may sleepwalk once and never again. Alternatively, it may occur repeatedly.
* Usually occurs in the first few hours of sleep.
* Wandering occurs with the eyes open. It is purposeless, and may be accompanied by muttering.

Causes
- Why a child should sleepwalk is not absolutely clear. Like a night terror, when a single event or moment

provokes terror, a single need or desire seems to provoke sleepwalking without the child ever fully awakening.

Treatment
- If your child repeatedly sleepwalks secure doors and windows, so they cannot be opened by the child as, rarely, accidents do occur. A child can negotiate stairs while sleepwalking.
- Do not awaken the child. This is not actually harmful but is not necessary and may lead to the child being puzzled and frightened to find themselves downstairs or in another room. It may in fact be very difficult to waken a sleepwalking child.
- Guide the child gently back to bed. Usually this is not difficult.

The Doctor
- It is rarely necessary to consult the doctor. If the problem becomes troublesome the doctor may prescribe a mild sedative.
- Stressful events that may be affecting the child should be explored in discussion, but often there are no unusual stresses or anxieties.

Wakefulness in children

Children have very variable sleep needs. From babies to adolescents, the average hours spent asleep quoted in books are only an example of what may happen. There are some children who appear to need much less sleep than others and usually it is pointless trying in vain to make a wakeful child sleep. Sleep problems with children do generally improve over a period of months. The problems may be simple, involving a demand for attention, or complex, involving a number of difficulties occurring from bedtime to early morning.

Symptoms
* The child may be very hard to settle at night, making continuing demands for yet another book, drink or ritual to be performed.
* The child may waken early and be wide awake and playful hours before either parent would consider rising.
* Continual demands may be made throughout the night for drinks, a cuddle or to go to the parents' bed.
* Symptoms are often more complex and difficult to manage if they form part of a larger behaviour pattern. This may be revealed by difficulties at school or during daytime activities.
* (See also **Night terrors**, **Nightmares**, **Sleepwalking**.)

Causes
□ Most commonly, there are no obvious precipitating factors causing a sleep problem. It may arise suddenly after a previous more convenient pattern has been established. It may cease as suddenly as it began.
□ Stresses and family problems may aggravate or lead to sleep problems in some children. In this case there may be other behaviour problems with the child.

Prevention
- Never use bed as a punishment, and never threaten to send a child to bed if he is being naughty.
- When a child is in bed avoid disturbance from brothers or sisters as much as possible.
- If the child needs a particular toy or teddy in bed with him, let him have it. Including a favourite toy in the ritual of going to bed is often helpful.
- Bed should be a pleasant and personal space for the child. It should be

associated with happy moments and objects the child likes best. The child should feel secure and relaxed in bed.
- When making the move from cot to a real bed, make a special moment of it. Try and make the new situation a promotion and a pleasure for the child.
- There are no rigid rules about a child needing to have a daytime nap. If it suits you to keep him up during the day, so he sleeps better at night, this is perfectly all right. A child will take all the sleep he needs if given a comfortable bed.
- Equally, if you need a rest, there is nothing wrong with the child being allowed to read or play in bed for a short time either before bedtime or during the day. Being in bed does not have to mean the child ought to sleep. If the child is happy it is fine to leave him playing.

Treatment
- The importance of being consistent and setting limits cannot be over-emphasised in the management of childhood sleep problems.
- If a child is making excessive demands for drinks these should be resisted. Sweet drinks should be replaced by water. It is important that all those involved with putting the child to bed adopt the same policy.
- Resist pleas from the child to come into your bed. It is very difficult to break this habit once it is established.
- When a 'going-to-bed' ritual becomes either too lengthy or elaborate it does no harm to set limits. A child quickly learns if you are consistent and do not give in to the increasing demands.
- Babies may cry at night, particularly when night feeds are discontinued, but it does no harm to leave them crying for a few minutes. If you always rush in at the first cry they are quick to learn they are on to a good thing.
- Older children having sleep difficulties may respond well to keeping a chart of the good nights, e.g. Marking them with a gold star. This may also help you to see when errors or inconsistencies in your plan to combat the problem occur.
- If the child has a potty nearby, and can see to use it, many children will be happy to do so without disturbing you. As they get older they may be able to use their own light to go to the toilet or get a drink.
- Leaving toys or activities around the child's bed in a special 'morning box' can often lead to a child playing contentedly alone before coming to the parents' room.
- As they learn to tell the time it does no harm to set a time before which children do not disturb you. At this age they can often amuse themselves happily. In fact, they often choose to sleep longer instead.
- Persistent sleep difficulties may force you to consult your doctor.

The Doctor
- Initially, the doctor may only offer advice on simple management.
- Family life will be discussed to see if there are other problems, or if a particular pattern of behaviour, on either your or the child's part, is exacerbating the problem. (It is not unknown for some children to be given coffee to drink before bedtime, which not surprisingly keeps them awake.)
- Sedative medicines may be prescribed, and should never be given without your doctor's advice. If these are used it is best to use them for a fixed period of five days, then cease them. Use over a prolonged period is at the risk of the child becoming dependent

on them. They are unlikely to be of lasting benefit.
- Where there may be severe sleep problems, or if the situation is causing considerable disruption to family life, seeking the help of a child psychiatrist can often yield considerable benefits. Your doctor can arrange this for you.

Soft spot

This small area at the front and top of your baby's head is a space between the bones. The skull bones are not fixed together at birth. This leaves spaces called fontanelles between them. The largest of these is the recognised soft spot. It shrinks in early life as the bones stick together. This is not an ailment but is a frequent cause of concern to parents.

Symptoms
* Often felt as a dip or hollow on the scalp.
* Often very obvious on a hairless baby.
* Sometimes pulsates with the baby's normal heartbeat.
* May be felt or seen as a raised lump on the scalp, particularly at times of screaming or when the head is tilted downwards.
* If sunken, can be an indication of dehydration and a lack of fluids.
* In rare situations when the baby is unwell, usually with fever, it may be continuously protruding and tense. This can be a sign of meningitis.

The Doctor
- Will often touch the fontanelle when checking an unwell baby, particularly if fever and/or vomiting and diarrhoea are present, leading to loss of fluids.
- Will observe it shrinking and finally going over the first eighteen months of life. It may persist longer, but is not a problem as the baby grows. If it is still present after eighteen months ask your doctor to check it for you.

Note
It is *not* a 'no go area' (see **Cradle cap**). Do not be afraid to touch, stroke or rub the area gently, or brush the hair. It is stronger than it looks and never a reason to avoid touching and enjoying the baby.

Speech difficulty

This is when there is a difficulty in pronouncing words clearly. It is present in a mild form in most children before school age. At this age it is not usually a true speech difficulty but a normal part of speech development. A problem may, however, develop and can persist into adult life. Many people have adopted elaborate ways of disguising their speech difficulty. It may not be noticeable in conversation but can be a source of great anxiety and hinder confidence. What may appear as a stutter or a stammer may in fact be dysfluency, which is a normal part of speech development. This occurs when a child is trying to express something (see below).

Symptoms
* The first part of a word or the first letter of a word may be repeated again and again.
* The speech seems to be held up or stuck on particular syllables or sounds.
* It may appear as if someone has 'lost their words'.
* It may lead to difficulty in either understanding or following a conversation.
* Sounds may be altered by poor voice production.

Causes

In children

- There may be inadequate vocabulary in a child's mind to allow him to express what he wishes to say. The resultant hesitation as he tries to express it impedes fluent speech.
- The brain may be working at a different speed from the mechanical ability to produce the appropriate sounds.
- This can be a normal part of language development.
- It can develop into a stammer as a way of attracting attention and making people listen.
- It can be caused by excitement and the rush to say something or be heard before a brother or sister.

In adults

- Persistence of a speech difficulty into adult life is usually because a way of speaking as a child has been carried through into adult life.

Treatment

- It is important before attempting to treat any speech difficulty to establish that hearing is normal.
- It is generally greatly underestimated how much can be done to help speech difficulties. Both in adults and children, speech therapists can help enormously.

In children

- You can help enormously by slowing down your own speech while reading. This allows the child to take in each word separately and better understand its meaning, pronunciation and context.
- Make time to listen to what your child is saying. Do not turn away when a sentence is half finished; hear the child out.
- Do not allow older brothers and sisters to repeatedly cut across a younger one's speech. This leads to a struggle to be heard which is not helpful for good speech development.
- Never 'give' children the word they are looking for; wait, and let them find it themselves.
- Try setting aside a few minutes to be alone with your child, allow him or her to choose an activity, pay attention to the activity but don't ever correct speech or pay particular attention to it. Thank the child for helping you play the game so he or she feels appreciated. Do this regularly.
- Avoid allowing a speech difficulty to become a focus of attention. Do not talk about it to young children, and avoid anything that either makes them conscious of it or allows them to feel you think they have a problem.

In adults

- Many adults do not realise the great help they can receive from speech therapists. It is never too late to take their opinion, and they may be able to remove a significant speech difficulty which is hindering everyday life or even job prospects.

The Doctor

- Can advise on whether you or your child should see a speech therapist, or if you should wait for normal speech development to take place as the child grows.
- If you are in any doubt as to whether your child has a speech problem it is much better to seek help early. This is because, like any habits we adopt, the sooner action is taken the easier it is to correct it.

Splinter

This refers to a small sliver of wood or other material penetrating the skin. It is rarely serious and can usually be removed by the simple procedure outlined below. If a splinter is a glass fragment or is near the eye it should always be dealt with by a doctor. If left alone and not removed splinters can cause infections.

Treatment

- First try to remove by pulling on the end of the splinter. You should pull in the line of the splinter, to avoid breaking it.
- If the end cannot be grasped:
  - sterilise a needle in a flame
  - break the skin over the end of the splinter
  - lift the end of the splinter nearest the surface upwards until it can be removed with tweezers
- If none of this succeeds, it is better to seek medical help than continue probing. Unsuccessful digging around can damage other tissues and make the eventual removal more difficult.
- If pain persists or swelling develops in an area where a splinter has been a problem, this may indicate either infection or the presence of another splinter which has not been noticed or removed earlier.

Sprains

Sprains are one of the commonest injuries. Their severity depends on the extent to which the structures around the joint are damaged. There is very little danger in a sprain unless the same joint is repeatedly strained, which may cause weakness. The ankle, for instance, may give way unexpectedly if it has been repeatedly strained. Common joints to strain are ankles, wrists, knees and fingers.

Symptoms

* Pain.
* Tenderness.
* Swelling.
* Discolouration.
* Loss of movement.
* It may be difficult to distinguish a bad sprain from a fracture. (See **Broken bones**.)

Causes

- All joints are surrounded by stabilising straps called ligaments.
- If a joint is pushed too far in one direction, or subject to too much weight, these straps will be either overstretched or broken.
- In a joint such as the ankle the ligaments are extremely strong and important in holding the various bones in the correct position. A clumsy movement can lead to your full weight forcing the joint in an odd direction, tearing the ligaments.
- When ligaments are torn there is damage to neighbouring muscles and bones. A fragment of bone may even be pulled off by a ligament. The swelling is due to the bleeding and release of body fluids into the injured area.

Prevention

- One of the commonest sprains is to the ankle. Unsuitable footwear, particularly for climbing or running, can make you more vulnerable to a sprain.
- If you are overweight or unfit the joints will be able to cope less well if subjected to exceptional pressures.
- Exercising and losing weight before an activity holiday, for example, can do much to avoid unnecessary sprains and injuries.

Treatment

- A sprain should be cooled immediately to minimise swelling and give pain relief. Cold water may be adequate, or a pack of frozen peas can mould itself well round a spained

joint (do not eat after refreezing).
- Raising the injured joint helps swelling to go down.
- Rest the joint as much as possible.
- The sprained joint should be firmly strapped up to provide support the ligaments are unable to provide, and decrease movements of the joint, so healing can take place.
- After a few days, exercise the joint gently to prevent stiffening, but do not bear weight or exert undue pressure on any sprained joint until healing is well advanced.

The Doctor
- If symptoms do not settle or the sprain is severe with a lot of swelling and joint deformity seek medical help.
- The doctor may arrange an X-ray if it is difficult to exclude the possibility of a broken bone.
- More rigid strapping or even plaster of Paris may be applied to a badly sprained joint.
- In unusual circumstances, where there is a severe tear of a ligament, it may be necessary to repair it at operation. This is occasionally done around the shoulder joint, for example (see **Shoulder pain**).

Squint

When the eyes do not appear to be looking in the same direction this is called crossed eyes or squint. It can be noticed in babies a few months old; it is always important and must be treated early. There may be others in the family who have had a squint. A squint in an adult usually means a childhood squint not adequately treated.

Symptoms
* A new baby often has difficulty focusing both his eyes for any length of time and so a false squint appears. If, after three months it persists, seek help.
* Some babies have large skin folds on the nose side of the eye. This can give a false impression of a squint; this impression is common in oriental babies.
* There are normally no complaints from the child, only an odd appearance noted by parents.

Causes
- Difficulty in focusing makes one eye 'move off' to a different place. The brain cancels one of the eye's image as with two images it would see double. The 'cancelled eye' moves away.
- Unequal eye muscles can pull one eye out of line.
- Longsightedness can lead to different images in one eye from the other. This can produce a squint.

Treatment
- Untreated, the bad eye loses its sight.
- Treated early, the bad eye can be made to work in partnership with the good eye.
- Parents can be surprised when the doctor advises covering the good eye. It makes the bad one do all the work, so gathering strength.
- It is more difficult to cover the good eye if treatment is delayed. This is because the vision in the bad eye weakens with time. The child may naturally then resist covering the good eye as it makes his life more difficult. It is therefore very important to seek early treatment.

The Doctor
- May show you and your child exercises to strengthen the bad eye.
- Spectacles may be prescribed to try and improve the vision of the bad eye so it goes on working correctly.

- Surgery to the muscles of the eye can pull the bad eye into line, correcting an imbalance in the muscles. This may require more than one operation.
- Sadly, children are too often prevented from having the benefit of squint correction due to illness or other family circumstances. The importance of early diagnosis and treatment cannot be over emphasised.

Sterilisation

Sterilisation, female

This is a more involved method of sterilisation than that available to men (see Sterilisation, male). Female sterilisation requires a general anaesthetic and a short stay in hospital. It provides effective contraception, although there is a very small chance of subsequent pregnancy. It has no effect on female hormones, the ovaries or the periods. The womb is left intact. It should be considered a permanent and irreversible form of contraception.

Before operation

Counselling before the operation is important to be sure that you understand the permanent nature of the operation and the very small chance of failure. You will be asked to sign a consent form for the sterilisation to be done.

The operation

- You will have a general anaesthetic; there is usually a quick recovery and you are home within twenty-four hours.
- A small incision about one inch long is made in the abdominal wall, through which a telescopic instrument can be inserted (called a laparoscope). Through this instrument it is possible to attach small clips to the tubes between the ovary and womb. These clips remain in place, effectively blocking eggs from reaching the sperm and sperm from reaching the eggs.
- Sterilisation may also be done while another operation is being carried out, but use of the laparoscope is the most common method.
- The operation may be difficult if you are overweight or have had previous surgery in the same part of the abdomen.

After operation

- You may have a feeling of being bruised inside.
- Stitches can be removed after around five to seven days.
- There is a small chance of a collection of blood forming, called a haematoma. This usually settles quickly.
- Before clips were used for sterilisation there was a greater risk of injury to other organs inside the abdomen. This is now rare.
- Intercourse without additional contraceptive precautions can take place as soon as you wish.
- Sterilisation reversal operations are very rare, and there is a poor rate of success. If pregnancy does occur following a sterilisation, or reversal of a sterilisation, there is a possibility that the pregnancy will occur outside the womb and will not develop. This is called an ectopic pregnancy and can lead to dangerous internal bleeding.

Sterilisation male (vasectomy)

Vasectomy is a simple operation that provides sterilisation for men. It is an increasingly popular method of contraception. As more people have this operation the myth of vasectomy affecting manhood is dispelled. Vasectomy has no effect on male hormones, nor on the quantity of fluid ejaculated. Normal or improved sex life can take place after vasectomy. The semen must be checked after the operation to ensure that it is sperm free; until it is, other contraceptive precautions must be used. The operation is a permanent form of sterilisation and no one should have a vasectomy unless they are absolutely sure they want no more children. It is virtually 100 per cent effective, although there is a very small chance of subsequent pregnancy, sometimes many years later.

Before operation
- Counselling before the operation takes place is important to ensure that you fully understand the irreversible nature of the operation and what will happen after the operation. You will be asked to sign a consent form.

The operation
- The operation is done under local anaesthetic. A small injection into the scrotum numbs the area.
- A small incision is made at the neck of the scrotum near the base of the penis. Through this incision a portion of the tube carrying sperm from testicle to penis is removed or sealed, so sperm cannot pass through it to the penis.
- This is rather like a simple plumbing procedure, and flow from one place to another is interrupted by removal of a portion of pipe.

After operation
- You will be advised to wear swimming trunks or a support for the few days following the operation, as there may be a dragging sensation in the testicles.
- You can often return to work the next day, unless your job involves heavy manual work.
- The stitches are usually absorbent and disappear on their own.
- Following the operation there may be some pain as the local anaesthetic wears off. This has been likened to a light kick on the testicles. It does not usually last long.
- There may be some bruising in the area, with discolouration. Occasionally there is a build-up of blood called a haematoma. This may resolve on its own or may require drainage, which can be done very easily by the doctor using a needle to draw off the fluid.
- Infection is uncommon but more likely if there is a haematoma. Infection usually settles on treatment with antibiotics.
- Occasionally there is a very rare complication of vasectomy, such as inflammation of the testicles, occuring shortly after operation. Also rarely, the sperm may reappear in the semen after a joint forms by itself between the two ends of the sperm-carrying pipe. This is extremely unusual, and the operation should be considered a safe form of contraception and irreversible.
- At least two semen samples will be required to check they are clear of sperm. The length of time before the fluid clears of sperm is variable. Usually after twelve to sixteen weeks the sample is clear and your doctor will advise you if it is safe to have intercourse without taking contraceptive precautions. Sometimes two clear semen samples are obtained well before twelve weeks.

Male or female sterilisation?
Both procedures should be considered irreversible. There is no doubt that vasectomy carries less risk and is a simpler procedure. Individual couples will make their own decision, but avoiding a general anaesthetic and hospital stay by choosing vasectomy is increasingly popular.

Stress

Stress is part of everyday life but at certain times may reach a level when it becomes difficult to cope. Tasks which could normally be completed without hesitation may become too difficult or too threatening to allow you to complete them. Stress may help you to perform well in interviews or exams; at other times it may be so intense you can't decide where or what to turn to.

Symptoms

* These are enormously variable but many are similar to those listed under **Anxiety**.
* In the long term stress may also cause exhaustion, tiredness and depression.
* Physical symptoms may frequently occur as a result of stress. The extent to which the mind causes these symptoms or whether they result from physical consequences of stress is often impossible to determine. Most people have experienced physical consequences of stress, such as indigestion or frequent bowel motions before a stressful event. These symptoms can often be exacerbated by other consequences of stress – for instance, loss of appetite leading to accumulation of more acid in the stomach because food is not eaten to absorb it, symptoms of indigestion being consequently more intense.

Causes

- The causes of stress are more numerous than can be sensibly listed. It is certainly true that everyone's response to stress is different. One person may be able to deal quite easily with a situation that might make another incapable of action.
- The effects of stress can be greatly exacerbated by poor general health. If you are tired, depressed or suffering from another illness, any stress may appear as the last straw.
- Keeping in good general health and avoiding dietary excesses or excesses of work or leisure activities can only help to enable everyday stress to be managed appropriately.

Prevention and Treatment

A number of factors can help in coping with a crisis or severely stressful situation.

- Concentrate on the 'here and now'. Do not brood on the past or try and plan for the future.
- Considering one problem at a time and advancing by taking action on one is better than allowing several problems to combine, preventing any positive action. Single out one area where you can take action and do so.
- Often listening to another person's viewpoint can give you a clue to the one area where you can take positive action. Other areas can wait, or follow after the first.
- When your area of action becomes clear, do act. Action is much healthier, and more likely to be of help in the long term, than storing up the problem because of fear of taking any action at all.
- Avoid being alone. Try joining a club or exercising. Continued solitude tends to cloud your ability to see your particular problems in perspective. If you cannot mix with others go for a run alone or visit a museum or exhibition. Often this distraction helps to put factors causing stress in perspective, enabling you to move forward.
- There is no point in 'crying over spilt milk'; holding grudges against individuals or situations is never helpful. Put past events, whatever the circum-

stances, behind you, though you may need to deal at some point with past psychological problems that have been buried (see below). Try to take action; not doing so because of grievances can only intensify the feeling of being 'hard done-by'.

- When away from your usual environment, whether it be travelling on the bus to work or while going for a regular walk, concentrate hard on what you see around you. Often, in the same way as going for a run or visiting a museum helps, this can give you momentary periods of relief from brooding on a persistent problem. Sometimes it is actually difficult to relax and you have to learn to impose on a daily routine a few moments when you deliberately think about something else.
- A daily routine can be helpful in providing a structure. It should not be abandoned because of stress. Use the security provided by a regular routine to allow you moments of quiet relaxation. Abandonment of a routine will only lead to further disorganisation of your thoughts and greater difficulty in deciding what takes priority.
- Crying and finding an outlet for anger is actually helpful, as is plenty of physical exercise.
- Follow the ideas listed for insomnia and sleep problems in adults. Avoid taking your problems to bed with you by concentrating on a distracting book before sleeping for example.
- If you are not managing, remember all the other people who do not manage either. You are never alone in coping with stress. Everyone at some stage in their lives feels completely overwhelmed. It is never too late, nor inappropriate, to seek help.

The Doctor

- Frequently, making an appointment to see the doctor – and knowing you have a fixed time to talk about your problems with a professional – is helpful in itself.
- List the problems to present to the doctor and explain as fully as possible all the circumstances affecting you.
- Often one or more consultations will be sufficient for you and the doctor to start to see and agree upon a way forward.
- If your stress has caused physical symptoms these can usually be quickly helped or treated. It may be that an acute period of stress has revealed underlying psychological difficulties which are unresolved. These do not have to be tackled now. Sharing them with the doctor can help you to put them temporarily aside in order to move forward, if that is the best course of action for you.
- In some instances further counselling sessions with the doctor, social worker or psychotherapist may be of great assistance. These may be continued over many months, but frequently allow you to resume normal living in the knowledge that you are taking positive action. This help will always be of assistance in coping with stress in the future.
- Persist in obtaining help with stress problems; do not let difficulties of access or fears of rejection put you off. Learning how best to handle your own emotions and cope with stress can be very painful but is always worth while.

Stretch marks

Stretch marks may appear anywhere that the skin is liable to stretching. They are particularly common in pregnant women and adolescent girls. They are of no significance and are in no way a danger. Their appearance can be distressing, and regrettably there is little that can be done about them.

Symptoms
* Red marks appear on the skin, which fade with time.
* The skin may return to almost its normal colour, or a flat, whiter skin may remain.
* This stretched line of skin may resemble flat scars.
* Stretch marks may be more noticeable in dark-skinned people.
* In pregnancy they may appear quite suddenly and unexpectedly.

Causes
* Stretch marks indicate that the elastic limit of the skin has been exceeded.
* If weight gain occurs, to such an extent that the skin cannot cope with the enlarged area, these marks will appear.
* The skin is no longer elastic in the area of the stretch mark, which may add to the scar-like, flat, appearance of the mark. Surrounding skin is more supple and elastic.

Treatment
* Once stretch marks have appeared they do not generally clear, though they may become less noticeable with time.
* Many attempts have been made to provide a cream which can increase the elasticity of the skin and avoid the marks occurring. These are particularly commonly used in pregnancy. They may well help to keep the skin looking and feeling healthy, though their exact value in avoiding stretch marks has not been proven.
* After marks have appeared, particularly after pregnancy, a lot can be done to maintain stomach muscle tone by exercising. Keeping the stomach wall in good shape can greatly diminish the unsightly appearance of stretch marks.

Stroke

When a blood vessel in the brain breaks or is blocked it damages the brain, causing a stroke. This commonly affects men or women in later life. The severity of the stroke varies enormously. There are strokes called transient attacks which last only a few minutes and cause no long-term disability. One-third of people suffering this kind of attack have no more. One-third continue to have them and recover. One-third will have a more serious stroke.

Strokes may leave people partly disabled through losing the use of an arm or a leg. It is also possible to be very badly disabled and be forced to use a wheelchair or, at worst, stay in bed. The outlook for people after a stroke is not always as catastrophic as people think. Even after a major stroke four out of five people can learn to walk with the aid of a stick or tripod.

Symptoms
In transient attacks
* Tingling.
* Inability to talk.
* Dizziness.
* Double vision.
* Numbness.
* Lightheadedness.
* Temporary loss of vision.

In minor strokes
* Loss of use of a hand or leg.
* Loss of speech.
* No loss of consciousness.
* Recovery more or less complete in one or two weeks.

In major strokes
* Weakness of one side of the body.
* Difficulty in getting about.

* Symptoms as above but persisting for longer.
* Emotional upset, ranging from mood changes to severe depression.
* Even patients severely affected at first can, with help, make a good recovery.

Causes
□ Anything interfering with the brain's blood circulation can cause a stroke – either a blockage from a blood clot or a breakage in the blood vessel wall, leading to internal bleeding.
□ These things are more likely to happen when there are:
  - narrow arteries
  - heart disease
  - high blood pressure
  - diabetes
  - an excess of fat
  - a family history of disease of the blood vessels

Prevention
- Strokes remain a major cause of death, third only to cancer and heart disease. The risk of having a stroke can be greatly reduced by:
  - treating high blood pressure
  - treating heart disease
  - avoiding smoking
  - avoiding being overweight

Treatment
- This is aimed at helping people back to as normal a life as possible as quickly as possible. A lot can be done.
- Many people may be involved: family and patient most importantly, doctors, occupational therapists, nurses, speech therapists, physiotherapists, social workers and health visitors, re-employment officers.
- Cigarette-smoking must be stopped.
- Weight must be kept down.
- Blood pressure must be treated.
- Alcohol should be taken only with caution (as effects can be exaggerated).
- Help should be given to achieve toilet, bathing, dressing and shaving care. This can do a great deal to encourage and maintain those who have suffered a stroke.
- Special adaptations (many can be arranged through the local authority) include:
  - toilets with rails, showers; bells and seats in showers; raised toilet seats; outward-opening doors; bath seats; non-slip mats
  - rails around the house and stairs
  - special cutlery available with large handles and combined knife/fork for one-hand use
  - mats to prevent plates slipping
  - gadgets for one-handed housework
- Occupation of the mind as much as possible, with interests as before, is essential.
- Encouragement and help to move about and exercise as much as possible is important.
- Patience and understanding from relatives is one of the most difficult and demanding aspects of strokes. The emotional outbursts and depression of people who have suffered a stroke can be an immense burden to both patients and their families.
- Speech disorders are common; encouragement to talk even when understanding is difficult is as important as formal speech therapy.
- Insomnia is not uncommon; during recovery your doctor can help.
- Depression is common. (See **Depression**.)
- Memory failure can be noted with personality change. Memory tends to pick up with time and many recover fully.
- It is always wise to take a doctor's advice.

☎ The Stroke Association, C.H.S.A. House, 123–127 Whitecross Street, London EC1Y 8JJ. Tel: 071 490 7999.

Sunburn

People of all ages can become sunburnt. The dramatic effects of the sun are often greatly underestimated and nasty sunburn can affect people quite unexpectedly. Because we see so little sun we are particularly poorly accustomed to coping with sun either in this country or on holiday. Sunburn is not usually serious, and a few simple precautions can prevent it.

Symptoms

* You can be severely sunburnt and not realise it until some hours later. This can lead to your staying out in the sun long after you should have covered up.
* Redness of the skin appears. Often this is only noticed when you have been indoors for some time.
* Showering can be very uncomfortable and may be the first sign of sunburn. The water feels as though it is burning the skin.
* Itching can be intense.
* Blisters may appear which subsequently burst and weep.
* Peeling follows as the damaged skin is shed. (See also **Heatstroke**.)

Causes

□ Over-exposure to the ultraviolet rays of the sun causes sunburn.
□ Any fair-skinned person is vulnerable; only olive- or black-skinned people can safely expose themselves to sun for long periods. Even if you have been abroad a lot, the first few days of sun after the usual British climate can have disastrous effects.
□ Sun oils and lotions can be responsible for exacerbating sunburn; many products actually cause you to burn more easily, but some contain sun blocks (See below).

Prevention

* It is particularly important to prevent sunburn in the very young and the elderly. Babies can burn very easily and after brief exposure to the sun. Always cover babies from bright sunlight at the beginning of a holiday; only gradually increasing their exposure to the sun over the first ten days or more.
* Covering with T-shirts and hats is normally essential until you are fully aware of how your skin will react to the sun.
* Remember that snow, sand and water all increase the extent to which you will burn in the sun. This is due to reflection of the sun's rays. Even during a short trip on the water you should always cover up.
* Use sun blocks, particularly on lips, nose, neck and shoulders. Sun blocks come in a range of strengths from one to fifteen. Most sun lotions and oils you see in chemists are in the very low number range around 3 to 8. For effective sun block you should ask for something nearer the ten to fifteen range; a virtually total block can be achieved by using number 15. A variety of good creams and oils are available, some of which can be obtained on prescription. Ask for a non-staining, water-based cream which will be easier and more pleasant to use. It is very advisable to use such a block on young children.
* After swimming it is normally necessary to repeat applications of a sun block.

Treatment

- When you are sunburnt it is essential to avoid further exposure to the sun.
- Applying a soothing cream or lotion to the affected area can ease discomfort; calamine lotion is very suitable. Cold water on a clean cloth is also soothing.
- A cold bath or shower may be helpful.
- Leave sunburnt areas exposed indoors but covered if outdoors. Blistering areas may require a light dressing. Air should always be allowed to reach the sunburnt surface.
- Paracetamol or aspirin may help discomfort.
- If a fever develops take immediate steps to reduce it and drink plenty of fluids. If it persists or worsens consider seeing the doctor as you could be at risk of developing heatstroke. (See **Heatstroke**.)

The Doctor

- It is not normally necessary to see the doctor for simple sunburn, unless it is very severe or a baby is affected.
- The doctor may prescribe other creams or lotions to soothe and prevent itching.
- He may provide dressings for blistered areas.
- He will also check for signs of sunstroke or heatstroke. (See **Heatstroke**.)

Tantrums

Tantrums occur when a child has an outburst of frustration during which he loses control and cannot be reasoned with. They can be very violent and alarming, not only for you but very much so for the child. Tantrums are extremely common, occurring in nearly three-quarters of all toddlers. They are part of the process of learning to cope with frustrations and becoming independent. They are not an example of a child being naughty, nor have they much to do with a child's temper. No matter how embarrassing or difficult a tantrum may be for you, it is helpful to remember that they start from a child's desire to try hard at something. They always improve with time, although, rarely, uncontrolled adult behaviour is effectively also a simple tantrum.

Symptoms

* The child suddenly takes up a position from which he can express his rage, stamping the foot, clenching the fist, turning red in the face and shouting.
* It may develop into rushing round the room, bashing into things.
* The child may bang objects against each other, or may start banging parts of his own body against the floor or wall – headbanging, for example.
* The child may hold his breath and start to go blue. This may be so extreme that the child loses consciousness; recovery is usually rapid. This is quite common. Sometimes little red spots come out on the child's face after a severe episode.

Causes

- The child is trying to control what goes on around them. Their inability to control events or to cope with things not going their way leads to frustration which erupts as a tantrum.
- The child is trying to be independent. In doing so, he has pride and a strong desire to try. Anything frustrating a child's efforts or desires may provoke a tantrum.
- If the child senses he is being rushed, hurried or pressurised a tantrum is more likely, the child fearing a loss of control and independence.

Prevention

- *Sometimes it is simply not possible to prevent tantrums*, but many situations arise where small adjustments can help avoid them.
- *Never give in as a consequence of a tantrum.* If children sense they can have their own way, which you have previously forbidden, by having a tantrum you will have much more difficulty in controlling them. At this point the tantrum becomes purposeful and it is much harder to stop it becoming a repetitive event.
- *Be tactful and allow the child to feel a certain amount of control.* Don't ask the child what he wants to eat, you decide, but leave it up to the child whether the food gets eaten or not. If you are going out and the child wants to walk but you want to use the buggy (usually because you are in a hurry), don't allow a confrontation to develop, take the buggy with you, but allow the child to walk initially. The child usually soon tires and either asks for the buggy or is easily tempted to use it. The same idea could be applied to a potential dispute over wearing a jumper or coat. Take it with you; the child is likely to be relieved to put it on very shortly after setting out. A common situation in which tantrums occur is on leaving a friend's house, or even the supermarket. The child plays a game with you to test his independence. If he senses he is going to lose control and be bundled out, a tantrum is likely. Make a game of leaving by asking him to show you the way to the bus or car; or let him pay the bus conductor or car park attendant. Usually the child's anticipation and excitement, created by being able to help, avoid a tantrum.
- *Putting yourself up a blind alley* by saying 'eat it or else', 'come', or you will do such and such, *is usually the worst possible approach*. The frustration and anger felt by the child at such loss of control can provoke a tantrum.
- *Even if you are in a rush, don't let the child sense it.* A child will continually want to test you. This frequently happens when it is time to get the child dressed. Few parents have not had children run away from them when they want to dress them. Sometimes it is fun, at other times it can be very irritating. It is important to join in the chase from time to time. If children are always met by the stony response of a humourless parent each time they try and play a game the frustration can develop into a tantrum. There are limits, but children have to learn these. It does no harm to enjoy occasionally what your child is trying to draw you into, and because you have joined in the child will usually be happier to cooperate in the end.
- *Toys that are too difficult for a child at a particular age can add to frustration and make tantrums more likely.* It is better to have no toy train than one that is so sophisticated the child cannot make it work or enjoy it.

Treatment

- Children having a tantrum will not hear you, so there is no point in shouting or scolding them. They are so absorbed and overwhelmed by their emotions that nothing you say will help until they start to calm down.
- Child feels very frightened and shocked, just as you are, by the strength of their emotions. It is best if they find everything unchanged when the tantrum ends.
- It is important that no damage occurs to the child, you or possessions

during a tantrum. If this happens they will be even more alarmed and impressed by the effects they can have.
- Stay as calm as possible throughout a tantrum.
- Hold a small child if possible. This may not only stop him hurting himself, but is very reassuring, the child feeling your support and, hopefully, calm presence as the tantrum passes.
- The importance of not letting a child have his own way after a tantrum, if you have previously suggested an alternative, is vital. As mentioned above, the tantrums must never be allowed to become the means of a child achieving a desire.
- If children are too old or too strong to be held, concentrate on preventing them injuring themselves and stay calmly nearby, leaving them to work out their anger, until the tantrum passes. It is better to leave children alone than to allow your own anger and frustration to explode.
- Older children and adolescents having tantrums have to learn to cope with frustration in a more controlled way. It is best to point out that their behaviour is not acceptable and explore together how the situation has arisen and possible solutions.

Teething

This describes the sometimes difficult time when a baby's teeth first emerge. It is never serious and not a reason for a baby to have high fever or diarrhoea and vomiting. The teeth can appear any time between six months and two years of age. During this time there are twenty teeth to come, so prepare yourself to be patient.

Symptoms
* More dribbling than usual.
* Chewing on anything and everything, from the baby's own fingers to the furniture.
* Bulges or lumps felt on the gums when you rub your finger on them.
* Visible angry red patches on the gums.
* Irritability.
* Being more clingy than usual.

Causes
□ Teething pain is caused by the discomfort of the first teeth bursting through the gums. Adults can sometimes remember the discomfort of erupting wisdom teeth, and, although less severe, teething must be jolly sore sometimes.

Treatment
This is aimed at comforting and reassuring the baby. The following measures can be taken to try and relieve the pain:
- Rubbing the gums with your finger can help.
- Allowing the baby to chew, though chewing on food such as hard rusks and carrots can lead to choking. Unless you are able to give the baby your undivided attention, choose teething rings or favourite toys. Always check for toxic paints or loose parts in toys.
- Some teething rings are sold which contain a special gel that can chill in the fridge. The cold ring soothes and numbs the pain.
- Avoid anything out of the freezer. Do not freeze teething rings or use ice, because this can damage the gum.
- Special gels are sold at the chemist, but care should be taken with these. Prolonged use of those containing anaesthetic can lead to an allergy to the gel itself. Prolonged or excessive use of gels containing aspirin can lead to overdose. Most doctors now advise against this type of gel. If a gel

is really felt necessary, Dentinox is one to try.
- Some gels (more often in other countries) contain sugar and/or alcohol – both definitely to be avoided!
- It is rarely necessary to give a fretful child paracetamol liquid. Before doing so you must be confident that there is no other illness causing the irritability. Regular doses given for teething must be avoided, as no medicine should be given unless really necessary.
- Cuddling, holding and talking to a teething infant can often do as much good as many of the above suggestions.

Note

It is important not to pass off an ill child as 'just teething'. In the first two years of life it is likely that a child may have an ear, throat or other infection at the same time as teething. High fever or greater irritability than usual, in association with other symptoms such as diarrhoea or pulling at an ear, should be checked by a doctor.

Temperature, raised

Having a raised temperature is usually a sign of infection. There are many causes of infection covered in this book, but, whatever the cause, the nursing of someone with a temperature is important. In children under five years of age it is essential to lower the temperature to prevent them having a fit. (See **Convulsions, febrile**.)

Symptoms

Adults

* Flushed appearance
* Aching all over.
* Headache.
* Sweating.
* Loss of appetite.
* Feeling cold.
* Other symptoms related to the illness such as cough, stomach upset, or those of flu for example.
* Temperature above normal.

Children

In children it may be more difficult to know if they have a fever. If any of the symptoms below occur you should take the temperature.

* Forehead hot to touch with the back of the hand.
* Flushed appearance.
* Irritability or unexplained crying.
* Feeding difficulty or loss of interest in food.
* Cough or runny nose.
* Rubbing ears or complaining of throat discomfort.

Treatment

A lot can be done to lower a temperature in order to make a child safer and more comfortable. The same measures adapted for adults are equally helpful. If children under six months have a fever it is wise to seek a doctor's advice before starting to give medicines.

- Remove layers of clothing. A light T-shirt and pants is normally adequate if the room is at normal temperature.
- One sheet as covering is normally sufficient; avoid adding extra blankets.
- Give plenty of fluids, particularly important as considerable additional fluid loss occurs when there is a fever.
- Regular doses of medicines such as paracetamol and, in adults, aspirin can also be used. Soluble or liquid preparations of these medicines are usually easier to take and may work more rapidly. Aspirin is no longer recommended for children under twelve years old.
- Sponging with lukewarm water can reduce temperature. This should be left on the skin to evaporate. Where feasible it is very effective, and often preferable, to use a bath of normal, or

slightly below normal, temperature. With children the effect of a pleasant bath in lowering temperature is often dramatic. The moist air may also help to relieve symptoms of congestion and cough. Do not use cold water or cold baths.
- Keep the room well ventilated but at normal temperature.

The Doctor
- If the reason for the temperature is not clear, or you are concerned, it is best to discuss symptoms with your doctor.
- In young children the cause of a fever should always be ascertained.
- If fever persists despite measures taken to reduce it, or if symptoms deteriorate, seek your doctor's advice.

Taking the temperature
A mercury thermometer or a special strip placed across the forehead can quickly tell you if the temperature is raised. Both are easy to use and easily available at chemists.

In children the thermometer should be placed for three minutes under the arm, rather than the mouth. Fever-strips on the forehead may be easier if the child is restless or if you have difficulty reading a mercury thermometer.

Normal temperature
Mouth 36–37°C. 96·8–98·6°F.
Underarm 35·6–36·7°C. 96–98°F.

Tension

Just as the problems posed by stress can cause psychological difficulties, making it difficult to decide on a course of further action, tension can cause physical difficulties which if left unattended can be very disabling.

Symptoms
* The commonest physical presentation of tension is headache. Muscles in the neck and over the head contract, causing pressure effects revealed as headache.
* Neck muscle tension may present as neck pain, or even tingling in the fingers and arms. Muscle tension pulls the neck bones together, causing nerves to be affected and leading to symptoms in the arms or hands.
* Tension may be reflected by altered activity in the stomach and intestines. The feeling of butterflies in the stomach may reflect acid in the stomach, built up because less food is eaten and tension prevents the stomach from emptying as efficiently as normal.
* Similarly, frequent bowel motions may be a reflection of tension in the intestines. Piles are commonly found after a period of increased tension. Contraction of the muscles around the back passage increases pressure and the likelihood of piles.
* Tension may be reflected in many other ways as it affects the body, e.g. preventing sleep or even leading to difficulty in swallowing.

Causes
□ See **Anxiety**, **Stress**.

Treatment
- Physical symptoms are often best treated by physical means. Exercising an affected area by repetitive movement, or contracting and relaxing affected muscles can be helpful. General exercise may also be helpful.
- Applying heat may be helpful. Hot-water bottles in a towel make good hot packs. Baths can also be helpful.
- Physiotherapists can often teach exercise or massage techniques which are helpful.
- Most importantly, the cause of

tension has to be addressed and removed. This can often be done by a simple change of timetable to allow yourself more time to make a journey or fulfil a commitment. Changing your daily routine slightly may have significant benefits in allowing you to relax.
- (See also **Anxiety** and **Stress** for suggestions on the treatment and management of factors which may lead to tension.

The Doctor
- If tension has caused physical symptoms the doctor may be able to prescribe a medication to relieve them, but the underlying tension will only improve when the cause is removed.
- Beta-blockers are often used for the treatment of physical symptoms of tension, such as shaking. They may also help other symptoms.
- Tranquillisers are likely to be of little long-term benefit and should be reserved only for very brief periods of treatment.
- In the long term, treatment of tension may require psychotherapy or counselling, which your doctor is able to arrange for you. Often, if physical tension is the predominant problem, a psychologist may be able to help by using relaxation techniques and a more physical approach to enable you to adapt more satisfactorily to situations that previously made you tense. Sometimes stress and anxiety management groups are organised, which can help you to learn ways of dealing with tension.
- For further information of dealing with tension and symptoms mentioned here, see the sections covering **Anxiety, Headache, Indigestion, Insomnia, Neck problems, Piles, Stress** and **Tranquilliser addiction.**

Testes problems

Problems considered here are:
    Swollen testicles
    Twisted testicles
    Undescended testicles

Swollen testicles

There are many causes of swollen testicles. The symptoms listed below help to distinguish them. They range in severity from resolving in a few days to requiring urgent treatment. Sometimes swellings are present at birth; in other cases they follow infections. Any unexplained swelling or problem with the testicles should be reported to your doctor at once.

Symptoms
* Swelling may be accompanied by severe pain, or may be painless.
* There may be a discharge from the penis, or pain on passing urine. If this occurs with a temperature it suggests infection.
* The swelling may come on within hours, or over several weeks.
* The swelling may be of the whole testicle, or its lining, or may be of a small area within or separate from the testicle.
* The swelling may contain blood, fluid, sperm or pus.

Causes
- Infection – including mumps and tuberculosis.
- Fluid – called a hydrocele.
- Blood – following an injury.
- Tumour – may start as a hard module or be first noted as a hard swelling.
- Varicose veins – said to be like a bag of worms.
- Twisting – see **Twisted testicles.**

Swelling due to infection
- The whole testicle is swollen and painful.
- There may be an infection with the same germs as cause a urine infection.
- The testicle is red, hot and tender.
- You may have a fever.
- There may be pain on passing urine, and a discharge from the penis.
- The symptoms come on within days of catching the infection.
- Inflammation of the testicle may follow mumps. (See **Mumps**.)
- Tuberculosis can also cause a gradual swelling, but there will usually be other signs of TB.

Treatment
- You should see your doctor early so the infection can be treated and the pain reduced.
- You will be asked to give a urine sample.
- Most infections will be treated by antibiotics.
- The pain will be helped by taking painkillers, wearing a scrotal support which can be bought from the chemist, or putting a pack of ice around the testicle.
- The inflammation following mumps is not helped by antibiotics, but the same types of pain relief will help. This is common after mumps in adults. There is a small risk of infertility following an attack in a man after puberty.
- Tuberculosis infection is rare in this country. It needs particular antibiotics as prescribed by a specialist.

Swelling due to fluid
- This may be present at birth (also referred to as a hydrocele).
- Fluid can pass down the tube through which the testicle passed a few weeks before birth, as the baby was developing.
- The fluid reduces when the baby lies down. When the tube closes as the baby grows, the fluid may disappear or it may be trapped around the testicle.
- Sometimes, in an adult, fluid may arise when there is inflammation in the testicle.
- The whole testicle appears swollen.
- There is no pain.

Treatment
- The fluid present at birth will often get better on its own. It is often better to wait to see what happens when the tube closes; a small operation may be needed to remove the fluid and tie off the tube. The adult form will need treatment according to the cause.

Swelling due to blood
- Following a kick to the scrotum the testicle may become rapidly swollen.

Treatment
- Because the pain is so severe you will usually go straight to a hospital. An urgent operation may be needed to save the testicle. This is distinct from simple bruising, when all that is needed is painkilling remedies.

Swelling due to tumour
- This is a relatively common cancer in young men.
- It occurs most often between the ages of twenty and forty.
- It is usually painless.
- It usually starts as a hard nodule.
- If left, the whole testicle gradually becomes swollen.

Treatment
- You are never wasting your time asking about a swelling on the testicle.

- Early treatment is very successful.
- Men should regularly examine their testicles, looking for a hard swelling which is usually painless.
- If there is any cancer the testicle will have to be removed. After this you will need to undergo courses of drug treatment.
- A plastic replica of the testicle can be inserted.

Swelling due to varicose veins
- The appearance is of many tubes (a bag of worms), rather like varicose veins in the leg. The swelling is warm but painless (varicocele).

Treatment
- An operation is advised. The warmth of the enlarged veins may decrease your fertility. It is a small operation, during which the abnormal veins are tied off.

Twisted testicles

A twisted testicle is an emergency. The twisting cuts off the blood supply to the testicle. It must be untwisted as soon as possible to preserve the testicle. It is fairly common, and can affect males of any age from birth to old age, but is most common in adolescence. This may occur without any provoking factors.

Symptoms
* There is sudden intense pain in the testicle.
* The pain may spread to the groin or lower abdomen.
* The testicle becomes swollen and very tender. You may feel sick or start vomiting.
* There is no pain on passing urine, unlike some other causes of painful testicle.

Causes
- The normal testicle hangs with its longest diameter in a vertical direction.
- A testicle that may twist lies with its longest diameter in a horizontal direction.

Treatment
- You need to see the doctor urgently if you suspect you may have a twisted testicle.
- He may attempt to untwist the testicle, especially if you are a long way from hospital. This is only a temporary measure, however, because the testicle must be untwisted and fixed in the correct position.
- This is done at operation under anaesthetic. It will bring great relief of pain and a full recovery provided it is done at once.
- The other testicle will be fixed in place at the same operation to prevent it twisting.

Undescended testicles

Testicles are formed within the abdomen of unborn babies and usually descend into the scrotum before birth. If not there at birth they may descend during the first year of life. In the scrotum the testicles are at a lower temperature, which is better for their development. After the first birthday, if they are still undescended, they are unlikely to come down on their own and an operation is usually needed.

Symptoms
* You may have noticed that the lump formed by a testis is only present on one side of the scrotum. This may have been noticed during your baby's first examination (lack of descent on both sides is less common).
* The scrotum is usually under-

developed on the same side.
* Testicles which are pulled back into the abdomen by a muscular reflex may be hard to distinguish from undescended testicles. They are called retractile testicles.
* The testicles normally retract out of the scrotum when the testicles are examined or exposed to cold. These testicles develop quite normally and do not need an operation.
* It is often easier to see if the testicles are in the scrotum when your child is relaxed in a warm bath.
* Your doctor may be able to push the testicles down into the scrotum.

Causes
☐ In most cases the child is otherwise normal.
☐ Undescended testicles are more common in premature babies, since they may be born before the normal descent of the testicles into the scrotum has taken place.
☐ Mumps does not make the testicles retract out of the scrotum.

Treatment
- You should go to the doctor if you think one or both testicles are undescended.
- The doctor will examine your child to distinguish between retractile or undescended testicles.
- If your baby is under one year old the doctor may ask you to come back for another check after the baby's first birthday, and may arrange for you to see a surgeon.
- To give the best chance of normal development, the testicles should be operated on before the age of three years. A brief stay in hospital will be required.
- Usually only a small cut in the groin needs to be made under general anaesthetic; if the testicle is stuck higher up in the abdomen a larger operation may be required.
- If an undescended testis is found in an older child the operation is still important.
- There is an increased risk of cancerous change in the testicle if it is left in the abdomen. Having the operation not only decreases the likelihood of this change, but allows the testicles to be regularly checked. It also helps to preserve the function of the testes in producing sperm.

Threadworms

These are white worms, about $\frac{1}{4}-\frac{1}{2}$ inch long, which live in the gut. They are surprisingly common in children, but are also frequently found in adults. They may be seen on the stool but do no harm and pose no danger. The infection may clear by itself, but if it causes symptoms usually requires treatment. It is easily passed to other people and repeated infections are common.

Symptoms
* Intense itching around the anus, often after the child is tucked up in bed and the warmth makes the worms come out of the anus to lay eggs.
* It can lead to a child waking at night, crying and frantic with distress due to the irritation around the back passage.
* In girls urine symptoms may be seen, e.g. a desire to go to the toilet but nothing comes. Girls are liable to this as their genitals expose them more easily to eggs and worms which irritate the urine passage. There may be discomfort around the urine passage and vagina (often mistaken for symptoms of a urine infection).

Causes
- Eggs laid at the back passage are picked up on scratching fingers, passed to the mouth and then swallowed.
- They are also passed to nightclothes, comforters, towels, even carpets, and then reach the mouth.
- Food can be infected with eggs from unwashed hands.

Prevention
- Washing hands and nails after wiping bottom.
- Washing hands before eating.
- Keep nails short.
- During treatment, daily changes of nightclothes and sheets can help.
- Tight fitting nightclothes may prevent scratching.

Treatment
- This has to be carried out with attention to the precautions listed, or re-infection can easily occur.
- Over-the-counter sachets of piperazine or a liquid called mebendazole (available on prescription) can be used.
- It is usual to treat all the family, although some doctors only treat those showing signs of infection.
- It is not uncommon to need to resume treatment on subsequent occasions.
- The medicines may cause loose motions, which helps to clear the infection.
- In pregnancy doctors may advise no treatment but scrupulous attention to prevention. The number of worms seems to decrease with time.

Thrombosis problems

Thrombosis occurs when blood forms a clot. A number of problems are caused by thrombosis, including strokes and heart attacks which are described elsewhere. Thrombosis can cause mild symptoms near the surface, called thrombophlebitis. More rarely, a thrombosis may form deeper in the leg, for example; this is called a deep-vein thrombosis. Both are considered below:

Deep-vein thrombosis
Thrombophlebitis

Deep-vein thrombosis

This is much rarer than thrombophlebitis and much more serious, as part of the clot may break off and cause a blockage in the arteries of the lungs. This can be fatal if it prevents the lungs from providing adequate oxygen to the body. A deep-vein thrombosis usually occurs in the legs, but it may also occur elsewhere, such as in the veins of the pelvis.

Symptoms
* Swelling of the leg in the area of the thrombosis, usually the calf or thigh. The whole leg may be affected and very painful.
* Oedema forms; this is a puffy swelling which you can indent with pressure from a finger.
* The veins on the surface of the leg may become more prominent, and the affected leg warmer to touch than the other one.
* There may be pain on certain leg movements and on pressure over the affected veins.

Causes
- Anything slowing the blood-flow through large veins may cause thrombosis. This is most commonly caused by lack of movement in the legs.
- Deep-vein thrombosis used to be common following operations, but now you are usually up and about

and keeping the legs moving very soon after recovering from the anaesthetic.
- Prolonged illness in bed puts you at risk of having a deep-vein thrombosis.
- Oestrogen, which is a hormone contained in some contraceptive Pills and some hormone treatments, may make you more susceptible to thrombosis. If you have a family history of deep-vein thrombosis you should not take the contraceptive Pill.
- Elderly people are more susceptible to thrombosis, as are those who are overweight.
- Rarely, clots from a superficial thrombophlebitis may lodge in a deep vein in the leg, causing deep-vein thrombosis.

Prevention
- Keep the legs moving. If you are confined to bed, keep your toes wiggling and move your legs as much as possible (pushing up and down on an imaginary peddle is a useful exercise to do in bed to keep the blood flowing well).
- If you are having an operation, special bandages or inflatable bags can be applied to your legs to keep the blood flowing more satisfactorily. Ask your surgeon about these before the operation is due.
- After an operation get up as soon as possible.

Treatment
- To diagnose a deep-vein thrombosis the doctor may have to arrange special tests, including X-rays to show the blood-flow in the veins.
- If you have a deep-vein thrombosis drugs can be given by injection and by mouth to prevent further clot formation. While taking them, you will have regular blood tests to establish the right dose of the drug. It is very important to take the drugs only as prescribed.
- Usually over two or more weeks the symptoms relating to the thrombosis settle. The drugs may be continued for several months.

Thrombophlebitis

This occurs often, and slightly more women than men are affected. The chance of thrombophlebitis occurring is greater if you have varicose veins. It is not usually serious, settling in one to two weeks.

Symptoms
* Redness of the vein.
* Tenderness.
* Itching.
* The vein stands out from the skin and may be hard, like a piece of thick string.
* If there is infection you may have a fever.

Causes
- Any injury or infection affects the inner surface of the vein, making it roughened and inflamed. Blood flowing through this vein is affected, and thrombosis may occur. The blood clots stick to the vein walls and cause thrombophlebitis.
- Having a needle or small plastic tube inserted in the vein while in hospital can injure the vein, causing a thrombophlebitis around the site of injury.
- Varicose veins cause turbulent and slower flow of the blood. The veins may also become inflamed. This combination of factors causes thrombophlebitis.

Treatment
- If there is no infection, or very mild infection, the body may be able to cope

alone and symptoms settle over one or two weeks.
- However, because there is a risk of infection spreading if it is not treated, and because it is often difficult to tell to what extent infection is present, you should always seek a doctor's advice.

The Doctor
- Will prescribe an antibiotic if there is infection. Aspirin is the most suitable painkiller.
- Bandaging the affected area may speed healing and prevent further clots forming. There is a convenient elastic stockinette available from chemists which is very suitable for legs and arms.
- If you are sitting or lying down it helps to keep your legs moving and elevated.

Thrush

This is an infection caused by a yeast called candida. It is common in babies and women but also affects men. It can lead to persistent nappy rash and can sometimes be seen in babies' mouths (see **Nappy rash**). Candida is found in the vagina even when healthy, but thrush occurs when the amount of candida becomes so great that it causes symptoms. It may last only a day or two or can persist for much longer, and it often returns. Although it is not a serious infection, its effects can be distressing.

Symptoms
In women
* White vaginal discharge.
* Itching.
* Red, sore vaginal skin.
* Uncomfortable skin around the entrance to the vagina.
* A hot feeling in the vagina.
* Pain on intercourse.
* It can also cause red, itchy, sore areas below breasts. (This can be helped by the same treatment as nappy rash.)

In men
* It can cause painful areas on the end of the penis.
* It can lead to a discharge and white patches below the foreskin.
* Pain and discomfort on intercourse is common.

Causes
- Anything that allows the candida to grow more freely can cause thrush.
- Tight jeans and nylon underclothing create a warm, moist atmosphere where candida flourishes.
- Antibiotics upset the balance of other substances in the vagina, allowing the candida to grow more and produce thrush.
- Injury to the skin caused by scratching, or intercourse when thrush is beginning, all make it easier for candida to grow.
- Being generally run down allows candida to grow more.
- Pregnancy leads to hormone changes, making thrush more common.
- The Pill does seem to make some people more prone to thrush, though it is not a reason for discontinuing it. Other causes are much more common and should be looked for first. If necessary, a change of Pill may be helpful.
- Diabetes makes people more susceptible to thrush.

Prevention
- Wear loose clothing.
- Avoid chemicals such as vaginal deodorants, disinfectants, bubble bath.
- Use a lubricant such a KY jelly or acijel, rather than risk breaking skin in the vagina if intercourse is uncomfortable.
- Eat natural yoghurt, especially at

times when you find you are prone to develop thrush.

Treatment

- Anti-yeast creams and pessaries are available which clear the infection quickly and simply. The cream, e.g. clotrimazole, is available without prescription; pessaries need a prescription.
- Although it does not always help, and can be messy, you can use natural yoghurt inserted into the vagina with the help of a tampon (filling the cardboard tube with yoghurt and pushing the tampon through the tube into the vagina).
- Many other remedies are talked about with variable effect, such as muslin compresses soaked in vinegar, or boiling up herbs or garlic and using the cooled water on a compress.
- Some people find they can prevent bad attacks by using yoghurt or other remedies early on.
- Acijel, no prescription needed, is a useful substance which helps to restore the normal balance in the vagina, thereby preventing thrush. It can also be used as a lubricant.

The Doctor

- May, on the first attack, take a swab test to be sure that candida is the cause of the problem. No candida on the swab test means that it is not thrush, and your doctor will advise you on appropriate treatment.
- May, on future attacks, prescribe pessaries and cream without an examination if you know your symptoms and feel confident you have thrush.
- May prescribe spare pessaries to keep for future attacks.
- May test your urine for sugar to see if you have diabetes.
- If you are prone to thrush, each time you are given antibiotics, which can cause thrush, ask for pessaries just in case.

Thyroid problems

The thyroid gland secretes a hormone which is essential to the normal functioning of the body. The hormone and its effects can be thought of as rather like the accelerator of a car, allowing only a certain amount of petrol to the engine. Pressing on the accelerator speeds up the car and the processes in the engine. Too much thyroid hormone speeds up the body. Conversely, too little petrol slows down, or eventually stops, the car. Too little thyroid hormone similarly slows down the body until eventually, and only rarely, coma develops.

The thyroid gland is situated in the neck near the adam's apple. It is shaped like the letter H, with the bar of the H straddling the windpipe. In some circumstances the whole gland may be swollen (described as a goitre) or a nodule may develop in the gland. Thyroid problems may also occur without any visible changes in the gland.

Problems considered here are:
Too little thyroid hormone
Too much thyroid hormone

Too little thyroid hormone

This can affect anyone, and is more common than having too much thyroid hormone. This condition is called hypothyroidism or myxoedema. It is commonest in middle-aged women.

Symptoms

* This condition has a slow onset over months or years.
* The whole body slows down.

- There is a feeling of exhaustion.
- Mental tasks become difficult.
- Aches and pains are common.
- The heart rate slows down.
- Constipation occurs.
- Despite eating less, there is weight gain.
- There is a continual feeling of cold even on a hot day.
- Hair becomes thin and dry.
- Skin is thickened and dry.
- Appearance becomes puffy and swollen (myxoedema).
- Voice deepens.
- Tingling in the fingers may be felt.
- Periods may become heavier and more frequent.

Causes
- This may occur for no known reason.
- It may follow treatment for an overactive thyroid gland (see below).
- Lack of iodine in the diet can cause this situation.
- The control mechanism of the thyroid gland may be upset, leading to decreased thyroid hormone production.
- Some babies are born with defective or absent thyroid glands. This is now sometimes checked at birth by routine blood tests. If undetected it can have serious consequences, delaying the baby's development. (Also called cretinism.)
- Rarely, too little thyroid hormone is found as part of a condition called Hashimoto's disease.

Treatment
- Whatever the cause, treatment is simple and effective. Tablets of thyroid hormone are taken for the rest of your life.
- Blood tests will be required to check that your hormone level has returned to normal while you are taking the tablets. Intermittent blood tests, perhaps every year, will be required to ensure that your needs for the hormone have not changed. The dose can easily be adjusted to provide the correct amount of hormone.

Too much thyroid hormone

There are several names to describe the situation where there is too much thyroid hormone: thyrotoxicosis, hyperthyroidism, toxic goitre, and Grave's disease. It occurs five times more often in women than men and is less common than the situation where there is too little thyroid hormone.

Symptoms
- Fidgeting and restlessness.
- Anxiety.
- Tiredness, but there is difficulty with sleeping.
- Shaking and trembling, especially on trying to write.
- Cold does not have an effect; summer clothes in winter may feel adequate.
- Sweating.
- Irritability.
- Palpitations and a fast heartbeat.
- Diarrhoea.
- Increased appetite, but weight is lost.
- Periods become infrequent or scanty.
- Neck swelling may appear.
- The eyes can be affected, becoming gritty, protruding and uncomfortable.

Causes
- The control mechanism affecting the production of thyroid hormone goes wrong, leading to its over-production. There may be overactivity of the whole gland, or of one nodule within the gland.

Treatment
- If you have symptoms of thyroid problems always see the doctor, as a simple blood test can quickly check for any abnormal hormone level.

The Doctor
- Blood tests will be carried out, not just to establish if the level of thyroid hormone is abnormal, but to monitor the effects of treatment.
- An anti-thyroid drug may be given which can sometimes, over a period of about eight weeks, effect a cure.
- A beta-blocking drug such as propranolol may be used to help relieve symptoms.
- If a cure is not effected by use of drugs, surgery may be considered. Frequently, removal of an overactive nodule or a large part of the gland can treat the illness.
- Treatment is also possible by taking a drink containing radioactive iodine, which concentrates in the gland and stops the overactivity.

Tics

Tics are repetitive movements, usually of the face, which occur most frequently around five to seven years old. Although tics may be irritating, they are harmless and generally go on their own. Up to a quarter of all children may have a tic at some stage between two and fifteen years old. Boys are three times more likely to be affected than girls. Often others in the family have been affected.

Symptoms
* Repeated gestures.
* Repeated blinking or grimacing.
* Repeated tossing of the head, rubbing the cheek, or sniffing.
* The gestures serve no useful purpose. Although movement may start in order to wave hair out of the eyes, the movement continues even when the hair is short.
* When a tic ceases another nervous habit may take its place.
* Often worse when tired, excited or anxious.
* There is a rare form of severe tic which may particularly involve the shoulders, limbs or trunk. It is characterised by severe jerking movements. If it is accompanied by explosive verbal outbursts it is called the Tourette Syndrome.

Causes
A number of different factors are thought to contribute to a tic developing.
- Hereditary factors: this is not clear cut but frequently both parent and child are or have been affected.
- Brain chemical and nervous factors: particularly in severe tics, which may persist into adult life, brain chemistry and nervous connections are thought to play a part.
- Family stress and pressures: it is thought that if a child is pressurised in a family situation a tic may be more likely to develop or persist.
- Other stress factors such as a change of school or teacher may accompany the development of a tic.

Treatment
- It is important to ignore a tic and to avoid a punitive approach which is typified by saying, 'Stop it or I will . . .'
- Relieving the child of stress, or supporting them through a difficult patch, is helpful.
- Mild tics usually disappear within a few weeks or months with this approach.
- Severe tics, including Tourette Syndrome (see above) will usually require the help of a doctor.

The Doctor
- May refer either the family, or individual, for counselling sessions. A combination of carefully noting when the tics occur, rewarding tic-free periods, and not mentioning the tics for prolonged periods, coupled with discussions with professionals, can be very beneficial.
- A drug called haloperidol has been found to help some very severe tics, but only a small minority of people become symptom-free due to this drug. There may also be unpleasant side-effects.

Tinnitus

Tinnitus is the medical term for ringing in the ear. This may be short-lived noise in the ear and not a sign of illness. Sudden bursts of tinnitus associated with vertigo and deafness are signs of Menière's disease (see **Vertigo**). A chronic, continuous noise often follows the loss of hearing which accompanies old age.

Symptoms
* The noise may be a high-pitched whine, like an untuned radio.
* There may be a buzzing, or a sound like machinery or rushing water.
* There may be deafness, especially for high-pitched sounds.
* The vertigo of Menière's disease is sudden and severe, and may cause a fall.
* An attack may cause vomiting.
* There may be a gradual loss of hearing.

Causes
- Tinnitus in old age is caused by deterioration in hearing. The nerves which sense high tones cannot detect them. The brain replaces this absence of sound with a buzz or whine.
- In Menière's disease there is excess fluid in the inner ear.
- Tinnitus may follow a perforated eardrum from a blow to the ear. This will improve, as the perforation heals.
- There are some very rare causes such as abnormal blood vessels.

Prevention
- Avoid damage to the ears from very loud noises.

Treatment
- Your doctor will usually be able to examine you and tell you that there is nothing seriously wrong, i.e. a tumour, or anything which will get worse. This may be enough to reassure you and many people can put up with the sound.
- Some people cannot bear the sound and need to try treatment. Unfortunately, this is not always very successful, particularly after old-age deafness.
- Your doctor may send you to an ear, nose and throat specialist. Your hearing will be tested and your ears examined for any serious or treatable cause. A masking device may be provided. This produces a noise which blocks out the tinnitus. Sometimes this helps. For some the noise of the device is worse than the tinnitus.
- The vertigo of Menière's disease can be treated by tablets, which your doctor can prescribe (see **Vertigo**). Menière's disease usually improves with this treatment.
- Sometimes the symptoms of tinnitus are very severe, and the specialist may consider an operation on the nerve to the ear. The price for relief from tinnitus and vertigo may be deafness.
- Some people benefit from acupuncture.
- Tinnitus can cause depression, in

which case anti-depressants may be needed and are sometimes very helpful.

☎ British Tinnitus Association, 105 Gower Street, London WC1E 6AH. Tel: 071 387 8033.

Tongue problems

There are various problems that can lead to painful or alarming tongues! The tongue is quite a complicated structure despite its rather crude appearance. If the troubles persist a dentist can often give more useful advice than a doctor.

Black tongue
The papilli, the little spots on the tongue become unusually long and dark-coloured. The cause is unknown. The treatment is to brush the tongue in any mouth rinse available from the chemist. Do this two or three times daily.

Furry tongue
A white or creamy surface to the tongue is usually due to an accumulation of bits of food, germs and cells from the tongue itself. This is usually seen during a period of illness. If it does not clear on regaining normal health try the treatment for **black tongue** above.

Patchy tongue
Areas on the tongue become a livid red, while the rest of the tongue remains normal. It can look like a red and pink map, which leads to its other name: geographical tongue. There is no treatment for this, but the patches tend to come and go, and will disappear in time. Avoiding spicy foods is all that can be done for any discomfort.

Shiny tongue
This is a smooth bright red tongue which gives discomfort when eating acid or spicy foods. It usually provides no cause for concern, clearing up quickly. If it persists a doctor should be seen; he may do a blood test to check you are not anaemic. This is also called Glossitis.

Ulcers on the tongue
See **Mouth ulcers**.

Tonsillitis

The tonsils are situated at the back of the mouth, forming a gateway which traps germs and prevents them penetrating to infect the body. When they are infected they become swollen and tonsillitis develops. Tonsils are lymph glands, a natural part of our defence system. They grow to reach a maximum size at around six or seven years old, thereafter shrinking. Every child usually has at least one bout of tonsillitis, and it may recur frequently. The number of attacks of tonsillitis decreases after seven years of age.

It is less common in adults, who usually suffer the symptoms of a sore throat or pharyngitis, which is a more generalised discomfort, less severe than tonsillitis. Since the introduction of antibiotics the dangers of tonsillitis have been enormously reduced. Previously, there was greater risk of heart or kidney damage due to certain types of bacteria which cause tonsillitis spreading to other parts of the body, particularly the heart or kidneys.

Symptoms
* Sore throat.
* Difficulty in swallowing.
* Fever, sometimes developing quickly and making children quite ill.
* Visible, red, swollen, angry-looking tonsils with or without white spots on them.
* Symptoms as for flu in adults. (See **Flu**.)

* Children may also:
  - complain of stomach pain
  - vomit or cough
  - have marked swelling of rubbery glands in the neck
  - have glandular swelling, persisting for weeks after an attack

Causes
- Bacterial or viral infection.
- The appearance of the tonsils gives little indication as to the type of infection.

Treatment
- This should initially be aimed at easing discomfort and controlling temperature.
- Simple painkillers such as paracetamol should be taken.
- Take sips of cool fluids and/or ice-cream.
- Bathing a child in a bath of usual temperature, or slightly cooler, can bring down the temperature very quickly.
- Adults should not smoke.
- Lozenges, mouthwashes or gargles from the chemist can be soothing.
- Adults can be greatly helped by soluble aspirin gargles (dissolve two in hot water, gargle and swallow, four times daily). Avoid in children under twelve.

The Doctor
- If symptoms persist for more than twenty-four hours and are not under control, a doctor's advice may be required.
- He can advise on whether antibiotics are necessary.
- In children other factors in the child's condition, such as a complicating ear or chest infection, may require antibiotics.
- A throat swab may be taken, particularly if the infections are recurrent, to ensure an appropriate antibiotic is given.
- In adults antibiotics are given less frequently nowadays, since the increasing importance of viruses in causing sore throats has been realised. In viral sore throats aspirin gargles are the best treatment.

Does my child need his/her tonsils removed?
A number of factors have led to a dramatic decrease in the number of tonsillectomy operations performed, including better living conditions, the use of antibiotics, understanding the importance of tonsils as part of our defence mechanism, and knowledge of the natural history of attacks of tonsillitis – which is gradually to decrease in frequency with age.

Some factors do indicate the need for removal of the tonsils, which is still a common operation:
- repeated attacks
- recurrent ear infections in association with sore throats
- breathing difficulties
- recurrent development of a quinsy, which is an abscess that forms during severe tonsillitis

Before a child's tonsils are removed it may be worth trying:
- a trial period of low-dose penicillin over a few months to prevent attacks
- checking the child's urine for infection, as occasionally this can be an important source of fever wrongly attributed to the throat

There is still a risk involved in tonsillectomy and the operation should not be undertaken lightly. (See also **Glandular fever**.)

Toothache

This affects all of us at some stage from the cradle to the grave, and you should always seek a dentist's help. It is rarely serious, but if left untreated can damage the tooth, other teeth and the gums. With modern dental treatments and the use of fluoride toothpastes the outlook is good for anyone suffering toothache.

Symptoms
* Stabbing pains.
* Sharp pain on contact with drinks, sweets, hot and cold foods.
* Jaw ache (intermittent throbbing).
* Earache.
* Difficulty in eating.
* Swollen gums.
* Swollen face.

Causes
- Intense sudden pain when acid produced by germs in a tooth cavity has broken through the tooth to reach the nerve.
- Tooth decay can kill the nerve and an abscess may form below, or around, the tooth. This swells as the germs increase in number and may finally come to a head as a gum-boil.
- Both these types of pain can be produced or exaggerated by eating.
- Wisdom teeth cause pain in two ways: firstly, by pushing against the back teeth from below before emerging; secondly, after emergence by struggling for room for themselves against the neighbouring tooth.
- With broken teeth, particularly if a nerve is exposed, the pain can be severe.

Prevention
- Plaque is a creamy-white paste that forms as a result of saliva and food mixing together. This is one of the major causes of dental problems. Avoid plaque building up by regular brushing.
- Fluoride treatment to teeth helps, but regular use of fluoride toothpaste should have the same effect.
- Regular dental check-ups are needed from three years onwards.
- There is now a treatment available which uses a resin to fill inaccessible cracks in children's teeth. This is of great benefit in preventing decay.

Treatment
- Sudden severe toothache, gum-swelling or tooth injury should be seen by the dentist as an emergency.
- Pain from infection may only subside when either the infection is drained and/or appropriate antibiotics started.
- Wisdom teeth can cause severe pain and may need to be extracted under local or, sometimes, general anaesthetic.
- While waiting to see the dentist the following measures may help:
  - painkillers taken regularly every four to six hours
  - hot-water bottle covered in cloth next to cheek
  - avoid local gels to gums

Tranquilliser addiction

Tranquillisers are among the most widely used drugs. They have been overprescribed by the medical profession, but there is now a much greater awareness of the dangers involved in the use of tranquillisers. They are still easily obtained – if not from doctors, from a variety of illegal sources. The addiction and difficulties they can cause is often made worse by the extent to which it is both unexpected and unwanted.

People's use of tranquillisers and their response to them varies enormously. The fact that reduction in use does cause withdrawal symptoms is now undisputed. The largest and most widely used group of these drugs are benzodiazepines. These drugs commonly have the letters 'azepam' as part of their generic name.

With the right approach to the problem and support from your family, friends and doctor, it is usually possible to cease or significantly reduce the use of this group of drugs. There is of course still a place for their use in specific situations. (See **Anxiety**.)

Symptoms

* Withdrawal after short-term use may cause no symptoms whatsoever.
* Withdrawal after prolonged or heavy usage may be accompanied by a wide range of symptoms including:
  - recurrence of anxiety symptoms
  - sleep disturbance, including insomnia and nightmares (see **Sleep problems**)
  - muscle spasms, tension and cramps
  - shaking
  - palpitations
  - flu-like symptoms
  - dizziness
  - oversensitivity to noise, lights and crowded places

Causes

- Withdrawal symptoms vary enormously, not only from person to person but according to the drug being used.
- Some benzodiazepine drugs appear to be much more addictive and have much worse withdrawal symptoms than others. One such drug, called lorazepam (Ativan), may cause severe difficulties. It has even been reported to induce, in some people, a fear of going out.
- The drugs have different effects partly because of the varying way in which the body can dispose of the drug once it has been taken. Every drug has a half-life – the time it takes for only half of the amount of drug taken to remain in the body – and some drugs build up more quickly in the blood stream than others.
- The chemical composition of the drugs is not exactly the same, and different drugs may have very varied effects when withdrawn.

Treatment

- It is always worth considering discontinuing the use of tranquillisers.
- It is better to take them as a short course and then discontinue them, rather than as a long-term measure. There are alternatives to taking tranquillisers, such as exercising or relaxation techniques. (See **Anxiety**.)
- When you have decided to come off tranquillisers you may find that you are not dependent on them and it is easier to stop than you expected.
- It is usually more difficult to stop suddenly, so try weaning yourself off slowly. This can be done by gradually reducing the number and strength of tablets. If a weaker strength is not available, it may be possible to halve the tablets or cut them up with a razor blade.
- Plan your withdrawal over several weeks and try and make it an even reduction. It is better to stop the reduction for a week or two than to reduce the dose too quickly and be obliged to increase it again.

The Doctor

- With the help of family and friends involved from an early stage it is usually possible to come off tranquillisers, but it is often important and helpful to include your doctor in the plan. One way of doing this is to avoid obtaining repeat prescriptions without seeing the doctor.
- The doctor can often help in drawing up an appropriate plan.
- He can also prescribe weaker tablets

or a different type to make the reduction possible.
- He may be able to put you in touch with groups concerned with tranquilliser addiction.
- He may advise or arrange for you to have access to relaxation techniques.

☎ MIND (National Association for Mental Health), 22 Harley Street, London W1N 2ED. Tel: 071 637 0741. (Can supply information on local support groups.)

Travel sickness

This is a feeling of nausea or actual vomiting brought on by movement. It is also called motion sickness as it occurs when our balance organ is receiving more messages from various movements than it can cope with. Just as funfair rides can make people sick, so the more gentle but equally confusing movements of a child's head in the back of a car can lead to travel sickness. It is very common in children but usually ceases in adolescence, only returning when movements are severe, such as at sea. Seasickness is caused by the same mechanism as produces travel sickness.

Symptoms
* Nausea.
* Actual vomiting.
* Feeling cold and clammy.
* Feeling faint and dizzy.
* Loss of appetite.

Causes
☐ As outlined above, if the brain is confused by movement it makes us feel sick.
☐ The balance organ is like a hollow sac filled with fluid. The level of the fluid and its position in the sac give us our balance. If the fluid is slopping around inside the sac the resulting confusion leads to travel sickness.

Treatment
- This is chiefly aimed at reducing the motion, which can often be greatly helped by simply propping a child's head against a pillow.
- Sleep is ideal, as motion is greatly reduced. A helpful side-effect of many travel sickness remedies is to cause drowsiness, which can be very helpful. You should not drive or try to work while taking these remedies.
- The stomach contents are important in adding to or minimising the problem. Do not travel on an empty stomach. It is best to travel shortly after a light snack, having eaten well more than three hours previously. On any long journey it is helpful to have snacks of biscuits and non-fizzy drinks.
- Distraction is essential. If there is one golden rule it is to avoid boredom and excessive tiredness. The contents of mum's handbag have averted many a bored child from becoming car sick.
- Avoid:
  – too much excitement before the journey, as this in itself can provoke sickness
  – cigarette smoke; choose non-smoking areas in public transport and don't smoke in cars
  – keep yourself warm, but the surroundings well ventilated
- If necessary, give one teaspoon of promethazine mixture to children below seven, and two if over seven years old. This can be obtained without prescription and is the most commonly given remedy if you visit the doctor. It is best given half to one hour before travel. As it may cause drowsiness, take advantage of this to wrap up children with blankets and pillows. If you are lucky you will enjoy the journey and they will not need the strong brown paper bags you should have taken with you.

Tremor

This is an uncontrollable shaking of part of the body, usually first noticed in the hands. Anyone may be affected by tremor but it is increasingly common as you grow older. Most people with tremor have no underlying disease, this being the most common movement problem known. It can also be one of the first symptoms of Parkinson's disease, which, although common, is not the most usual cause of tremor. In more than half of those affected there is a family history of others who have have 'the shakes' or a tremor.

Symptoms

* Usually begins in both hands, but may start in the head, one hand, legs, voice or chin.
* Can be disabling and embarrassing.
* Writing and drinking may become difficult.
* Tremor worsens with stress, anxiety and fatigue, but may improve with relaxation. Alcohol in many patients stops the tremor, sometimes completely. It can, however, also cause tremor (see below).
* Tremor which is absent if you are resting makes Parkinson's disease less likely.

Causes

- The causes of ordinary tremor, also called physiological or essential tremor, are unknown.
- A number of factors may make an ordinary tremor worse, such as:
  - anxiety and stress (see **Anxiety**, **Stress**)
  - thyroid problems (see **Thyroid**)
  - withdrawal from certain drugs, including beta-blockers and tranquillisers
  - alcohol may cause tremor to worsen, as may withdrawal from alcohol
  - some drugs, particularly those used in epilepsy and some anti-depressants, may enhance tremor
- Ordinary tremor is 100 times more common than Parkinson's disease in the forty- to fifty-year-old age group, and about 10 times more common in the over-sixties.
- Parkinson's disease has a number of distinguishing features from ordinary tremor:
  - the tremor is present when the affected limb is at rest, e.g. on the arm of a chair
  - there is often a degree of stiffness and slowing of movement
  - there may be continuous rubbing together of the thumb and forefinger
  - tremor diminishes when the hand is put into action
  - movement while walking will diminish, leading to a shuffling gait and arms held stiff instead of swinging
* Tremor may very rarely be caused by other brain or nerve disease, but usually there will be other signs of the illness.

Treatment

* Ordinary tremor can often be tolerated, and may need no urgent treatment if you are under the age of fifty and symptoms are mild. If the tremor worsens, or you have further symptoms of Parkinson's disease such as stiffness and slowing of movement, consult your doctor.

The Doctor

* Will carry out an examination to try and distinguish between ordinary tremor and Parkinson's disease. Blood tests may be necessary to detect any underlying problem, e.g. thyroid trouble, which could be making the tremor worse.

- Ordinary tremor, which is a nuisance either at work or socially can be greatly helped by treatment with propranolol, a beta-blocker drug. If you have asthma this may be made worse by propranolol, in which case a drug called primidone may help.
- If the reason for the tremor is not clear, it may be necessary to see a doctor specialising in these problems (a neurologist). Using special tests, including carefully recording the tremor on machines, it is possible to distinguish between different causes of tremor.
- Drugs used for Parkinson's disease may make ordinary tremor worse.
- Parkinson's disease may be treated by a number of different drugs. These particularly help symptoms of stiffness and immobility. They are not very helpful in controlling the tremor of Parkinson's disease. Some have unpleasant side-effects.

☎ The Parkinson's Disease Society, 22 Upper Woburn Place, London WC1H 0RA. Tel: 071 383 3513.

Ulcers

There are two different kinds of ulcer which may give pain in the upper part of the abdomen. If you are told you have an ulcer, this may either be in the stomach itself or in the tube into which food is passed from the stomach, called the duodenum. Ulcers in both places are called peptic ulcers; they are related to the acid and juices used in digestion. A stomach ulcer is also referred to as a gastric ulcer, an ulcer in the duodenum as a duodenal ulcer.

Some of the characteristics of these ulcers are different, so they are considered separately. A stomach ulcer may rarely show changes of cancer, for example, whereas a duodenal ulcer is always benign. Both ulcers may persist and lead to scarring around the exit of the stomach, which leads to vomiting and difficulty in emptying the stomach. This is called pyloric stenosis.

Considered here are:
Duodenal ulcers
Stomach ulcers

Duodenal ulcers

The food enters the duodenum as it leaves the stomach. It is thought that the acid from the stomach can cause an ulcer in the duodenum by injuring its surface. Duodenal ulcers are about half an inch across and can cause severe pain. They are not very dangerous and do not change into cancerous ulcers. Often they heal with time, but if persistent may lead to bleeding, causing anaemia. Sudden heavy bleeding may occur, leading to vomiting blood or black stools. This is much commoner from duodenal ulcers than gastric ulcers. Very rarely, the ulcer may cause an actual hole in the wall of the intestine, leading to internal bleeding and peritonitis; this is called a perforated ulcer. Hospital attention is then needed at once. Duodenal ulcers are common in young and middle-aged people. Men are four times more likely to be affected than women.

Symptoms
* These are similar to those described for stomach ulcers. It may be impossible to tell from the pain whether the ulcer is in the duodenum or in the stomach.
* Typically, someone with a duodenal ulcer wakes in the early hours of the morning with pain in the top of the tummy, which is relieved by milk and biscuits.

Treatment
- Stop smoking, which aggravates the symptoms through its effects on the stomach.
- Stop drinking alcohol.
- No special diet is required, but eat slowly and rest afterwards. (See **Indigestion**.)
- Food in the stomach helps to absorb acid and prevent it exacerbating the duodenal ulcer. Eat frequent small meals.
- Try antacid medicines from the chemist. Liquids are generally more effective than tablets and best taken shortly after food.

The Doctor
- Will advise on how and when to eat meals in relation to your lifestyle.
- Other antacid medicines may be prescribed.
- A drug to block the secretion of acid will be prescribed. (See **Stomach ulcers**.)
- Investigations to confirm the presence of a duodenal ulcer will be arranged. (See **Stomach ulcers**.)
- Surgery is not commonly carried out for duodenal ulcers. If it is, a procedure to cut the nervous supply to the stomach responsible for acid secretion is more common than removal of part of the stomach. This is because the side-effects of partial stomach removal can be very troublesome, including diarrhoea, weight loss, dizziness and trembling after eating.
- Drugs can usually provide good healing and control of duodenal ulcers. They may be continued over a long period, after healing has taken place to prevent recurrence.

Stomach ulcers

These occur equally often in men and women, are about one inch across and respond well to treatment. They are not usually serious, although prolonged bleeding from such an ulcer may cause anaemia; sudden severe bleeding can produce shock and require urgent medical attention at hospital. There is a small chance of cancerous change in stomach ulcers, but most heal satisfactorily. As you grow older there is increasing likelihood of developing a gastric ulcer.

Symptoms
* Burning, gnawing pain in upper part of stomach. May also be felt in the chest.
* Pain is different from that described under indigestion as its relationship with food is more variable and unpredictable. There may be pain-free periods; at other times pain may occur shortly after or many hours after eating.
* There may be loss of appetite and consequent loss of weight.
* Vomiting may occur.

Causes
- Exactly why a stomach ulcer should occur is not clear. The bile and juices from the duodenum may irritate the stomach lining, but many other factors are thought to be important. It is not necessarily acid in the stomach itself that causes an ulcer.
- Smoking is well known to make you more likely to have a stomach ulcer and interfere with healing.
- Alcohol exacerbates stomach ulcers.
- Medicines containing aspirin are also likely to provoke stomach ulcers, particularly if taken in large quantities.
- Eating irregular and hurried meals makes you more likely to develop stomach ulcers. (See **Indigestion**.)

Treatment
- Resting when ulcers are painful, preferably in bed, helps them to heal.
- Small, frequent meals should be taken.
- Stop smoking, alcohol, and tea and coffee.
- Try antacid medicine and tablets from the chemist.

The Doctor
- If pain persists for more than a couple of weeks, or is severe, see the doctor.
- The doctor will arrange for a number of tests, to confirm the presence of an ulcer.
- A barium meal X-ray examination may be arranged. This involves drinking a white liquid, which reveals the shape of the stomach lining when the X-rays are taken.
- A gastroscopy or endoscopy may be arranged. During this examination you are mildly sedated with a tranquilliser drug and may not remember anything of it. An anaesthetic spray is used on the back of the throat and you are able to swallow a long, thin tube which carries a light and telescope down the throat and into the stomach. Samples of juices from inside the stomach and duodenum can be removed through this tube. Pieces of an ulcer can also be removed e.g. to look for cancer changes.
- Blood tests to look for anaemia and check how your liver is working may be done. The liver is quick to respond to too much alcohol, for example, and knowledge of your drinking having reached a level to bring about liver changes is important in attempting treatment of any ulcers present.
- The doctor may arrange stool examination to check for the presence of blood, which can be a sign of bleeding from an ulcer.
- You will be prescribed antacids and special drugs which block the acid secretion of the stomach (called H2 receptor blocking drugs). These drugs have dramatically altered the ability and success of doctors in treating ulcers. There are few side-effects and treatment may be continued over several months or more.
- Surgery is now much less commonly performed. It involves removal of part of the stomach. Although this may provide a cure, it is not without side-effects. Much more commonly, correct use of drug treatment and regular supervision to ensure healing of the ulcer is sufficient.

Umbilical problems in the newborn

At birth the umbilical cord is divided between two clamps. The clamp on the end of the umbilicus next to the baby is then replaced by a small plastic clip; alternatively, a simple band or piece of sterile string may be used. This prevents bleeding. A number of usually minor problems can occur around the umbilicus.

Symptoms
* The cord normally dries up, shrivels and drops off after a few days. If it is knocked off after a few days this does not usually matter as it will come off soon anyway.
* Infection can appear around the umbilicus; this may appear as a red inflamed area or a whitish-yellow discharge. There may be yellow spots on the skin. Seek treatment from your midwife or doctor immediately if you think there may be an infection.

* When the umbilical cord has dropped off there may be persistent weeping and blood-staining noticed on the nappy. Unless infected, this is not usually serious and settles quickly (see below).
* Some days or weeks after birth a small fleshy lump, called an umbilical granuloma, may appear at the umbilicus. This sticks out of the tummy button like a little pink tongue. It can be easily dealt with and is of little significance (see below).
* A hernia may appear at the umbilicus (see **Hernia, umbilical**).

Causes
☐ Infection is generally caused by germs (bacteria) picked up from the surroundings or from people.
☐ Why an umbilical granuloma appears is not clear.

Prevention
● Keeping the umbilicus clean, particularly until the cord has dropped off, is of great importance. This should be done using cottonwool and surgical spirit. Convenient alternatives are small medical wipes which come in sealed sachets, presoaked in a suitable cleansing spirit. These can be bought at the chemist or may be issued by the hospital. Antiseptic powder is also available to keep the area clean.
● When the umbilical cord has dropped off, simple washing at bathtime is usually quite sufficient.
● If there is persistent non-infected discharge or bleeding, keep the area clean with wipes and washing. This usually ceases after one or two weeks.

Treatment
● Signs of infection described above must be treated to prevent the baby developing a generalised infection, which can be very serious.
● The health visitor or midwife can usually treat an umbilical granuloma. This is done by touching it with a small wooden stick which has a chemical called silver nitrate on it. This seals off the granuloma and makes it shrink down until it is no longer visible. Sometimes more than one treatment is necessary.

The Doctor
● Will advise on umbilical problems and may take a swab test to check for infection.
● Antibiotics will be prescribed if infection occurs.

Urine infection

If germs enter the normally germ-free urine passage they can spread to the bladder, kidneys and pipes in between. They grow well in the warm urine, and if left untreated cause the symptoms of general infection and cystitis (see **Cystitis**). Urine infections should always be treated, as they can damage the kidney, which is a delicate and vital structure. They are much commoner in women but may also occur in men. Sometimes others in the family are affected, which may reflect a particular shape of the urine passage that makes family members more liable to develop infections. Urine infections usually clear up quickly with appropriate antibiotics. If the urine infection is in the kidney it is called pyelonephritis.

In adults

Symptoms
* These may be those of cystitis. (See **Cystitis**.)

* They may occur without cystisis symptoms, but with high fever or a combination of symptoms including:
  - tummy pain
  - backache
  - groin ache
  - high fever
  - vomiting
  - nausea
  - sweating
  - pain on passing urine

Causes

- The commonest cause is a particular germ called *e.coli*, which is normally present in the gut. If it gets into the urine passage it can cause problems.
- Other germs may lead to infection. This makes testing the urine before treatment kills the germs very important. It is only by identifying the germ that the right antibiotic can be chosen if the first antibiotic does not work.
- Having catheters inserted into the bladder when in hospital and during childbirth can introduce germs to the bladder.
- Other important factors leading to urine infection are mentioned in the sections on **Cystitis, NSU, Pelvic infection**.

The Doctor

- Treatment should be preceded by your doctor sending a urine sample to a laboratory for identification of the germ responsible for the infection.
- Antibiotics will be given, the choice depending on the kind of infection.
- As treatment is usually started before the laboratory results are available, it occasionally has to be changed if it is discovered that the antibiotic chosen would have no effect on the particular germ found.
- If you are not improving on an antibiotic, it is important to consult your doctor.
- If infections are repeated or prolonged, kidney damage can result. To check for this, and for any particular tendency towards infection, an X-ray may be requested. This X-ray may reveal a piece of pipework that allows urine to collect or pass the wrong way, causing infections and possible damage to be more likely. The X-ray is called an intra-venous urogram or pyelogram (IVU or IVP).
- The section on **Cystitis** lists some useful tips to help relieve symptoms.

In children

Adults may have several episodes of urine infection without undue concern, but children should not have urine infections. Any child with a urine infection should be seen by a doctor who has experience of treating this problem. This is because the urine passages are delicate, and injury through childhood infections can cause damage affecting the kidney in adult life.

Symptoms

* These may be the same as those listed for adults, but only one or two may occur.
* Urine infections in childhood can go unsuspected and only be revealed when a child is not growing properly. Children failing to gain weight will often have their urine checked, particularly if there is no other reason to explain why they are not growing adequately.
* Cystitis symptoms in children, such as soreness on passing urine, are more likely to be due to local irritation or infection (see **Foreskin problems**) than urine infection.

Treatment

- This is as for adults, but X-ray investigation is more usual.
- Treatment may be prolonged over a

period of several years to prevent infections, particularly if X-ray tests show a tendency towards infection or kidney damage.

Vaginal problems

Problems considered here are:
   Vagina, dry
   Vagina, swelling at the entrance
   Vaginal discharge
   Vaginal irritation
Problems considered elsewhere are:
   Absence of orgasm
   Genital warts
   Gonorrhoea
   Painful intercourse
   Pelvic infection
   Thrush

Vagina, dry

Symptoms
* Intercourse becomes painful or uncomfortable.
* Local irritation is felt.

Causes
☐ Lack of secretions prior to, and during, intercourse. This may occur due to a lack of sexual arousal because of a difficulty in technique or over-hasty intercourse in anxious circumstances. There may be a sexual problem such as impotence in your partner, lack of orgasm or pain on intercourse. (These problems are described under **Sexual problems**.)
☐ Alteration of hormone levels for a variety of reasons, including illness, may lead to a dry vagina.
☐ Following pregnancy, hormone levels alter and the level of sexual arousal may also alter.
☐ After the menopause there is a lack of oestrogen in the vagina, which leads to fewer secretions and potential irritation.

Treatment
● Lack of secretions during intercourse is a common problem which can be immediately helped by the use of a lubricant such as KY jelly, available from chemists. Taking more time over foreplay prior to penetration of the penis into the vagina often helps the vagina to be sufficiently lubricated. Stimulating the clitoris with fingers, or during oral sex, usually helps. If a problem with a dry vagina persists see the doctor.

The Doctor
● Can often discover the problem by examination or by taking a smear test which gives information about the level of hormones in the vaginal cells.
● May prescribe a lubricant, or if there is a lack of oestrogen may prescribe pessaries containing oestrogen, or creams such as dienoestrol. This is only normally necessary after the menopause. Treatment with oestrogen creams or pessaries should be limited to the minimum amount needed to improve the situation. Use the cream or pessary as instructed. This usually involves daily treatment for one to two weeks, followed by treatment only once a week, or as necessary. Excessive use of oestrogen treatment in the vagina can lead to side-effects.
● If you continue to have problems you may consider seeking help from a family planning clinic or psychosexual counselling service. Access to this does not have to be via your doctor. Addresses of your local family planning clinics are in the phone book; they can put you in touch with any counselling you may need.

Vagina, swelling at the entrance

Swelling around the entrance to the vagina is common. This area is called the introitus.

Symptoms
* Both lips of the vagina may be swollen.
* A localised swelling may appear, which can be red, hot and painful. It may discharge pus.
* Sores may appear with some swelling around them.
* Irritation may be intense. (See **Vaginal irritation**.)

Causes
- Bruising from vigorous intercourse causes swelling, which usually settles quickly.
- Infections in the vagina or surrounding skin can cause swelling at the introitus; usually there will be other symptoms of infection, such as discharge or pain. (See **Vaginal discharge**.)
- Local sensitivity or allergy may cause swelling. (See **Vaginal irritation**.)
- A Bartholin's cyst occurs when one of the glands around the introitus becomes infected and swells up. These glands normally secrete a lubricating substance on to the skin surface just inside the lips of the vagina. If the glands become blocked and infected, a painful swelling may build up on one side. This has some of the characteristics of a large boil.

Treatment
- Local vaginal infections are treated with pessaries or creams; some infections may require antibiotics. (See **Vaginal discharge**, below.)
- If you have a persistent swelling or think you may have a Bartholin's cyst, see your doctor as soon as possible so treatment can be commenced.

The Doctor
- Will examine you and may take swab tests for infection before starting any treatment.
- May prescribe antibiotics to try and reduce a Bartholin's cyst. Unfortunately, this may not always produce a satisfactory response and a simple operation may be required to drain the cyst and the collection of pus within it.
- If the swollen Bartholin's cyst recurs repeatedly after antibiotic treatment a larger operation may be performed to try and prevent the problem recurring. This may involve a general anaesthetic and a stay in hospital for a few nights. You will be sent home with instructions on how to clean and dress the affected area.

Vaginal discharge

Some vaginal discharge is normal. The amount varies greatly from person to person and also with changes in natural hormone levels. If you have vaginal discharge that is excessive, itchy and foul-smelling consult the doctor.

Symptoms
* Vaginal discharge may be clear, white, greenish-yellow or brownish.
* Bleeding may occur.
* The amount of discharge may vary considerably due to a number of factors, including severity of infection and stage of the menstrual cycle.
* There may be associated symptoms such as pain, bleeding or irritation.

Causes
☐ Discharge may be normal and caused by:
- natural changes due to hormones, particularly noticeable mid-cycle
- changes of pregnancy, when discharge is usually heavier
- altered hormones caused by taking the contraceptive Pill, or other hormone treatment

☐ Infection in the vagina may be due to:
- thrush (see **Thrush**)
- infection (see **Pelvic infection**)
- Trichomonal vaginitis, an infection caused by a tiny organism called trichomonas; the symptoms are similar to thrush but the discharge is usually unpleasant – smelly and greenish-yellow in colour; it is highly infectious and your partner is also likely to be infected

☐ Cervical problems can cause discharge:
- cervical erosions on the neck of the womb can cause discharge or may bleed after intercourse
- see **Cervical problems**

☐ Bleeding may appear as discharge, which can be due to:
- pregnancy (see **Miscarriage**)
- normal menstruation or some irregularity in the cycle (see **Periods**)

☐ Tampons or contraceptive sponges if left in the vagina or forgotten may cause vaginal discharge, which is usually foul-smelling.

Treatment
If the cause of discharge is abnormal treatment is usually simple and effective.
- Infections can be treated by a course of tablets or vaginal pessaries. It may be necessary for your partner to have treatment. See your doctor for treatment of infective vaginal discharges.
- Cervical problems at the neck of the womb are usually easily dealt with. (See **Cervical problems**.)

The Doctor
- Can remove any tampons or sponges you did not know were in the vagina.
- Will take swabs to check if infection is the cause and prescribe appropriate treatment.
- May refer you to a gynaecologist if discharge or bleeding persists and cannot be explained or treated.

Vaginal irritation

Apart from infection, vaginal irritation may occur due to a variety of often unsuspected causes. This irritation is often focused around the entrance to the vagina and the surrounding lips. This area is also called the vulva.

Symptoms
* Itching.
* Inflamed red skin.
* Bleeding and marks from intense itching.
* Associated discharge of infection.
* Other skin problems elsewhere.
* Pain on intercourse.
* Bladder control may be affected, particularly in the elderly.

Causes
☐ Infections can cause irritation.
☐ Sensitivity to vaginal douches or deodorants is common.
☐ Sensitivity to spermicides is also common.
☐ Vulval warts can cause irritation. (See **Warts, genital**.)
☐ After the menopause there is a decrease in the level of hormones. (See **Vagina, Dry**.)
☐ White patches of skin called leukoplakia may develop. These are asso-

ciated with a slightly increased risk of cancer of the vulva.
- Some drugs, including antibiotics which may cause thrush, can cause irritation.
- In diabetes there is an increased likelihood of vaginal irritation.

Treatment
- Avoid all vaginal preparations, including talcum powder, douches or deodorants. These are unnecessary.
- Use a lubricant during intercourse if necessary. (See **Vagina, dry**, above.)
- Avoid scratching the area and keep it clean, washing with plenty of water and simple non-perfumed soap. Do this twice a day, using a shower on the area if possible.
- A soothing, simple, moisturising cream may be helpful. Aqueous cream from the chemist is suitable.

The Doctor
- Can advise on the cause of the irritation and prescribe treatment for infection, and a cream to decrease irritation.
- Often a change of spermicide or method of contraception is possible.
- In post-menopausal women a cream containing oestrogen may be prescribed. (See **Vagina, dry**, above).

Varicose veins

When veins on the legs become distended, twisted and prominent they are described as varicose. It is an extremely common problem, affecting three times more women than men. Half of all those with varicose veins have parents who have had the same problem. They are not serious, but are a cause of considerable discomfort and can lead to unpleasant complications such as ulceration. Being tall, overweight and pregnant puts you at risk, as does standing all day at work without moving much.

Symptoms
* First sign is usually seeing the veins appear bluer and larger than normal.
* These go on to enlarge and cause discomfort and pain, particularly when standing.
* The veins themselves can be tender.
* They are commonly on the calf muscles and the inside of the leg, anywhere from ankle to groin.
* They also appear elsewhere, particularly around the anus, where they are called haemorrhoids (see **Piles**). In pregnancy they may also appear around the vagina.
* Skin discolouration may be seen.
* Irritation and itching is often intense.
* Symptoms may be worse before and during periods.
* The feet may be swollen and shoes therefore tight.
* Symptoms may be caused by complications, such as:
  - varicose eczema
  - ulceration
  - thrombophlebitis and deep-vein thrombosis
  - bleeding if injured – if this happens raise leg as high as possible, wherever you are, and apply a firm dressing such as a clean handkerchief until the bleeding stops

Causes
- Blood has to reach the feet, which it does by the pumping action of the heart and gravity. It then has to come back to the heart, but there is no suction action to the pump. To flow uphill the blood has to be squeezed in the veins by muscles. There are one-way valves in the veins, which only

allow the blood to flow upwards to the heart. Varicose veins are caused by these valves being damaged or absent. The poor valve system in varicose veins allows the veins to distend as they fill up with blood, because it is not being moved upward to the heart.

- Various things can make varicose veins more likely:
  - prolonged standing – if we are not moving about our muscles don't squeeze the veins and so it is more difficult to move the blood uphill to the heart
  - pregnancy – the enlarging womb squashes and narrows the veins, making it more difficult for blood to come up from the legs to the heart; the increased amount of blood in the veins damages the valves, making varicose veins more likely

Treatment
- With small varicose veins, resting as much as possible with the feet up helps.
- Taking a more active role at work and changing tasks so that prolonged standing is avoided is worth trying.
- Don't scratch areas of irritation.
- Wear support tights or stockings.

The Doctor
- May be able to help by prescribing stockings, or dressings and ointments to decrease itching.
- X-ray tests may be necessary to reveal the pattern of veins in the legs.
- Surgery and/or injections may be helpful.
- The vein may be removed. This is not as bad as it sounds, and does not involve long incisions but several little ones, through which a long wire hook is inserted to pull out the veins below the skin. This is called stripping the vein.
- A chemical may be injected into particular veins to stop blood getting into those veins. This does not always work and is not suitable for all veins, particularly those higher up the leg.
- You can expect to be wearing bandages or stockings for six weeks after surgery and to be off work for about a month.
- Unfortunately, despite treatment, varicose ulceration can still occur and about one in ten people have a recurrence of varicose veins in later life.

Verrucas

Many people have spent hours with their feet either soaking in bowls of liquid or having their feet dug about quite unnecessarily because of verrucas. These are no more than a simple wart which, because of its position on the sole of the foot, is pushed flat into the skin. In themselves they do not generally cause as much in the way of symptoms as the hard skin which may develop around them. Many myths surround verruca treatment, including soaking a potato in vinegar and applying twice daily to the wart. This, like so many other treatments, false or real, is unnecessary as they will always go away by themselves.

Symptoms
* Hardened, flat area of skin.
* Varying size from one spot to a cluster which is merely several warts together.
* White or brown colour.
* Pain on walking, but often painless.
* As seen for warts, if the verruca is cut, black splinter-like spots can be seen in it; these are blood vessels and

help to distinguish verrucas from corns. (See **Corns**.)

Causes
- Viral infection. (See **Warts**.)

Treatment
- No treatment is recommended for children under five. If the children are older, and the verruca has been present for more than six months, treatment should only be carried out if there is considerable pain and discomfort.
- Local paints can be applied as for warts on the hands. (See **Warts**.) These should be applied after a bath, the skin and the verruca being rubbed with a pumice stone, followed by the application of a special plaster.
- Many people now believe this can do more harm than good. Your doctor may advise you to do nothing, but wait for the natural disappearance of the verruca.
- If necessary, painful, persistent or large verrucas can be dealt with by one of the other treatments mentioned for **Warts**.

Are they infectious?
- Although they are most likely to be picked up in changing rooms or swimming baths from bare feet, many skin doctors think they are not as infectious as once feared.
- Thousands of children have been prevented from swimming because of verrucas, but most schools now do *not* prohibit swimming if you have a verruca.
- Some insist on waterproof plasters, but the extent to which these are effective – or stay on – is variable.
- Routine screening of children for verrucas is unnecessary.

Vertigo

This means a particular type of dizziness with a sensation of spinning, when the whole room seems to move around; it is different from light-headedness. There are many different causes. Although some of these are serious, it is usually a short-lived disturbance of balance which clears up completely.

Symptoms
* It feels as if you or the room are spinning. This is the same feeling as when you have been turning in rapid circles and suddenly stop.
* Depending on the cause, there may be other symptoms, including deafness, ringing in the ears, vomiting, falling over, weakness.
* Vertigo may be brought on by lying down and then getting up, or turning the head suddenly.
* It may follow a head cold or head injury.

Causes
- Viral infection of the balance organ:
  - the dizziness starts suddenly
  - no head position is comfortable
  - it may go on for weeks, but will usually gradually improve over ten days or so
  - shingles is one particular viral infection which may cause vertigo
- Vertigo on lying down or getting up:
  - may follow a head cold or mild head injury
  - may only happen in certain positions, e.g. head tilted backwards
  - commonest in middle age
  - gets better after several weeks or months
- Vertigo on turning head round:
  - commonest in elderly people with arthritis in the neck

- narrow blood vessels are kinked as the head turns
- blood flow to the balance area of the brain is reduced (see **Neck problems**)

□ Menière's disease:
- sudden severe vertigo with deafness and ringing in the ear (see **Tinnitus**)

□ Drugs:
- especially those for epilepsy
- also some antibiotics, aspirin and alcohol

□ Migraine:
- accompanied by typical headache

□ Epilepsy:
- vertigo may precede a rare form of fit

□ Multiple sclerosis:
- there will already be other signs, such as weakness, numbness or blurred vision

□ Brain tumour:
- this is a very rare cause of vertigo; there will usually be other signs of nerve damage and the symptoms will persist without any improvement

Treatment
- Although most cases are not serious, and full recovery will take place on its own, you should see your doctor as some of the causes of vertigo are serious.
- The unpleasant symptoms can be relieved by tablets. These should not be taken with alcohol, as this increases the drowsiness they can cause. Avoid driving or operating machinery if taking tablets for vertigo.
- A neck collar will be provided if the vertigo is caused by turning the head. This prevents kinking of narrowed blood vessels.
- If the symptoms are caused by drugs, these will be changed or reduced.
- If there are signs of nerve damage, specialist help may be sought from a neurologist, who can investigate for serious causes.

Viral illness

Increasingly, doctors are using the words 'viral illness' to describe a number of different complaints. Germs causing infections may be either viruses or bacteria. Bacterial infections are treated by taking antibiotics. Viral infections cannot be treated, antibiotics having no effect on them. In many viral infections, particularly in children, antibiotics will however, be described. This is because it is usually impossible to tell immediately whether a virus or a bacteria, is responsible for the infection. The body's own defence mechanisms normally cope adequately with viral infections, and recovery takes place regardless of any antibiotics.

The important role of viruses in causing so many infections has only recently come to be understood. The fact that the body normally copes with minor viral infections adequately is illustrated by the normal recovery from a common cold (see **Colds**). The fact that treatment aimed at viruses is difficult can be seen with the problems involved in treating the AIDS virus. In some special instances, such as the herpes virus, treatment has been developed which is effective. This drug, called acyclovir, helps in the treatment of this particular infection, but for the vast numbers of other viruses there is no treatment. (See **AIDS, Colds, Flu, Genital herpes, Shingles**).

Symptoms
* Some viruses produce a regular pattern of symptoms. Examples discussed elsewhere are measles, mumps, chicken pox and herpes infections.

* Viruses may also produce symptoms of conjunctivitis, hepatitis, meningitis, tonsillitis and glandular fever. All these conditions are also discussed elsewhere.
* Less specific symptoms caused by viruses include:
  - cold symptoms (see **Colds**)
  - fever for twenty-four hours
  - stomach and bowel upsets (see **Gastroenteritis**)
  - a wide variety of rashes (see **Rashes**)

Causes

□ There are at least twenty different families of virus which commonly cause symptoms in this country. For each family of virus there may be as many as a hundred or more related viruses.

□ When you have been infected with a virus you do develop some immunity to that particular virus in the future. This partly explains why older people have fewer colds and viral infections than children.

Treatment

● Because there is no specific treatment for viral infections, treatment must be aimed at the symptoms.
● Most of the above illnesses, their symptoms and treatment, are described elsewhere.
● Of all the measures taken to treat viral infections in children the most important factors to consider are:
  - control of fever to avoid fits (see **Convulsions, febrile**)
  - control of body fluids to avoid dehydration, particularly in gastroenteritis (see **Gastroenteritis in infants**)

The Doctor

● If an adult or child has an infection which cannot be positively identified as either bacterial or viral in origin, an antibiotic may be prescribed, depending on the circumstances. Use of an antibiotic may prevent a simple throat infection being complicated by a later ear infection, for example.
● In adults it may be appropriate to await the improvement likely with a viral infection, or possible worsening of a bacterial infection, before starting to take antibiotics.
● Laboratory tests can identify viruses, but these are not as widely available as tests to identify bacteria. The tests to identify viruses may take longer to complete, by which time the illness is often over. Some tests, e.g. looking at fluid from skin blisters, use powerful microscopes to identify at once the virus causing the illness. Unfortunately, identification of the actual virus will continue to have little effect on treatment until satisfactory medicines to deal with viral infections are developed.

Post-viral syndrome

A few people suffer an extremely debilitating illness following viral infections. This may have a number of different features, including muscle pains, extreme tiredness and lethargy. Depression may be profound. It may last a variable amount of time but some may still feel unwell one year later. The exact nature and best treatment for this group of symptoms is not established.

Vitamin deficiency

Most people in this country eat a diet which contains adequate vitamins. Except in certain specific circumstances vitamin deficiency is very unlikely to occur, and even marginal vitamin deficiency should not be treated by taking vitamin pills. A varied diet of fresh food provides all the vitamins that are required and can rapidly correct most mild deficiencies. Excessive use of vitamins, in particular vitamins A and D, can have serious consequences.

Symptoms

* Do not usually occur until deficiency is well advanced.
* Vitamin B deficiency can lead to numbness and pain in hands and feet.
* Vitamin C deficiency can lead to coarse skin, internal bleeding, stiff limbs, bleeding gums (scurvy).
* Vitamin D deficiency can lead to rickets; other bone changes may occur in adults and the elderly (note: excesses of vitamin D are dangerous).

Risk groups

Some people are undoubtedly more at risk than others. Those at risk include:
- Those on special diets.
- Vegans.
- Elderly people on inadequate diets.
- Faddists.
- Premature infants, especially if weight was below 1.5 kg at birth.
- Dark-skinned infants not exposed to adequate sunlight.
- Those with difficulty absorbing vitamin B12 due to stomach abnormalities or following stomach operations. This leads to pernicious anaemia (see **Anaemia**). (The liver normally contains nearly three years' supply of vitamin B12.)
- Anorexics.
- Alcoholics.
- Vagrants.

What is an adequate diet?

- A diet which is varied and contains fresh fruit and vegetables, dairy products, eggs, meat or fish, and wholemeal cereals will contain adequate vitamins.
- The preparation of food is important; prolonged boiling or warming destroys vitamins. Mashing destroys vitamin C as air reaches it. Prolonged storage also decreases vitamin C content. Never boil green vegetables in water containing sodium bicarbonate; although this preserves colour, it destroys most of the vitamins.
- Potatoes are an important source of vitamin C. Boil and eat them with their jackets on, as the vitamin C is just below the skin.
- The Chinese way of eating is an excellent way of ensuring a good supply of vitamins, pieces of meat serving as a garnish for quantities of cereals and vegetables.

Treatment

Treatment with vitamin supplements should be limited to the following situations:

● *Pregnancy*. Folic acid deficiency is unusual in pregnancy but may occur where there is an inadequate diet. Folic acid is frequently given with iron preparations (see **Pregnancy problems**). Women who have previously had a child with a neural tube problem, e.g. spina bifida, can reasonably take multi-vitamins – starting about twenty-five days before planned conception until about ten weeks of pregnancy. Whether this has a preventive effect is the subject of a large-scale study taking place currently.

● *The newborn*. Vitamin D may be required if a breast-fed child is deprived of sunlight (Abidec 0.3 mls daily would be suitable.) Vitamin E need only be given to premature infants weighing below 1.5 kg. Artificial feeds are required by law to

contain enough vitamins for the baby's needs. Goat's milk is deficient in folate.
- *Infants*. Breast milk contains sufficient vitamins to cover most needs in infancy. Vitamin K is sometimes given at birth by injection; this may help in the prevention of bleeding problems.
- *Children*. Small supplements of vitamin D may be necessary for children who are exposed to little sunlight, who are severely handicapped and housebound, or children taking certain drugs for convulsions. (Asian children eating chapattis may also need supplements of calcium (see **Bowlegs**.)) Overdoses of cod-liver oil or halibut-liver oil can be dangerous. It is not required if the diet is adequate.
- *Adults*. Very few adults require regular vitamin supplements, but they should be considered in the risk groups mentioned above.

The Doctor
- May prescribe vitamins, but can only do so when there is a potential or actual deficiency.
  - May arrange blood tests, e.g. to establish deficiency of vitamin B12. Stomach operations may lead to difficulty in absorbing vitamin B12. This is due to the absence of a chemical called 'intrinsic factor', which is needed to help absorption of vitamin B12. Its absence leads to pernicious anaemia.
  - Certain drugs prescribed for other conditions (e.g. tuberculosis or epilepsy) may lead to vitamin deficiency. Your doctor will prescribe vitamins to prevent the deficiency if necessary.

Vomiting

This is the process by which stomach contents are expelled through the mouth. In small children it can be dangerous as it may lead to excessive loss of fluids, leading to dehydration. In adults vomiting is rarely dangerous unless the vomit is inhaled. The most frequent causes of vomiting are not serious, but vomiting may indicate a more serious illness almost anywhere in the body.

Causes
- If there is an irritant or unpleasant substance in the stomach vomiting will occur. Alcohol excess or food poisoning are common examples. (See **Alcoholism**, **Gastritis**, **Gastroenteritis**.)
- Vomiting is common in children. It may happen as part of an infection, such as gastroenteritis, or occur with a heavy cold or cough. It may be seen with ear or throat infections. (See **Colds**, **Ear problems**.)
- In both adults and children more serious illness such as meningitis, urine infection or intestinal problem may cause vomiting. (See **Appendicitis**, **Ulcers**, **Urine infection**.)
- Disturbance of the balance organ through motion or infection may cause vomiting. (See **Travel sickness**.)
- Drugs may cause vomiting, both when prescribed and when abused. Glue-sniffing may also cause vomiting. (See **Drug abuse**, **Glue-sniffing**.)
- Liver problems, gallstones and kidney stones may cause vomiting. (See **Gallstones**, **Jaundice**.)
- Pelvic infection, pregnancy and gynaecological problems may cause vomiting. (See **Pelvic infection**, **Pregnancy problems**.)
- Headaches may be accompanied by vomiting. (See **Head injuries**, **Migraine**.)

- Cancer in the brain or elsewhere may cause vomiting.

Treatment
- The dangers of dehydration and inhalation when someone is vomiting should always be considered. This is particularly true of young infants, who may become dehydrated rapidly. Always seek a doctor's advice if vomiting is prolonged or fluids cannot be replaced. (See also **Diarrhoea**.)
- Treatment of separate causes of vomiting is not considered here.
- Treatment of the person who is vomiting may be helped by adapting the following tips to the particular circumstances:
  - most people prefer to be left alone
  - water can be taken after vomiting to rinse out the mouth
  - have a sponge or tissue to hand to wipe the mouth and chin
  - dispose of vomit quickly to avoid the smell causing further distress
  - if a vomiting person is drowsy ensure the head is lower than the body and lie them on their side to avoid inhalation of vomit
  - avoid solid food but encourage water or weak fruit drinks to be drunk in sufficient quantities to replace lost body fluids

The Doctor
- Will attend to the cause where appropriate (see above).
- Anti-vomiting drugs may be given by injection, suppository, or tablets. They may work either by affecting the brain or by altering the way the stomach empties. Often the vomiting settles on its own without the medicines being required.
- Anti-vomiting drugs are not normally given to infants or children, treatment being aimed at the cause.
- As you recover from vomiting, avoid alcohol or foods that may have started it. Keep to foods you know will settle on your stomach well. Boiled rice (perhaps flavoured with lemon or beef extract), bananas, stewed apples without sugar, and bread, may all be suitable. Stick to water or very weak drinks. Avoid coffee and tea initially. Flat, clear drinks are usually better tolerated than fizzy ones.

Warts

These are small, harmless growths that appear on the skin. Often appearing suddenly, they are unsightly but not, in any way, a danger. Many myths surround warts and their treatment. They do not lead to cancer, nor does swinging a cat in a churchyard make them go away. They do, however, go away by themselves, although it may take up to two years. Sometimes interfering with warts is more likely to spread them than cure them. They are common in children but rare beyond forty-five years of age; wart-like growths appearing after this age should be checked by your doctor.

Symptoms
* Common warts often appear on the hands.
* They may spread to produce crops of warts on several fingers and both hands; knees are often also affected.
* They vary in size from pinheads to large peas.
* Little black spots looking rather like splinters can often be seen in the wart. These are blood vessels, which can be seen more easily if the wart is shaved.

Causes
- Viral infection.
- The body fights viral infections and in

doing so builds up resistance to infection. It is thought that this may explain why warts are less common as we grow older.
- You may have caught the wart anything from one to six months or more before it appears.
- They are passed by touch or contact with shed skin.

Treatment
- They will go by themselves eventually. In children and young adolescents it is often best to wait for them to go naturally.
- If a treatment is made necessary by the appearance, teachers or teasing friends there are several methods to choose from.
- Start with a wart paint, and try one containing salicyclic acid first, as these are generally more effective:
  - avoid normal skin – this can be protected with vaseline
  - do not use on face or on genital warts
  - can be combined with gentle abrasion, but not such as to produce bleeding, to improve appearance
  - treatment if started will sometimes have to be continued daily for more than eight weeks to make a significant impression on the wart

The Doctor
- Often older children can have other treatments available from the doctor. These may not be suitable for the young as they can be painful. They include:
  - freezing – your general practitioner or skin doctor may be able to do this
  - burning – can be painful and unpleasant
  - scraping – only suitable for some warts
- All these treatments may need to be repeated as warts recur or new ones appear.
- Always remember that warts will go by themselves, so the smooth white stone, in a plain brown paperbag, at the crossroads, on the night of a full moon, may not be necessary.

Warts, genital

These are small cauliflower-like growths that appear anywhere around the genital area in men or women. They are ordinary warts but you should always see your doctor for advice. They are infectious but not serious. If you have genital warts you will usually be advised to have a cervical smear each year. This does *not* mean that genital warts cause cervical cancer, merely that more changes are seen on the smear tests of those who have had genital warts than others.

Symptoms
* They vary in size from small dots or lumps in the skin to larger growths.
* They often grow rapidly to form clusters like a bunch of tiny grapes.
* Pregnancy often makes their growth even more rapid.
* They can be uncomfortable or painful.
* They may recur even after treatment. Partners' warts must be treated at the same time.
* They can be itchy.

Causes
- Genital warts are a viral infection.
- They are infectious, usually being spread by touch.
- (See **Warts**.)

The Doctor
- Can organise effective treatment and should always be consulted.
- Paints of podophyllin applied twice

weekly and left on for four to six hours are usually effective (prescription required). However:
- care has to be taken with normal skin, protecting with vaseline if necessary
- overuse of paints applied by yourself or others can cause skin reactions
- do not use podophyllin in pregnancy
- Freezing or other techniques (see **Warts**) can also be used. If the warts are numerous and widespread a general anaesthetic is, rarely, needed.

Whooping cough

This is a highly infectious disease of the breathing passages caused by bacteria. It affects babies and children under five most severely. Older children may also catch it. The illness can last for up to four months from first symptoms to recovery. Many babies need to be in hospital, and a few die each year. Whooping cough can be prevented by immunisation. There are epidemics every few years, when many more children are infected. The outbreaks have been much worse since people became hesitant about having their children immunised.

Symptoms
* Symptoms begin one or two weeks after contact.
* The diagnosis is uncertain during the runny-nose stage.
* This consists of a dry cough, cold and temperature. It lasts for two weeks and is the most infectious stage.
* The coughing stage lasts for another six weeks or even longer.
* There are many coughing spasms each day, which may last for up to half a minute.
* The child struggles to cough up plugs of sticky mucus.
* The face goes bright red and the eyes bulge.
* Vomiting is common and the child may become dehydrated.
* The coughing is ended by the typical whoop, a high-pitched sound as the child suddenly breathes in. Small babies do not produce it.
* Afterwards the child is exhausted.
* Little pinprick spots may appear in the face and eyes, which are not important in themselves.
* Brain haemorrhages are rare but serious, and may cause paralysis or even death.
* Lack of oxygen due to breathing difficulties may cause bad fits.
* The lungs may be infected with other germs causing pneumonia, and long-term lung damage may occur.
* The strain of coughing may cause hernias which need operation in later life.
* The child normally gets better over another two to six weeks.

Causes
- Most cases, and all severe cases, are caused by one specific germ.
- There is life-long immunity to this after one attack.

Prevention
- Immunisation is normally given as a course of three injections, starting from around three months and usually completed within the first year of life. Some degree of protection is afforded by each injection.
- Widespread immunisation is needed to wipe out the infection. This is the only protection available to small babies and children who cannot be immunisation because of contraindications like epilepsy.
- Small babies are not protected by their mothers having had whooping cough, and are also most at risk.

- Isolate a child with whooping cough during the infectious period. This is from seven days after contact until three weeks after coughing spasms start.
- An antibiotic, erythromycin, can be given to infants in contact with whooping cough. This helps prevent disease and it can be given during the catarrhal phase to reduce severity.
- It is of no use once coughing spasms start.

Treatment
- Contact your doctor, as this can be a serious infection.
- Your doctor will decide if your child needs to be in hospital.
- All newborn babies and most small babies need to be in hospital.
- Severe attacks in hospital will require oxygen, tube-feeding and physiotherapy to help with breathing.
- Keep the room at constant warm temperature to reduce coughing attacks, and humidify the air. (See **Croup**.)
- Give plenty of warm drinks.
- If pneumonia develops, antibiotics will be given.
- If your child has a fit, call your doctor or go to the hospital at once. After immediate treatment for the fit, your child will need to remain in hospital.

Wrist pain and tingling fingers

The commonest cause of wrist pain and tingling fingers is called carpal tunnel syndrome. The carpal tunnel is the narrow passage between the wrist bones and the skin. The nerves to the hands pass through this passage. Swelling in the tunnel leads to pressure on the nerves and consequent symptoms. It is common in pregnancy due to fluid retention, and may also occur frequently in middle-aged women, especially around the menopause. It is not usually serious, but the pain can be severe. Effective treatment is available if it does not clear on its own.

Symptoms
* Pain felt in the the wrists and shooting up the arms.
* Tingling and numbness, particularly affecting the thumb and first and second fingers.
* Pain is often worst at night, and may be relieved by shaking the hands.
* Both hands may be affected.
* If persistent and severe, weakness of the thumb may develop.

Causes
- Swelling inside the carpal tunnel may be caused by fluid retention. The fluid accumulates inside the tunnel and exerts pressure on the nerve as it passes to the hand.
- Repetitive use of the wrist joint may exacerbate carpal tunnel syndrome.

Treatment
- It may clear on its own without any specific treatment.
- If troublesome in pregnancy, it usually resolves after childbirth.
- A splint or strapping applied to the wrist may help. This can be worn at night if not practical during the day.
- If severe, seek help from your doctor.

The Doctor
- May prescribe a diuretic to decrease fluid if there is fluid retention.
- A steroid injection may help, particularly if there is local swelling due to an inflammation in the tendons. (See **Shoulder pain**.)
- An operation is possible to slit the

encircling tissue that forms the tunnel. This relieves the pressure on the contents of the tunnel. It can be very effective, but is only usually carried out if symptoms are extremely persistent.

Index

Note: Page numbers in bold type refer to main entries

A

abdomen *see* stomach
abdominal migraine, 149
abdominal operation for hysterectomy, 131
abnormal cervical smear, 49–51
abortion, **179–80**
  and PID, 163
abscesses
  in breast tissue (mastitis), **37–8**, 39
  and drug abuse, 80
  in mouth and gums, 27
    and sinusitis, 200
  see also boils
absence seizures, 89
ACCEPT (Addictions Community Centres for Education, Prevention, Treatment and Research), 7, 81
aches and pains
  and anxiety, 14
  and colds, 55
  in joints and muscles, and glandular fever, 108
  and raised temperature, 220
  and too little thyroid, 230
acne, **1–2**
  see also boils; hair problems; skin problems
acute bronchitis, **44–5**
  and cough, 64
  see also cough(s); pneumonia
acute cholecystitis (gallbladder infection), 102
addiction *see* drug(s), addiction; tranquilliser addiction
adenoids, **2–3**
  and glue ear, 84
  and infection of middle ear, 85
  see also cough(s); glue ear; tonsillitis
adolescence
  and anorexia nervosa, **12–14**
  and breasts, **41–2**
  and school refusal, **190–1**
  and stretch marks in girls, 213–14
  and twisted testicles, 224
  see also puberty
agaraphobia and anxiety, 15
aggression
  and alcoholism, 5
  and drug abuse, 79
  and hyperactivity, 129
  towards baby, 23
AID (artificial insemination by donor), 137
AIDS (acquired immune deficiency syndrome), **3–5**
  and drug abuse, 80
  and ear-piercing, 82
  and pneumonia, 172
  testing for, 4
  as viral illness, 250
AIH (artificial insemination by husband), 137
A1 Anon Family Groups, 7
alcohol
  and bad breath, 27
  for cold hands and feet, 56
  and duodenal ulcer, 240
  and headache, 116
  and hiatus hernia, 125
  and hoarseness, 128
  and impotence, 191–2
  and indigestion, 135
  and infertility, 135
  and irritable colon, 138
  and jaundice, 141
  and nightmares, 203
  and palpitations, 162
  and stomach ulcer, 240
  for tremor, 238
  see also alcoholism
Alcohol Concern, 7
alcoholism, **5–7**
  and confusion, 60
  and dementia, 73
  and gastritis, 103
  and high blood pressure, 34
  and jaundice, 141
  and liver damage, 141
  and vitamin deficiency, 252
  and vomiting, 253
  see also alcohol; headaches; tranquilliser addiction
Alexander technique for backache, 26
allergies, **7–8**
  and asthma, 19, 20
  and bites and stings, 32
  and blisters, 33
  and conjunctivitis, 60, 61
  and ear-piercing, 82
  and gastroenteritis, 104
  and hayfever, 114–15
  and hyperactivity, 129
  and itching, 139
  and painful intercourse, 193–4
  and rashes, 186
  and shock, *see* anaphylactic shock
  see also asthma; eczema; gastroenteritis; hayfever; hives
alopecia (patchy hair loss), 112
Alzheimer's disease (pre-senile dementia), **72–4**
Alzheimer's Disease Society, 74

amenorrhoea (absence of periods), **166**
amnesia (memory loss)
  and dementia, 72
  and head injury, 117
anaemia, **8–10**
  and duodenal ulcer, 239
  and heavy periods, 168
  and hysterectomy, 131
  and jaundice, 141
  and palpitations, 162
  pernicious, 9
  and pregnancy, **174–5**
  sickle-cell, 9
    and gallstones, 102
  and stomach ulcer, 240
  and vitamin deficiency, 252
  see also arthritis; constipation; periods; pregnancy problems; ulcers
anaesthetic, general, for repair of broken bones, 42
anaphylactic shock, 196
  and stings, 33
  and severe allergic reaction, 8, 115
anger
  and bereavement, 28
  and drug abuse, 79
  and mania, 144
angina (heart pain in chest), **10–11**
  and cramp, 67
  and heart attack, 119–20
  see also blood pressure, high; obesity; stress
animal bites and stings, **32–3**
ankle(s)
  broken, 43
  sprain, 208
  swelling, 12
    and chronic bronchitis, 45
    and heart failure, 121
    and high blood pressure, 35
    and PMT, 181
    see also arthritis; pregnancy, problems; thrombosis; varicose veins
anorexia nervosa, **12–14**
  and amenorrhoea, 166
  and vitamin deficiency, 252
  see also bulimia nervosa
anti-social behaviour and hyperactivity, 129–30
anus (back passage)
  and cystitis, 70
  infections, and gonorrhoea, 110
  itching, 139
  stinging, tingling, itching and genital herpes, 106
  unexplained bleeding from, and cancer, 47
anxiety, **14–16**
  and alcoholism, 6
  and baby blues/post-natal depression, 22
  and breast development in adolescence, 42
  and depression, 74
  and high blood pressure, 33–4
  and hyperactivity, 130
  and indigestion, 134
  and menopause, 148
  and migraine, 150
  and nightmares, 203
  and school refusal, 190
  and painful intercourse, 194
  and sleep problems, 201
  and stress, **212–13**
  and tension, 221
  and too much thyroid, 230
  and tranquilliser addiction, 236
  and tremor, 238
  see also blood pressure, high; depression; school refusal; sleep problems; thyroid
apathy and bereavement, 28
appendicitis, **16–17**
  and gastroenteritis, 104
  and vomiting, 253
appendix, grumbling, 17
  see also colon, irritable
appetite
  decreased/loss of
    and anaemia, 9
    and baby blues/post-natal depression, 23
    and cancer, 47
    and depression, 74
    and drug abuse, 79
    and flu, 97
    and glandular fever, 108
    and glue sniffing, 109
    and heart failure, 121
    and heatstroke, 122
    and mumps, 153
    and raised temperature, 220
    and rheumatoid arthritis, 18
    and stress, 212
    and travel sickness, 237
    and stomach ulcer, 240
  increased, with weight loss, and too much thyroid, 230
arm(s)
  aching, and flu, 97
  broken, 43
  jerking of, and epilepsy, 89–90
  pains in
    and alcoholism, 6
    and backache, 24
    and heart attack, 119
  pins and needles in, 170
  -pits
    fungus infection in, 22
    sweat rash and itching, 140
  rashes, 186
  and scarlet fever, 188
  swelling under, and glandular fever, 108
arteries
  furring up of, and angina, 10, 11
  and high blood pressure, 33
  narrow, and stroke, 215
arteriosclerosis, 67
  and heart attack, 120
Arthritis and Rheumatism Council, 19
Arthritis Care, 19
arthritis (joint diseases), **17–19**

260

and anaemia, 9
and ankle-swelling, 12
and dislocation, 78
and finger swelling, 187
and gastritis, 103
of hip, and limp, 142
in neck, and vertigo, 249
and NSU, 159
and obesity, 160
osteo- (wear-and-tear), **17–18**
and psoriasis, 184
rheumatoid (inflammatory), **18–19**
and shoulder pain, 197
in spine, and pins and needles, 170
and swelling, 88–9
artificial feeds for babies, and constipation, 61
Asians
 and Mongolian blue spots, 30
 and rickets in children, 37
asphyxia and fits, 90
Association for Post-Natal Illness, 23
Association of Breast-feeding Mothers, 40
Association of Continence Advisors, 133
asthma, **19–22**
 and allergy to pollen, 8
 and beta-blocking drugs, 16, 35
 and cough, 64
 and eczema, 86
 and flu, 97
athlete's foot, 22
aura, migraine, 150

B

babies/infants, problems and illnesses
 abdominal migraine, 149–50
 anaemia in pregnancy, 174
 anxiety of mother, 15
 asphyxia, 90
 bedwetting in reaction to arrival of, 28
 birthmarks on, **30–2**
 bottle-fed, and gastroenteritis, 104–5
 bowlegs in, 37
 breast-feeding problems, 40
 breathing problems and bronchiolitis, 44
 bronchiolitis, **43–4**
 cataracts, 49
 chicken pox, 52, 53
 clicky hips, **126–7**
 colds, 54
 colic, **57–8**
 comforters, **58–9**
 congenital dislocation of hips, **126–7**
 constipation, 61, 105
 convulsions, febrile, **62–4**
 cradle cap, 66
 croup, **67–8**
 diarrhoea, 78
  see also gastroenteritis in infants
 epilepsy, 90
 episiotomy, **91–2**
 eye infection and gonorrhoea, 110
 fits, 90
 foreign body in nose, **98–9**
 foreskin problems, **98–101**
 gastroenteritis, **104–6**
 glue ear, **83–4**
 groin hernia, 123–4
 hair loss, patchy, 112
 Hirschsprung's disease, 62
 impetigo, **132**
 infection of middle ear, 85
 irritable hip and limp, 142–3
 jaundice, **141–2**
 knock knees, 142
 measles, **145–6**
 meningitis, **146–7**
 mouth ulcers, **152–3**
 mumps, **153–4**
 nappy rash, **155–6**
 pneumonia, **171–3**
 premature, low vitamin stores in, 37
 prevention of obesity, 161–2
 raised blood pressure in pregnancy, 175–6
 rickets, 37
 risk of catching AIDS during pregnancy and birth, 4
 scarlet fever, **188**
 soft spot, 206
 speech difficulty, 206–7
 squint, 208–9
 sticky eyes, 61, **93–4**
 tantrums, **217–19**
 teething, **219–20**
 umbilical hernia, **124–5**
 umbilical problems, **241–2**
 unborn, and German measles, 107–8
 undescended testicles, **224–5**
 viral illness, 97, 251
 vitamin deficiency, 252–3
 wakefulness, **204–6**
 whooping cough, **256–7**
 see also childbirth; pregnancy problems
baby blues, 22–3, 74
 see also post-natal depression
back
 -ache, **24–6**
  and arthritis in spine, and pins and needles, 170
  and chicken pox, 53
  and cystitis, 69
  and flu, 97
  and prolapsed disc (slipped disc), 24, 26
  and sciatica (nerve pain, a.k.a. sciatica), 24, 26
  and urine infection, 243
  see also arthritis; neck, stiff and painful
 Mongolian blue spots on lower, 30
 pain
  and gallstones, 102
  and gastritis, 103
  and painful periods, 167
 passage see anus
Back Pain Association, 26
bacterial infection, **35–6**, 55, 82
 see also boils; ear-piercing

261

BACUP (British Association of Cancer United
    Patients), 48
bad breath, 26–7
  see also mouth ulcers; tonsillitis; toothache
balanitis (infection of tip of penis), 99
  and painful intercourse, 193
baldness, 113
Bartholin's cyst
  and painful intercourse, 193
  and vagina, swelling at entrance, 244
bat ears (protruding ears), 83
bed
  -bugs, 32
    crabs, 65–6
    scabies, 187
  rest for backache, 25
  -wetting (enuresis), 27–8
    see also incontinence
bee stings, 32
behaviour problems
  and deafness, 71
  and dementia, 73
  and drug abuse, 79
  and hyperactivity, 129–30
  tantrums, 217–19
belching
  and hiatus hernia, 125
  and indigestion, 134
bereavement, 28–30
  and amenorrhoea, 166
birth see childbirth
birthmarks, 30–2
  brown (simple), mole, 30
  café au lait spot, 30
  Mongolian blue spots, 30
  port wine stain, 31
  stork mark (salmon patch), 31
  strawberry naevus (*cavernous haemangioma*),
    31–2
bites, 32–3
  and blisters, 33
  insect, 32–3
    and hives, 127
  and stings, 32–3
black tongue, 233
bladder problems
  and backache, 24, 25
  and bedwetting, 27–8
  incontinence, 132–3
  inflammation of (cystitis), 69–71
  urine infection, 242–4
  and vaginal irritation, 246
bleeding
  birthmarks/moles
    brown (simple) mole, 30
      cancer, 47
    strawberry naevus (*cavernous haemangioma*), 31–2
  cancers, 9
  and circumcision, 99–100
  cracked nipple from breast-feeding, 40, 41
  cuts, 68–9
  duodenal ulcers, 239–40
  after intercourse and cervical erosion, 52
  between periods and cervical erosion, 52

and foreign body in nose, 99
internally (subarachnoid haemorrhage) and
    headache, 116
menstrual, see periods
miscarriage, 151–2
nosebleeds, 159–60
post-menopausal
  and cancer, 47
  and cervical cancer, 51
  and cervical erosion, 52
and rash, 186
rectal, and piles, 168–9
and stomach ulcers, 240–1
ulcers, 9
unexplained
  from back passage, and cancer, 47
  from urine passage, and cancer, 47
and vaginal discharge, 246–7
of varicose veins, 247
see also blood; cuts; haemorrhage; wounds
blisters, 33
  from burns, 46, 47
  from chicken pox, 53
  from chilblains, 53–4
  from cold sores, 56–7
  from eczema, 86–7
  from genital herpes, 106
  from rashes, 186
  from shingles, 195–6
  from sunburn, 216
bloating
  and irritable colon, 138
  and PMT, 181
blocked duct, in breast-feeding, 40
blood
  AIDS from infected, 4
  and anti-arthritic drugs, 19
  blister and painful nails, 155
  changes in, from chemotherapy, 48
  and cuts, grazes and wounds, 68–9
  loss and head injury, 118
  pressure, high (hypertension), 33–5
    and alcoholism, 6
    and angina, 11
    and ankle-swelling, 12
    and anxiety, 14
    essential hypertension, 34
    and fits, 63
    and headache, 116
    and obesity, 160
    in pregnancy, 175–6
    secondary hypertension, 34
    and stroke, 90
    see also pregnancy problems
  pressure, low, and shock, 196
  production problems (anaemia), 8–10
  in saliva, and cancer, 47
  sugar and diabetes, 75–7
  supply limited
    to muscles (angina), 10–11
    to skin, and chilblains, 53
  supply to hands and feet sensitive to cold,
    55
  and swollen testicles after injury, 222–3

262

transfusion
  and AIDS, 4
  and jaundice, 141
vessel(s)
  blood clot in, and heart attack, 120
  changes, and migraine, 150
  and cramp, 67
  disease
    and high blood pressure, 34
    and stroke, 215
  malformations and birthmarks, 32
  narrowing of, 67
  stroke from blockage/breakage of, in brain, **214–15**
body fluids, loss of
  from burns, 46–7
  from heatstroke, 122
body temperature system, upset by heatstroke, 122
boils, **35–7**
  and acne, 1
  and drug abuse, 80
  in ear canal, 81
  staphylococcus food poisoning, 104
  and styes, 94–5
  see also abscesses
bone(s)
  broken, **42–3**
  disease and bowlegs, 37
  infection (osteomyelitis), and limp, 142–3
boredom and glue sniffing, 109
bottle-fed babies and gastroenteritis, 104–5
bowel problems
  alteration of regular pattern, and cancer, 47
  constipation, 61–2
  diarrhoea, 77–8
  impairment of control, backache, 24, 25
  irritable colon, **138–9**
bowlegs, **36–7**
  and knock knees, 142
brain
  cancer in, and vomiting, 254
  chemical factors in
    and anorexia nervosa, 13
    and hyperactivity, 129
    and tics, 231
  damage/injury
    and alcoholism, 6
    at birth and deafness, 71
    and epilepsy, 90
    and head injury, **117–18**
  dementia, 73
  haemorrhage and whooping cough, 256
  infection of linings *see* meningitis
  inflammation
    and fits, 63
    and measles, 145–6
  and shock, 196
  and stroke, 214–16
  tumours
    and confusion, 60
    and dementia, 73
    and epilepsy, 90
    and fits, 63, 90

  and headache, 117
  and vertigo, 250
breast problems, 37–42
  and adolescence, **41–2**
  blocked duct, 40
  cancer
    lumps, 38–9
    screening for, 48
  discomfort and menopause, 148
  engorgement, 40–1
  feeding, **39–41**
    and amenorrhoea, 166
    and asthma, 20
    and colic, 57
    and epilepsy, 91
    and gastroenteritis, 105
    and irregular periods, 165
  infection (mastitis), **37–8**
  lumps, **38–9**
    in puberty, 41
  milk, risk, of catching AIDS through, 4
  tenderness
    in adolescence (pubertal mastitis), 41
    and PMT, 181
breath, bad, **26–7**
  see also mouth ulcers; tonsillitis; toothache
breathing problems
  and acute bronchitis, 45
  and adenoids, 2
  and AIDS, 3
  and allergy, 8
  and anaemia, 9
    in pregnancy, 174
  and angina, 11
  and ankle swelling, 12
  and anxiety, 14–15
  and asthma, **19–22**
  and bronchiolitis, 43–4
  and chronic bronchitis, 45
  and croup, 67–8
  and heart attack, 120
  and heart failure, 121
  and hives, 127
  increased (hyperventilation), **130**
  and palpitations, 162
  and pleurisy, 171
  and pneumonia, 172
  and poisoning, 173
  and shock, 196
  and tantrums, 217
British Association for the Hard of Hearing, 72
British Deaf Association, 72
British Diabetic Association, 77
British Epilepsy Association, 91
British Heart Foundation, 35
British Migraine Association, 151
British Pregnancy Advisory Service, 180
broken bones, **42–3**
  and sprain, 208
  and swelling, 88
bronchiolitis, **43–4**
bronchitis, **44–5**
  and asthma, 19

263

bronchitis Contd.
   and colds, 54, 55
   and cough, 64
   and flu, 97
   and measles, 145
   and pleurisy, 171
   see also cough(s); pneumonia
Brook Advisory Centre, 180
bruising, see skin, bruising
bulimia nervosa, 14
   see also anorexia nervosa
bunions, **45–6**
   and bursitis, 89
   see also corns
burning
   bites and stings, 32
   cold sores, 56
burns, **46–7**
   blisters, 33
   and shock, 196
bursitis, 46
   and elbow pain, 88
   of knee (housemaid's knee), 89
   and shoulder pain, 89
   and swollen elbow, 89
buttocks, Mongolian blue spots on, 30

C

café au lait spot, 30
Cancer Research Campaign, 48
cancer(s), **47—8**
   of brain and vomiting, 254
   of breast
      lumps and, **38–9**
      screening for, 48
   of cervix, **51–2**
      screening for (smear test), 48, 49–51
         abnormal, **49–51**
   and cough, 64
   of intestine, and jaundice, 141
   Kaposi's sarcoma, and AIDS, 3
   leukaemias, 48
   of lymph glands, 48
   of mouth, and alcoholism, 6
   of oesophagus, and alcoholism, 6
   of pancreas, and jaundice, 141
   of prostate gland, 47, **181–2**
      see also prostate
   and shingles, 195
   of stomach, and indigestion, 134
   of testicles, **223–4**
   of throat, and alcoholism, 6
   treatment for
      chemotherapy, 48
      and chicken pox, 52
      radiotherapy, 48, 52
   of vulva, 247
   see also tumours
candida and thrush, 228–9
carbuncle, 35
   see also abscesses; boils

carcinogenics, 47
carcinoma in-situ, 50
carpal tunnel syndrome, 257
CAT scan for fits, 63
cataracts, **48–9**
   see also diabetes; German measles
catarrh
   and allergy, 8
   and colds, 54
   and pneumonia, 172
cavernous haemangioma (birthmark, strawberry
      naevus), 31–2
cerebro-spinal fluid, loss of and head injury,
   118
cervical problems, **49–52**
   abnormal smear, **49–51**
      see also genital herpes; genital warts
   cancer, **51–2**
      screening for, 48, 49–51
   discharge
      cervical cancer, 51
      cervical erosion, 52
   erosion, 52
   and hysterectomy, **130–2**
   and irregular period, 165
   and miscarriage, 152
   removal of cervix and womb, and cervical
      cancer, 52
   and vaginal discharge, 246
   see also vaginal problems
cervical spondylosis (stiff, painful neck), **156–8**
chalazion (swelling inside eyelid), 95
cheeks
   painful, and sinusitis, 200
   swollen, and mumps, 153
chemotherapy for tumours, 48
chest
   aching, and cough, 64
   bubbly noise and heart failure, 121
   heart pain in
      angina, **10–11**
      and heart attacks, 119
      and heart failure, 121
      and palpitations, 162
   infections
      and asthma, 20
      and bronchiolitis, 44
      and bronchitis, 44–5
      and chicken pox, 53
      and meningitis, 147
      and pneumonia and confusion, 60
   spots on, and chicken pox, 53
   tightness in, and asthma, 19
chicken pox, **52–3**
   and itching, 139
   and pneumonia, 172
   and rashes, 186
   and shingles, 196
chilblains, **53–4**
   see also cold hands and feet
childbirth
   and AIDS, risk of babies catching, 4
   anaemia and haemoglobin production prob-
      lems at, 9

and baby blues/post-natal depression, 23, 74
and bowlegs, 37
and brain injury and deafness, 71
and clicky hips/congenital dislocation of hips, 126–7
and deafness, 71
and episiotomy, 91–2
and forceps delivery, 30
and genital herpes, 106–7
having several children at young age, and cervical cancer, 51
and incontinence, 133
lack of oxygen at (asphyxia), 90
manic depression following, 144–5
and painful intercourse, 193
and PID, 163
and piles, 169
skin blemish at see birthmarks
and sticky eyes in infants, 94
thinning of hair in mothers after, 113
children's illnesses and problems
alopecia (patchy hair loss), 112
baby blues/post-natal depression, 23
bat ears, 83
bedwetting, 27–8
bereavement, 29
bowlegs, 36–7
chicken pox, 52–3
colds, 54
cold sores, 56
colour blindness, 58
comforters, 58–9
constipation, 61–2
convulsions, febrile, 62–4
coughs, 65
cradle cap, 66
croup, 67
deafness, 71
diabetes, 76
ear ache, 81
eczema, 86
epilepsy, 89–91
flat feet, 97
foreign body in nose, 98–9
fungal infection, 112
glue ear, 83–4
hair pulling, 112
headlice, 118–19
hyperactivity, 128–9
impetigo, 132
infection of middle ear, 85
irritable hip, and limp, 142
knock knees, 142
limp, 142–3
measles, 145–6
mouth ulcers, 152–3
mumps, 153–4
night terrors, 202
poisoning, 173–4
prevention of obesity, 160–1
raised temperature, 220
rashes, 186
rickets, 37
scarlet fever, 188

schizophrenia, 188
school refusal, 190–1
sleepwalking, 203–4
slipped femoral epiphysis, 143
speech difficulty, 206–7
tantrums, 217–19
threadworms, 225–6
tics, 231–2
tonsillitis, 233–4
travel sickness, 237
urine infection, 243–4
vitamin deficiency, 253
wakefulness, 204–6
whooping cough, 256–7
wry neck, 158
see also babies; infants
chills and heart attack, 120
chlamydia
and NSU, 159
and PID, 163
cholesterol
and angina, 11
and gallstones, 102
cholecystectomy (removal of gallstones), 102
chronic bronchitis, 44–5
and cough, 64
see also cough(s)
cirrhosis (permanent liver-scarring) and alcoholism, 6
cigarette smoke
and chronic bronchitis, 45
and cough, 64
see also smoking
circulation problems
and chilblains, 53–4
and confusion, 60
and cramp, 66–7
in legs, and heart failure, 122
Raynaud's disease see cold hands and feet
circumcision, 99–100
claustrophobia and anxiety, 15
clef palate and glue air, 84
clicky hips and congenital dislocation of hips, 126–7
coccyx, swelling over and heart failure, 121
coxsakie infection, and rash, 186
coffee
and insomnia, 201
and palpitations, 162
coils (intra-uterine contraceptive devices, IUCDs) and heavy periods, 168
cold, feeling
and raised temperature, 220
and too little thyroid, 230
and travel sickness, 237
cold hands and feet (Raynaud's disease), 55–6
and high blood pressure, 35
see also chilblains
colds, 54–5
and acute bronchitis, 44–5
and asthma, 20
and bronchiolitis, 44

colds *Contd.*
  and croup, 68
  and flu, 97
  and German measles, 107
  and headache, 116
  and infection of middle ear, 85
  and measles, 145
  and nosebleeds, 159
  and pneumonia, 172
  and sinusitis, 200
  and raised temperature, 220
  and vertigo, 249
  as viral illness, 250
  and whooping cough, 256
cold sores, **56–7**
  and genital herpes, 106
  and mouth ulcers, 153
colic, **57–8**
colitis and allergy, 8
collarbone, broken, 43
colon, irritable, **138–9**
  and grumbling appendix, 17
colour blindness, 58
coloured phlegm and acute bronchitis, 44–5
colposcopy, 50
coma
  and head injury, 117
  and measles, 146
  and meningitis, 147
comforters, **58–9**
  and colic, 57
Compassionate Friends, The, 30
conceiving difficulties, *see* infertility
concentration decreased/poor
  and alcoholism, 5
  and anxiety, 14
  and hyperactivity, 128–9
  and mania, 144
  and menopause, 148
concussion and head injuries, 117
condoms to reduce risk of AIDS, 4
conductive deafness, 71
cone biopsy, 51
confusion, **59–60**
  and anaemia, 9
  and drug abuse, 80
  and fainting, 96
  and heart failure, 121
  and pneumonia, 172
  and poisoning, 173
  and shock, 196
  in taking Pill, and irregular, unexpected periods, 165
conjunctivitis, **60–1**
  and allergy, 8
  and foreign body in eye, 92
  and general swelling of eyelids, 93
  and sticky eyes in infants, 93–4
consciousness, loss of
  and diabetes, 76
  and epilepsy, 89
  and glue sniffing, 109
  and poisoning, 173
  and shock, 196
  temporary, *see* fainting
  see also coma; concussion; fainting
constipation, **61–2**
  and anaemia, 10
    in pregnancy, 174
  and anorexia nervosa, 12
  and appendicitis, 16
  and drug abuse, 80
  and gastroenteritis in infants, 105
  and irritable colon, 138–9
  and painful intercourse, 194
  and too little thyroid, 230
contact dermatitis
  and eczema, 86
  and itching, 140
convulsions, febrile, **62–4**
  and measles, 146
  and scarlet fever, 188
  and raised temperature, 62–4, 220
coping difficulties
  and baby blues/post-natal depression, 23
  and drug abuse, 79
CORDA (Coronary Artery Disease Research Association), 121
corns, 46, 64
  see also bunions; verrucas; warts
Coronary Prevention Group, 121
cosmetic surgery (plastic surgery) and birthmarks, 31, 32
cough(s), **64–5**
  and acute bronchitis, 44–5
  and adenoids, 2
  and AIDS, 3
  and asthma
    brought on by exercise, 20
    repeated nightly, 19
  and backache, 24
  and broken ribs, 43
  and bronchiolitis, 44
  and cancer, 47
  and chronic bronchitis, 45
  and colds, 54
  and croup, 67–8
  dry, and acute bronchitis, 45
  and flu, 97
  and glue sniffing, 109
  and groin hernia, 123–4
  and incontinence, 132
  and measles, 145
  and para-umbilical hernia, 124
  and pleurisy, 171
  and pneumonia, 172
  and raised temperature, 220
  and tonsillitis, 234
  wet, 64
  wheezy, 64
  whooping, *see* whooping cough
crabs (pubic lice), **65–6**
cradle cap, 66
  and soft spot, 206
cramp, **66–7**
croup, **67–8**
  and measles, 145–6
Cruse-Bereavement Care, 29

crying
  and eye problems, 92
  and nappy rash, 155
and wakefulness in children and babies, 205
cuts, 68–9
  in birthmarks, 30, 31
  and head injury, 118
  see also bleeding
cystic fibrosis and pneumonia, 172
cystitis, 69–71
  and incontinence, 133
  and urine infection, 242–3
cyst(s)
  breast lumps, 39
  infected and painful intercourse, 193
  meibomian (swelling inside eyelid), 95

D

dandruff, 113–14
  and itching, 140
deafness, *see* ear problems
death
  from AIDS, 3
  from anaphylactic shock, 8
  and bereavement, 28–30
  from broken neck or spine, 43
  from burns, 47
  from cancer, 47, 48
  from drug abuse, 80
  from glue sniffing, 109
  from heart attack, 120
  from meningitis, 147
  from pre-senile dementia, 74
  from shock, 196
deformity and broken bones, 42
dehydration
  and gastroenteritis, 104
    in infants, 104–6
  and whooping cough, 256
delirium tremens (DTs) and alcoholism, 6
dementia, 72–4
  and confusion, 60, 72–4
  and incontinence, 133
  pre-senile (Alzzheimer's disease), 72–4
  senile, 72–3
dental problems, *see* teeth
dental treatment and sinusitis, 200
deodorants, sensitisation to and itching, 140
depression, 74–5
  and alcoholism, 6
  and anxiety, 14
  and bereavement, 28
  and birth
    mild, short-term (baby blues), 22–3, 74
    post-natal, 23, 74
  and dementia, 73
  and drug abuse, 79
  and high blood pressure, 34
  and incontinence, 133
  manic-, 144–5
  and menopause, 148
  and PMT, 148

  and school refusal, 190
  and shingles, 195
  and sleep problems, 201
  and stress, 212
  and stroke, 215
  winter, 75
dermatitis
  contact- and eczema, 86
  and skin allergies, 8
    and ear-piercing, 82
detachment, and baby blues/post-natal depression, 23
development, slow, and deafness, 84
dhobie itch (groin itching), 22
diabetes mellitus, 75–7
  and bedwetting, 27
  and cataracts, 49
  and confusion, 60
  and fainting, 96
  and fits, 63
  insulin-dependent, 75–6
  non-insulin dependent, 76
  and obesity, 160
  and stroke, 215
  and thrush, 228
  and vaginal irritation, 247
diaphragm weakness and hiatus hernia, 125
diarrhoea, 77–8
  and appendicitis, 16
  and constipation, 61
  and gastritis, 103
  and gastroenteritis, 103–4
  and irritable colon, 138
  and measles, 145–6
  and painful periods, 166–7
  and too much thyroid, 230
diastolic blood pressure, 33
diet
  and acne, 1
  and allergies, 8
  and anaemia, 9, 10
    in pregnancy, 174
  and arthritis, 18
  and bad breath, 27
  and constipation, 61, 62
  and diabetes, 76
  and diarrhoea, 77
  and eczema, 87
  and gastritis, 103
  and gastroenteritis, 104
  and heart attack, 121
  and heavy periods, 168
  and hives, 127
  and hyperactivity, 129
  and indigestion, 134
  and irritable colon, 138
  and measles, 146
  and migraine, 150
  and mouth ulcers, 153
  and nappy rash, 155–6
  and obesity, 160–2
  and piles, 169
  and sickness in pregnancy, 177
  and sleep problems, 201

267

diet *Contd.*
  and stress, 212
  and vitamin deficiency, **252–3**
  and vomiting, 254
  obession with, *see* dieting, excessive (anorexia nervosa), **12–14**
  see also bulimia nervosa
digestion, chronic, and rickets, 37
discharge
  cervical
    and cervical cancer, 51
    and cervical erosion, 52
  and itching, 139
  and miscarriage, 151
  nasal, foul-smelling, from foreign body, 99
    see also nose, runny
  from penis and swollen testicles, 222
  from stye, 94–5
  from urethra and NSU, 159
  vaginal, 245–6
dislocation, **78–9**
  of hips, 126
  and shoulder pain, 197
  and swelling, 88
  see also arthritis
dizziness
  and ear wax, 81
  and fainting, 96
  and heart attack, 120
  and heatstroke, 122
  and hyperventilation, 130
  and neck, stiff and painful, 156
  and stroke, 214
  and tranquilliser addiction, 236
  and travel sickness, 237
  and vertigo, 249
  see also vertigo
double vision
  from stiff and painful neck, 156
  from stroke, 214
Down's syndrome and glue ear, 84
dreams
  vivid, and bereavement, 28
  see also nightmares; sleep problems
dressings for cuts, 68–9
drink problems *see* alcoholism
driving and angina, 11
drop attacks, and stiff and painful neck, 156–7
drowsiness
  and antihistamine tablets, 33
  and drug abuse, 79
  after epileptic fit, 90
  and headache, 116
  and head injury, 118
  and measles, 145
  and meningitis, 147
  and mumps, 154
  and shock, 196
drug(s)
  abuse, **79–81**
  and confusion, 60
  and poisoning, 173
    solvents *see* glue-sniffing, 79
  addiction, 6, **79–81**

  alcoholism, **5–7**
  tranquilliser, 7, **235–7**
  and alcoholism, **5–7**
  and amenorrhoea, 166
  and anaemia, 10
  and anxiety, 15–16
  -taking, infected equipment and AIDS, 4, 5
  and constipation, 61
  and gastroenteritis, 104
  and depression, 74
  and hives, 127
  and impotence, 192
  and incontinence, 133
  and irregular periods, 165
  and itching, 140
  and jaundice, 141
  and nightmares, 204
  and palpitations, 162
  poisoning, **173–4**
    and fits, 63
  and rash, 186
  and sleep problems, 201
  and tremor, 238
  and vaginal irritation, 247
  and vertigo, 250
  and vomiting, 253
  withdrawal, *see* drug(s), addiction
DTs (delivium tremens) and alcoholism, 6
duodenal ulcers, bleeding and anaemia, 9
dust, inhaled
  and asthma, 20
  and chronic bronchitis, 45
  and cough, 65
dyskaryosis, mild (CIN 1), 50
dysplasia, 50
  mild (mild dyskaryosis, or CIN 1), 50
  severe (carcinoma in -situ, or CIN 3), 50

E

ear problems, **81–6**
  deafness, **71–2**
    and glue ear, 71, 83–4
    and ear wax, 81–2
    and infection of middle ear, 85
    and inflammation of outer ear, 85
    and tinnitus, 232
    and vertigo, 249
  ear ache, 81
    and colds, 54, 55
    and measles, 145
    and toothache, 81
  ear-piercing, **82–3**
    and AIDS, 4
  ear wax, **81–2**
  and enlarged adenoids, 2–3
  foreign body in, 83
    and deafness, 71
  glue ear, 2, 3, **83–4**
    and adenoids, 2
    and deafness, 71, 83–4
    and earache, 81
    and infection of middle ear, 85

see also glue ear; tonsillitis
infection of middle ear, 85
  and measles, 145
  and meningitis, 147
inflammation of outer ear (canal), 85–6
  see also boils
protruding (bat ears), 83
tinnitus, 232–3
eczema, 86
  and asthma, 19
  and dandruff, 114
  and hayfever, 114
  and itching, 139, 140
  and skin allergies, 8
    and ear-piercing, 82
  seborrhoeic, 66
EEG (electroencephalogram) for fits, 63
ejaculation, premature, 194–5
elbow
  and broken arms, 43
  joint and gout, 111
  pain, 87–9
  pins and needles at, 170
  psoriasis, 185
  swollen (olecranon bursa), 88–9
  'tennis', 87–8
  see also neck problems; shoulder, pain
elderly people's illnesses/problems
  broken bones, 42
  cancer of prostate, 181–2
  confusion, 59–60, 72–3
  cramp, 66–7
  deafness, 71
  deep-vein thrombosis, 226–7
  dislocated hip or thigh, 78–9
  ear wax, 81–2
  flu, 97–8
  heart attack, 120
  hiatus hernia, 125
  incontinence, 133
  neck problems, 156–8
  osteo-arthritis, 17–18
  pneumonia, 171–3
  senile dementia, 72–3
  shingles, 195–6
  tinnitus, 232
  tremor, 238–9
  vertigo, 249
  vitamin deficiency, 252
emotional problems/upsets
  and amenorrhoea, 166
  and asthma, 20
  and constipation, 61
  and dementia, 72
  and fainting, 96
  and hyperventilation, 130
  and irritable colon, 138
  and PMT, 180–1
  and school refusal, 190
  and shock, 196
  and stroke, 215
  and sickness in pregnancy, 177
  and tantrums, 217–19
encephalitis, 146

and headache, 116
Endometriosis Society, 137
endometriosis
  and painful intercourse, 194
  and painful periods, 169
energy, loss of, and depression, 74
enuresis (bedwetting), 27–8
  see also incontinence
epilepsy, 63–4, 89–91
  and confusion, 60
  and fainting, 96
  and vertigo, 250
episiotomy, 91–2
  and painful intercourse
essential hypertension, 34
exercising
  for anxiety, 15
  and arthritis, 17, 18
  and asthma, 19
  and cramp, 67
  for heart attack, 121
  and heart failure, 121
  for high blood pressure, 35
  and incontinence, 132
  for obesity, 161
  obsessive, and anorexia nervosa, 12
  pain during, and angina, 11
  after repair to broken bones, 42–3
  and sleep problems, 201
  strenuous and heatstroke, 122
exhaustion
  and baby blues/post-natal depression, 23
  and gout, 111
  and heatstroke, 122
  and infertility, 135
  and mania, 144
  and migraine, 150
  and shingles, 195
  and stress, 212
  too little thyroid, 230
eye problems, 92–6
  cataracts, 48–9
  and cold sore virus, 56
  conjunctivitis, 60–1
    and allergy, 8
  and high blood pressure, 34
  iritis, 49
  itching see itching, eyes
  -lashes, swellings amongst (styes), 94–5
  -lid(s)
    general swelling of, 93–4
    pallor of, and anaemia, 9
    stork mark on, 37
    foreign body in, 92–3
    swelling inside, 95
  pressure on (glaucoma) and headache, 116
  protruding and too much thyroid, 230
  redness, 92–4
    and German measles, 107
    and measles, 145
  on skin outside, 95
  soreness around, and glue sniffing, 109
  squint, 209–10
  sticky, in infants, 61, 93–4

269

strain and headache, 116
sunken, in dehydration of infants, 105
swollen, from hayfever, 114, 115
watering, 92–3
   from foreign body
   from hayfever, 114
yellow from jaundice, 140–1

F

face
  and cradle cap, 66
  and cuts, 68
  neuralgia and headache, 116
  red and whooping cough, 256–7
  red spots on, and German measles, 107
  swelling
    and hives, 127
    and toothache, 235
  tic, 231–2
fainting, **95–6**
  and anaemia, 9
  and diabetes, 76
  and tantrums, 217
  and vertigo, 249
  see also coma; concussion; consciousness, loss of
faintness
  and heart attack, 120
  and heatstroke, 122
  and hyperventilation, 130
  and shock, 196
  and travel sickness, 237
  see also weakness
Families Anonymous, 81
family
  and anxiety, 15
  arguments and anorexia nervosa, 13
  help from
    with baby blues/post-natal depression, 23
    with bedwetting, 28
    with bereavement, 28, 29
    with drug abuse, 80–1
    with hyperactivity, 129
    with manic-depression, 144–5
    with schizophrenia, 189
  planning, 178–80
  problems
    and school refusal, 190–1
    and tics, 231
    and wakefulness in children, 204
  therapy for anorexia nervosa, 13–14
Family Planning Clinics, 180, 193
fatigue *see* tiredness
fatness, fear of (anorexia nervosa), **12–14**
  see also bulimia nervosa
fear
  feeling of, and palpitations, 162
  and night terrors in children, 202
  of separation from parents, and school refusal, 190
feeding problems in infants
  and hyperactivity, 128–9

refusal
  and dehydration, 105
  and meningitis, 147
  and pneumonia, 172
feet
  arthritis in, 17
  athlete's foot, **22**
  blisters on, 33
  bunions, **45–6**
  chilblains, **52–3**
  cold, **55–6**
    and anti-hypertension drugs, 35
    and beta-blockers, 16, 35
  corns, **64**
  flat, 97
  ganglions on, 101
  infection from splinter, and limp, 142
  in-growing toenails, 138
  itching, 139
  misshapen, and bunions, 46
  muscle spasms and hyperventilation, 130
  pain and flat fleet, 97
  sweat rash, 139
  swelling, **12**
    and varicose veins, 247
  tingling and anaemia, 9
  verrucas, **248–9**
  see also toes
female sterilisation, 210
fertility, techniques to aid, **137**
  see also infertility
fever, **220–1**
  and acute bronchitis, 45
  and AIDS, 3
  and ankle-swelling, 12
  and appendicitis, 16
  and bad breath, 27
  and breast infection, 37
    and breast lumps, 39
  and chicken pox, 53
  and colds, 54
  and cold sores in children, 56
  and convulsions, **62–4**, 89
  and cough, 64
  and croup, 68
  and cystitis, 69
  and gastroenteritis, 104
  and general swelling of eyelids, 93
  and German measles, 107
  and glandular fever, 108
  and headache, 116
  and heatstroke, 122
  and hoarseness, 128
  and infection of middle ear, 85
  and inflammation of prostate, 184
  and measles, 145
  and meningitis, 147
  and mumps, 153
  and nappy rash, 155
  and nightmares, 203
  and palpitations, 162
  and PID, 163
  and pleurisy, 171
  and pneumonia, 172

scarlet, **188**
and shingles, 195
and sunstroke, 217
and swollen testicles, 223
and thrombophlebitis, 227
and tonsillitis, 233–4
and urine infection, 243
fibres and chronic bronchitis, 45
fibro-adenosis (lumpy breasts), 39
fibroids, **96–7**
and heavy periods, 168
and hysterectomy, 131
and infertility, 136
finger(s)
broken, 43
chilblains on, **53–4**
cold, **55–6**
and beta-blocking drugs, 16
and herpes, 140
nails *see* nail problems
ring stuck on, **187**
swelling of, and PMT, 181
thrush affecting fingertips, 140
tingling in
and too little thyroid, 230
and wrist pain, **257–8**
see also hands
fits
and asphyxia, 90
and brain inflammation, 63
and brain tumour, 63, 117
convulsions, febrile, **62–4**, 89
delirium tremens (DTs), and alcoholism, 6
drugs to stop, and rickets, 37
epileptic, *see* epilepsy
and headache, nausea and vomiting, 117
and head injury, 63, 89
and low blood sugar, 63
and mealses, 146
and meningitis, 147
and poisoning with drugs or lead, 63
and raised blood pressure, 63
and sprain, 208
and strokes, 90
flashing lights and migraine, 150
flat feet, **97**
and knock knees, 142
flatulence and irritable colon, 138
flea-bites, 32
flu (influenza), **97–8**
and acute bronchitis, 45
and cough, 64
and genital herpes, 106
and glandular fever, 108–9
and hoarseness, 128
and pneumonia, 172
and raised temperature, 220
symptoms of, and tranquilliser addiction, 236
and tonsillitis, 233–4
vaccination, 98
as viral illness, 250
see also viral illness; vitamin deficiency
fluid(s)

loss/shortage
and burns, 46
and heatstroke, 122
retention
and ankle-swelling, **12**
and blisters, 33
and bunions, 45
and menopause, 148
and pleurisy, 171
and swollen testicles, **222–3**
and wrist pain and tingling fingers, **257–8**
see also swelling
folic acid deficiency and anaemia, 9–10
in pregnancy, 174
Food and Chemical Allergy Association, 8
food poisoning
from berries, 173
from boils, 36
and gastroenteritis, **103–4**
forceps delivery and temporary bruising, 30
foreign bodies
in ear, **83**
and deafness, 71
in eye, **92–3**
and conjunctivitis, 60, 61
inhaling and croup, 68
in nose, **98–9**
foreskin problems, **99–101**
balanitis (infection of tip of penis), **99**
circumcision, **99–100**
and painful intercourse, 193
para-phimosis, **100**
phimosis (tight foreskin), **100–1**
and thrush, 228
freezing treatment for cervical changes, 50–1
friction
and blisters, 33
and boils, 36
and bunions, 45–6
and burns, 46
frustration and tantrums, 217–19
fungal infections
athlete's foot, **22**
infected nails, **154–5**
itching, 140
patchy hair loss, 112, 113
rash, 186
thrush *see* thrush
furry tongue, 233

G

gallbladder
and gallstones, **101–2**
infection (acute cholecystitis), 102
and obesity, 160
gallstones, **101–2**
and indigestion, 134
and jaundice, 141
and vomiting, 253
see also anaemia; jaundice
ganglions, **101**
gastric flu, 103

gastritis, 103
  and alcoholism, 6
  and vomiting, 253
  see also arthritis; indigestion; ulcer, stomach
gastroenteritis, 103–4
  and food poisoning, 103–4
    see also appendicitis; diarrhoea; vomiting
  in infants, and diarrhoea, 78
    see also constipation; soft spot
  and viral illness, 251
  and vomiting, 253
genetic factors
  and anorexia nervosa, 13
  and bunions, 46
  and hyperactivity, 129
genital herpes, 106–7
  and abnormal cervical smear, 50
  and cervical cancer, 51
  and hayfever, 115
  and painful intercourse, 193–4
  as viral illness, 250
genital warts, 255–6
  and abnormal cervical smear, 50
  and cervical cancer, 51
German measles (rubella), 107–8
  at pregnancy
    and cataracts, 49
    and deafness, 71
    and rash, 186
GIFT (gamete intra-fallopian transfer), 137
glandular fever, 108–9
  and depression, 74
  and liver damage and jaundice, 141
    see also tonsillitis
glandular problems
  adenoids, 2–3
  swollen, and AIDS, 3
glaucoma and headache, 116
glue ear, *see under* ear problems
glue sniffing (solvent abuse), 79, 109–10
  and confusion, 60
  and poisoning, 173
  and vomiting, 253
    see also drug abuse
gonorrhoea, 110–11
  and PID, 163
  and sticky eyes at birth, 94
gout, 111
  and frozen shoulder, 198
  and rheumatoid arthritis, 18
    see also rheumatoid arthritis
grand mal (major epileptic fit), 89–91
Grave's disease *see* thyroid problems, too much thyroid
grazes and cuts, 68–9
greasy hair, 114
grief and bereavement, 28–9
gripe water and colic, 58
groin
  ache, and urine infection, 243
  hernia, 123–4
  itching (dhobie itch), 22
  and scarlet fever, 188
  swelling in, and glandular fever, 108

grommets and adenoids, 3, 83–4
guilt
  and bereavement, 28
  and depression, 74
gum(s)
  blistered, from cold sores, 56
  disease, 27
  swollen, and toothache, 235
  and teething, 219–20

H

haemoglobin, anaemia and difficulty in production of, 9–10
haemolytic jaundice, 141
haemophilia and AIDS, 4
haemorrhage and miscarriage, 151–2
haemorrhoids (piles), 168–9, 247
hair
  on café au lait spot (birthmark), 30
  care of, 1
  cradle cap, 66
  fine downy on skin, and anorexia nervosa, 12
  and headlice, 118–19
  and itching scalp, 140
  loss, 111–13
    alopecia, 112, 113
    baldness, 113
    and chemotherapy, 48
    fungal infection, 112
    general, 113
    patchy, 112–13
    thinning, 113
  problems, 113–14
    dandruff, 113–14
    greasy, 114
    unwanted, 114
      see also acne; skin problems
  pulling, 112
  thin and dry, and too little thyroid, 230
hallucinations
  and alcoholism, 6
  and bereavement, 29
  and depression, 74
  and drug abuse, 80, 109
  and glue sniffing, 109
  and night terrors in children, 202
hands
  blisters on, 33
  cold
    and anti-hypertension drugs, 35
    and beta-blockers, 16, 35
  itching, and contact dermatitis, 140
  loss of use in minor stroke, 214
  muscle spasms and hyperventilation, 130
  and nails *see* nail problems
  painful joints, and German measles, 107
  and rheumatoid arthritis, 18
  and scabies, 140
  tingling, and anaemia, 9
  trembling, and alcoholism, 6

272

see also fingers
hangovers, 7
  and headache, 116
  see also alcoholism
hayfever, **114–15**
  and allergy to pollen, 8, 114–15
  and asthma, 19
  and conjunctivitis, 60, 61
  and eczema, 86
  and hives, 127
  and itching, 139
head
  -banging and tantrums, 217–19
  colds, *see* colds
  injury, **117–18**
    and confusion, 60
    and dementia, 73
    and fits, 63, 89
    and headache, 116
    and vertigo, 249
    and vomiting, 253
  jerking of, and epilepsy, 89–90
  -lice, **118–19**
    and itching, 140
  pain and headache, 116
  spots on, and chicken pox, 53
headaches, **116–17**
  and allergy, 8
  and anxiety, 14
  and chicken pox, 53
  and colds, 54
  and flu, 97
  and German measles, 107
  and head injury, 118
  and heatstroke, 122
  and high blood pressure, 34
  and meningitis, 147
  and menopause, 148
  and migraine, **149–51**
  and mumps, 153–4
  and neck, stiff and painful, 156
  and painful periods, 167
  and palpitations, 162
  and pre-eclampsia, 176
  and raised temperature, 220
  and scarlet fever, 188
  and sinusitis, 200
  and tension, 221
  and vomiting, 253
head banging and tantrums, 217–19
headlice, 118–19
  see also head, injury; migraine
Health Publications Unit, 39
hearing
  aids and deafness, 71–2
  problems and dementia, 73
  see also ear problems
heart
  attacks, **119–21**
    and confusion, 60
    and high blood pressure, 34
    and shock, 196
    and thrombosis, 226

  see also angina; heart, failure; shock; thrombosis
  -beat
    rapid and anxiety, 14, 16
    slow and too little thyroid, 230
  -burn
    and hiatus hernia, 125
    and indigestion, 134
    and sickness in pregnancy, 177
  conditions
    and flu, 97
    and palpitations, 162–3
  disease
    and high blood pressure, 34
    and obesity, 160
    and stroke, 215
  failure, **121–2**
    and ankle swelling, 12
    and beta-blocking drugs, 16
    and confusion, 60
    and heart attack, 120
    see also thrombosis
  pain in chest (angina), **10–11**
  palpitations, **162–3**
    and anaemia, 9
    in pregnancy, 174
    and angina, 11
    and anxiety, 14
    and high blood pressure, 34
    and hyperventilation, 130
    and menopause, 148
    and too much thyroid, 230
    see also menopause; thyroid
  and scarlet fever, 188
  strain on, and chronic bronchitis, 45
  and tranquilliser addiction, 236
  X-rays for angina, 11
  see also blood pressure; strokes
heatstroke, **122–3**
  and sunstroke, 216
hernia, **123–6**
  groin, **123–4**
  hiatus, **125–6**
  umbilical, **124–5**
  and whooping cough, 256
hepatitis (liver inflammation)
  and alcoholism, 6
  and jaundice, 140–1
hepatitis B
  in drug abuse, 80
  in ear-piercing, 82
  and jaundice, 141
hereditary spherocytosis, and anaemia, 9
herpes, genital, *see* genital herpes
herpes simplex
  type 1 (cold sores), 56
  type 2 (genital herpes), 106
herpes zoster (chicken pox virus), 53, 196
hiatus hernia, **125–6**
  and indigestion, 134
  and sickness in pregnancy, 177
high blood pressure *see* blood pressure, high

273

hip(s)
  arthritis in, 17, 18
  dislocated
    clicky and congenital (affecting children), 126–7
    and limp, 142–3
    non-congenital (affecting elderly), 78–9
  joint replacement, 18
  pathological fracture in, 42
Hirschsprung's disease, 62
HIV I and II viruses, and AIDS, 3–4
hives (a.k.a. urticaria; nettlerash), 127–8
  and rash, 186
hoarseness, 128
  and colds, 54
  and croup, 67–8
hormone(s) changes and problems
  and amenorrhoea, 166
  and baby blues/post-natal depression, 23
  and breast development in adolescence, 41
  and dry vagina, 244
  and heavy periods, 168
  and high blood pressure, 34
  and infertility, 135–6
  and irregular, unexpected periods, 165
  and migraine, 150
  and miscarriage
  and Pill causing ankle swelling, 12
  and PMT, 181
  and sickness in pregnancy, 177
  and vaginal discharge, 246
  replacement therapy, 149
  thyroid, see thyroid problems
hot flushes
  and menopause, 148
  and raised temperature, 220
house dust mites, allergy to, and asthma, 20
household products
  poisoning from, 173
  sensitisation to, and itching, 139
housemaid's knee (bursitis of knee), 89
hunger pain and indigestion, 134
hydrocele and swollen testicles, 222
hygiene problems
  and dementia, 73
  and scabies, 187
hymen, tight, and painful intercourse, 193
Hyperactive Children's Support Group, 130
hyperactivity, 128–30
hyperemesis (severe sickness in pregnancy), 178
hypersensitivity, 7
  see also allergies
hypertension see blood pressure, high
hyperthyroidism see thyroid problems, too much thyroid
hyperventilation
  and anxiety, 14
  see also anxiety; blood pressure, high; palpitations
hypomania, 144
hypothermia and confusion, 60
hypothyroidism, 229
hysterectomy, 130–2
  and amenorrhoea, 166
  and cervical cancer, 52
  and fibroid removal, 97
  see also cervical problems; fibroids; menopause; periods
Hysterectomy Support Group, 132

I

icepacks
  for backache, 25
  for bites and stings, 32
Imperial Cancer Research Fund, 48
impetigo, 132
impotence, 191–3
  and dry vagina, 244
  and premature ejaculation, 194–5
  see also orgasm, absence of
incontinence, 27, 132–3
  and dementia, 73
  see also bedwetting; constipation; cystitis; dementia; prostate problems; stroke; urine infection
indigestion, 134–5
  and allergy, 8
  and duodenal ulcer, 240
  and gastritis, 103
  and hiatus hernia, 125
  and iron, 10
  and stomach ulcer, 240
  and stress, 212
  and tension, 221–2
  see also gallstones; hernia, hiatus; pregnancy problems; ulcers
infants, see babies/infants problems and illness
infarct and heart attack, 120
infertility, 135–7
  and fibroids, 96
  and infrequent periods, 164–5
  and PID, 163
  techniques to aid, 137
  see also fibroids; pelvic infection; periods; testes problems
infectious mononucleosis see glandular fever
inflammation
  of the outer ear (canal), 85–6
    see also boils
  of temple artery (temporal arteritis) and headache, 116
inflammatory joint disease
  gout, 18
  rheumatoid arthritis, 18–19
influenza, see flu
in-growing toenails, 137–8
injury
  blood loss after, and anaemia, 9
  and manic depression, 145
  and pleurisy, 171
  and shock, 196
  strain, and backache, 24
  swelling after, 12
  and thrombophlebitis, 227
insect bites
  and hives, 127

and itching, 139
and stings, **32–3**
insomnia
 in adults, *see* sleep problems in adults
 in children, 204–6
Institute of Behavioural Therapy, 16
insulin-dependent diabetes, 75–6
 new developments in treatment, 77
intestines
 cancer of, and jaundice, 141
 inflammation of, *see* gastroenteritis
 injury to and groin hernia, 123
intestinal disease and incontinence, 133
intoxicated behaviour, and glue sniffing, 109
in-vitro fertilisation (IVF), 137
iritis, 49
iron-deficiency anaemia, 9
 in pregnancy, 174
irritability
 and alcoholism, 5
 and baby blues/post-natal depression, 23
 and bedwetting, 28
 and diabetes, 76
 and drug abuse, 79
 and gastroenteritis in infants, 105
 and glue sniffing, 109
 and hypomania, 144
 and nappy rash, 155
 and painful periods, 167
 and PMT, 181
 and teething, 219
 and too much thyroid, 230
irritable colon, **138–9**
 see also constipation
irritable hip, and limp, 142–3
irritation
 and scabies, 187
 vaginal, **246–7**
 and varicose veins, 247
itching, **139–40**
 anal, and threadworms, 225–6
 eyes
  and conjunctivitis, 60
  and foreign body, 92
  and hayfever, 114
 generalised, 139
 hives, 127–8
 and jaundice, 140
 limited, 139–40
 in rashes, 186
 skin
  and allergy, 8, 82
  and athelete's foot, 22
  and bites and stings, 32–3
  and cancer, 47
  and chilblains, 53
  and chicken pox, 52–3
  and cold sores, 56
  and conjunctivitis, 60
  and crabs, 65–6
  and ear-piercing, 82
  and eczema, 86–7
  and fungal infection, 112
  and genital herpes, 106
  and genital warts, 255
  and headlice, 118–19
  and moles, 30
   indicating possible cancer, 47
  and psoriasis, 186
  and sunburn, 216
  and thrombophlebitis 227
  and thrush, 228
  and vaginal irritation, 246
  and varicose veins, 247
 see also eczema; hair problems; hayfever; thrush
IVF (in-vitro fertilisation), 137

J

jaundice, **140–2**
 and gallstones, 102
 and glandular fever, 108
 and vomiting, 253
 see also alcoholism; anaemia
jaw
 ache, and toothache, 235
 dislocated, 79
 joint problems and headache, 116
 pain in
  and earache, 81
  and heart attack, 119
 swelling of gland around (mumps), **153–4**
jealousy and alcoholism, 6
jellyfish stings, 32
jerking movements, severe tics and verbal outbursts (Tourette Syndrome), 231
joint problems
 aching
  and flu, 97
  and glandular fever, 108
 and allergy, 8
 big toe, and gout, 111
 dislocation, **78–9**
 painful
  and German measles, 107
  and menopause, 148
 sprain, **208–9**
 swollen, and arthritis, 187
 and tendonitis, 199
 see also arthritis

K

Kaposi's sarcoma (a skin cancer) and AIDS, 3
kidney(s)
 disease causing high blood pressure, 24
 and obesity, 160
 problems
  and ankle-swelling, 12
  caused by high blood pressure, 34
 and scarlet fever, 188
 and urine infection, **242–4**
knee(s)
 arthritis in, 17
 bursitis (housemaid's knee), 89

knee(s) *Contd.*
    joint, and gout, 111
    knock, **142**
        see also bowlegs
    and psoriasis, 185
    sprain, 208

L

laryngitis
    and colds, 54, 55
    and cough, 65
    and croup, 68
    and hoarseness, **128**
laughing and incontinence, 132
laxatives
    and anorexia nervosa, 12
    and appendicitis, 17
    and constipation, 62
lead poisoning and fits, 63
legs
    aching, and flu, 97
    bow-, **36–7**
    broken, 43
    circulation in and heart failure, 122
    cramp in, **66–7**
    deep-vein thrombosis, **226–7**
    and dhobie itch, 22
    jerking of, and epilepsy, 89–90
    knock knees, **142**
    limp, **142–3**
    loss of use in minor stroke, 214
    pains in
        and alcoholism, 6
        and backache, 24
    rashes, 186
    sciatica in, 26
    swelling, 12
    varicose veins, **247–8**
leukaemia(s), 48
    and anaemia, 10
    and chicken pox, 52
    and pneumonia, 172
leukoplakia, **246–7**
lice, *see* headlice
lies, telling, and glue-sniffing, 109
lifting
    and backache, 24, 25
    and groin hernia, **123–4**
light, causing pain
    in meningitis, 147
    in migraine, 150
    in mumps, 154
    in tranquilliser addiction, 236
lightheadedness and stroke, 214
limp, **142–3**
    see also arthritis; gout; hips; splinter
lip(s)
    blue
        and chronic bronchitis 45
        and pneumonia, 172
    cold sores around, 56
    mouth ulcers on, **152–3**

purple, and epilepsy, 89
-reading and deafness, 72
lipomas, **143–4**
liver
    changes to, and alcoholism, 7
    congestion and heart failure, 121
    infection and jaundice, 140
    inflammation (hepatitis), and alcoholism, 6
    scarring (cirrhosis), and alcoholism, 6
low blood sugar, *see* diabetes
lumps
    breast, **38–9**
        in puberty, 41
    hives, **127–8**
    lipomas, **143–4**
    tumours, 47
        removal of, 48
        see also cancer(s)
    unexplained appearance of, and cancer, 47
lung problems/infections
    asthma, **19–22**
    and broken ribs, 43
    bronchiolitis (of small airways), **43–4**
    bronchitis, and early damage from measles or
        whooping cough, 45
    cancer, 64
    and colds, 54, 55
    and cough, **64–5**
    deep-vein thrombosis, **226–7**
    fluid in and heart failure, 121
    pleurisy, 171
    pneumonia, **171–3**
        and AIDS, 3
    TB and cough, 64
    whooping cough, **256–7**
lymph glands
    cancer of, 48
    enlarged, by genital herpes, 106
    swelling of
        and breast infection, 37
        and German measles, 107
        and mumps, 154
        and tonsillitis, **233–4**

M

malaria and liver damage, and jaundice, 141
male sterilisation (vasectomy), **210–11**
malnutrition and pneumonia, 172
manic depression, 74, **144–5**
MASTA (Medical Advisory Services for Travellers Abroad), 5
mastitis (breast infection), **37–8**
measles, **145–6**
    and acute bronchitis, 45
    and conjunctivitis, 60
    German, *see* German measles
    and infection of middle ear, 85
    and pneumonia, 172
    and rash, 186
    see also convulsions, febrile; croup; diarrhoea
medicines and nightmares, 203
meditation for anxiety, 15

meibomian cyst (swelling inside eyelid), 95
memory loss *see* amnesia
Menière's disease
   and tinnitus, 232
   and vertigo, 250
meningitis, 63, 146–8
   and deafness, 71
   and epilepsy, 90
   and fits, 89
   and general swelling of eyelids, 93
   and headache, 116
   and head injury, 117
   purple rash, 186
   and soft spot, 206
   see also soft spot
meningococcal meningitis, 147
   and rash, 186
menopause, 148–9
   and abnormal cervical smear, 50
   and amenorrhoea, 166
   bleeding after, and cancer, 165
   dry vagina after, 244
   and hysterectomy, 131
   infrequent periods before, 165
   and manic-depression, 144–5
   and palpitations, 162
   post-
      bleeding
         and abnormal cervical smear, 49
         and cancer, 47, 51
         and cervical erosion, 52
      and self-examination for breast lumps, 39
   and vulval itching, 139
   and wrist pain and tingling fingers, 257
   see also sleep problems
menorrhagia (heavy periods), 167–8
menstruation
   and infertility, 135
   tension before, *see* premenstrual tension (PMT)
mental disturbances/illness
   anorexia nervosa, 12–14
   anxiety, 14–16
   baby blues/post natal depression, 22–3
   confusion, 59–60
   dementia, 72–4
   depression, 74–5
   and drug abuse, 79–80
   schizophrenia, 188–90
middle ear, infection of, 81, 85
   and measles, 145
migraine, 149–51
   and allergy, 8
   and headache, 116
   and pins and needles in arm, 170
   and vertigo, 250
   and vomiting, 253
   see also headaches
Migraine Trust, 151
MIND (National Association for Mental Health), 189
miscarriage, 151–2
   and heavy periods, 168
   and PID, 163
   and vaginal discharge, 246

Miscarriage Association, 152
moles
   birthmarks, 30–2
   brown (simple), 30
   changes around, indicating possible cancer, 47–8
   see also breast lumps
Mongolian blue spots (birthmark), 30
mood changes, unpredictable
   and drug abuse, 79
   and glue sniffing, 109
   and hyperactivity, 129
   and manic-depression, 144–5
   and stroke, 215
morning sickness in pregnancy, and indigestion, 134
motorcycle accidents and head injury, 118
mouth
   abscesses in, 27
   bile or acid tastes in
      and hiatus hernia, 125
      and indigestion, 134
      and sickness in pregnancy, 127
   blistered from cold sores, 56
   cancer of, and alcoholism, 6
   dry, and dehydration in infants, 105
   hanging open, and adenoids, 2
   pale patch around, and scarlet fever, 188
   soreness around, and glue sniffing, 109
   thrush in, and AIDS, 3
   ulcers, 152–3
      and allergy, 8
      and bad breath, 27
   uncomfortable, and anaemia, 9
multiple sclerosis and vertigo, 250
mumps, 153–4
   and meningitis, 147
   and swollen testicles, 222–3
mumps meningitis, 154
muscle
   aches and pains, and glandular fever, 108
   cramps and heatstroke, 122
   disease, and alcoholism, 6
   spasms (tetany)
      and backache, 24–6
      and cramp, 66–7
      and hyperventilation, 130
      and tranquilliser addiction, 236
      and wry neck, 158
   sprain, and limp, 143
myxoedema, 229

N

nail problems, 154–5
   infected, 154–5
   in-growing toe-, 137–8
   painful, 155
   psoriasis, 185
   unsightly, 155
   see also psoriasis

277

nappy
  discomfort on changing and clicky hip/congenital dislocation, 126
  rash, **155–6**
  and thrush, 228–9
  see also thrush
nasal discharge *see* nose, runny
National AIDS Helpline, 5
National Association for the Childless, 137
National Childbirth trust, 23
National Eczema Society, 87
National Schizophrenia Fellowship, 189
nausea
  and anxiety, 14
  and appendicitis, 16
  and chemotherapy, 48
  and drug abuse, 80
  and fainting, 96
  and flu, 97
  and gastroenteritis, 103
  and headache and brain tumour, 117
  and heart attack, 120
  and hernia, 123
  and indigestion, 134
  and irritable colon, 138
  and migraine, 150
  and sickness in pregnancy, 176–7
  and travel sickness, 237
  and urine infection, 243
neck problems, **156–8**
  arthritis
    of spine and pins and needles, 170
    and vertigo, 249
  broken, 43
  and elbow pain, 88
  and fainting, 96
  and shoulder pain, 197
  stiff and painful, **156–8**
    and backache, 26
    and ear ache, 81
    and headache, 116
    and heart attack, 119
    and meningitis, 147
    and mumps, 154
    and tension, 221
    see also gout; shoulder pain
  stork mark on nape of, 37
  swelling, and too much thyroid, 230
  swollen lymph glands in
    and German measles, 107
    and glandular fever, 108
    and tonsillitis, 233–4
  trapped nerves, and headache, 116
  wry, **158**
needles, infected and shared
  and AIDS, 4, 80, 82
  and hepatitis B, 80, 82
  see also drug abuse; ear-piercing
nerve(s)
  damage
    and fits, 64
    and head injury, 118
  deafness, 71–2

pain (sciatica, aka neuralgia), 24, **26**
problems and alcoholism, 6
nervousness
  and high blood pressure, 33–4
  and menopause, 148
  tics, **231–2**
  upsets and bedwetting, 27
nettlerash (urticaria hives), **127–8**
neuralgia (nerve pain sciatica), 26
  facial and headache, 116
night
  attacks of heart failure, 121
  cramps, 67
  -mares, *see under* sleep problems
  terrors in children, *see under* sleep problems
nipple, cracked
  and breast-feeding problems, **40–1**
  and breast infection, 38
noise(s)
  and deafness, 71
  and headache, 116
  hearing strange, and migraine, 150
  oversensitivity to, and tranquilliser addiction, 236
  and tinnitus, 232
non-insulin-dependent diabetes, **76**
non-specific urethritis, *see* NSU
nose
  adenoids, 2–3
  blocked intermittently, and hayfever, 114
  -bleeds, **159–60**
  blowing
    and colds, 55
    and cough, 65
  catarrgh
    and allergy, 8
    and colds, 54
  cold sores around nostrils, 56
  foreign body in, **98–9**
  runny
    and acute bronchitis, 44–5
    and adenoids, 2
    and allergy, 8
    and bronchiolitis, 44
    and colds, 54
    and cough, 64
    and flu, 97
    and hayfever, 114–15
      and measles, 145
      and pneumonia, 172
    and sinusitis, 199–200
  soreness around, and glue sniffing, 109
  stork mark on bridge of, 30
  swabs for boils, 36
NSU (non-specific urethritis), **158–9**
  and cystitis, 71
  and gonorrhoea, 110
  and sticky eyes at birth, 94
  and urine infection, 243
numbness
  and backache, 24, 25
  and chilblains, 53
  and bereavement, 28

and dislocation, 78
and hyperventilation, 130
and migraine, 150
and neck, stiff and painful, 156
and pins and needles, 170
and stroke, 214

O

obesity, 160–2
  and angina, 11
  and hiatus hernia, 125
  and high blood pressure, 34
obsessive dieting (anorexia nervosa), 12–14
obstructive jaundice, 141
oedema in leg, and deep-vein thrombosis, 226
oestrogen and deep-vein thrombosis, 227
olecranon bursa, see elbow, swollen
orbital cellulitis, 93
orgasm
  absence of, 191
  and dry vagina, 244
  and premature ejaculation, 194–5
  see also impotence
osteo-arthritis, 17–18
  and backache, 24
  and dislocation, 78
  and slipped disc, 26
osteomyelitis and limp, 142–3
osteophytes, 157
otosclerosis, 71
outer ear, inflammation of, 81, 85–6
ovarian problems
  ovarian disease and removal of ovaries and womb (Wertheim's hysterectomy), 131
  and painful intercourse, 194
Overeaters Anonymous and Women's Therapy Centre, 14
overeating and induced vomiting (bulimia nervosa), 14
overweight
  fear of being, see anorexia nervosa
  and hiatus hernia, 125
  and para-umbilical hernia, 124
overwork and infertility, 135
  see also work-related problems
oxygen
  and bronchitis, 45
  and croup, 68
  lack of
    at birth (asphyxia) and fits, 90
    to heart and heart attack, 120
    and pneumonia, 172
    and shock, 196
    and whooping cough, 256

P

palpitations, 162–3; see heart, palpitations
pancreas, cancer of, and jaundice, 141
panic attacks and anxiety, 14
papilloma, 95

papular urticaria, 127
paralysis
  and broken neck or spine, 43
  and dislocation, 78
  and head injury, 118
  from stroke, 214–16
paranoia
  and alcoholism, 6
  and schizophrenia, 189
para-phimosis, 100
parasites, and scabies, 187
para-umbilical hernia, 124–5
Parkinson's disease and tremor, 238–9
Parkinson's Disease Society, 239
patchy tongue, 233
pathological fracture (breakage of thinning bones), 42
pelvic infection (PID), 163–4
  and cystitis, 71
  and gonorrhoea, 110
  and heavy periods, 168
  and infertility, 136
  and irregular periods, 165
  and NSU, 158
  and painful intercourse, 194
  and painful periods
  and urine infection, 243
  and vaginal discharge, 246
  and vomiting, 253
  see also appendicitis; NSU
pelvic inflammatory disease and gonorrhoea, 110
pelvis and deep-vein thrombosis, 226
penis, problems and disorders, 99–101
  blisters on, from genital herpes, 106
  discharge and swollen testicles, 222
  impotence and, 191–2
  inflammation of, and painful intercourse, 193
  milky discharge and gonorrhoea, 110
  pain at base of, and inflammation of prostate, 184
  penile infections and gonorrhea, 110
  and thrush, 228
  see also foreskin problems
perennial rhinitis (year-long hayfever), 114–15
periods, 164–8
  bleeding between, and cervical erosion, 52
  and cold sores, 56
  heavy (menorrhagia), 167–8
    and anaemia, 9
    and fibroids, 96
    and too little thyroid, 230
    see also hysterectomy; thyroid problems
  and hysterectomy, 131
  infrequent, 164–5
    and too much thyroid, 230
    see also infertility
  irregular, 165
    and infertility, 135–6
    and unexpected, 165
    see also cervical problems; pelvic infection
  and menopause, 148–9
  none, 166
    and anorexia nervosa, 12
    see also menopause; thyroid problems

279

painful, 166–7
  and fibroids, 96
  and painful intercourse, 194
  and vaginal discharge, 246
  and varicose veins, 247
  see also fibroids; pelvic infection
  and PMT, 181
  and self-examination for breast lumps, 39
  upset by drug abuse, 80
perforated ulcer, 239
peritonitis
  and appendicitis, 16
  and duodenal ulcers, 239
pernicious anaemia, 9
  see also anaemia
personal/ity problems
  and alcoholism, 5, 6
  and drug abuse, 79–80
  and glue sniffing, 109
  and hyperactivity, 129
Perthes disease, and limp, 143
petit mal, 89
pharyngitis, 233
phimosis, 100–1
phlegm, coloured
  and acute bronchitis, 44–5
  and pneomonia, 172
phobias and anxiety, 14–15
Phobic Action, 16
physical fitness, lack of, and palpitations, 162
piles, 168–9
  and anaemia in pregnancy, 174
  and constipation, 61
  and painful intercourse for homosexuals, 193
  and tension, 221
Pill, the (contraceptive)
  and acne, 2
  and amenorrhoea, 166
  and cervical erosion, 52
  confusion in taking, and irregular, unexpected periods, 165
  and premenstrual tension, 180–1
  and thrush, 228
  and vaginal discharge, 246
pins and needles, 169–70
  and diabetes, 76
  and Raynaud's disease, 55
  see also backache; neck problems; wrist pain and tingling fingers
plaque, build-up of, and bad breath, 27
plaster casts for broken bones, 42–3
plastic (cosmetic) surgery
  and bat ears, 83
  and birthmarks, 31, 32
pleural effusion, 171
pleurisy, 170–1
  and pneumonia, 172
  see also bronchitis; pneumonia
PMT *see* premenstrual tension
pneumocystis carnii pneumonia, and AIDS, 3
pneumonia, 171–3
  and AIDS, 3
  and chicken pox, 53
  and cough, 64

and measles, 145
and pleurisy, 171
and whooping cough, 256
  see also acute bronchitis; cough; pleurisy
pneumothorax, 171
poisoning and over-dosage, 173–4
  see also drug abuse; glue sniffing
poliomyelitis as infant (infantile paralysis) and limp, 142
pollen, allergy, to
  and asthma, 20
  and hayfever, 8, 115
  and hives, 127
polyps at cervix and irregular period, 165
port wine stain (birthmark), 31
POST (peritoneal ovum and sperm transfer), 137
post-natal depression, 23, 74
  and manic depression, 144–5
  mild, short-term (baby blues), 22–3, 74
  see also depression
post-viral syndrome, 251
posture
  poor
    and backache, 24–5
    and headache, 116
  unusual, and pins and needles, 170
pot belly, and alcoholism, 6
pre-eclampsia (raised blood pressure in pregnancy), 175–6
pregnancy problems, 174–8
  and abnormal cervical smear, 50
  and AIDS, 4
  and amenorrhoea, 166
  anaemia, in, 9, 10, 174–5
    see also anaemia; constipation; piles; varicose veins
  and ankle-swelling, 12
  and cervical erosion, 52
  and chicken pox, 53
  and constipation, 61
  and dry vagina following, 244
  and finger swelling, 187
  and genital herpes, 107
  and genital warts, 255
  German measles, 107–8
    and cataracts, 49
    and deafness, 71
  and hair loss, 111
  and hiatus hernia, 31
  and indigestion, 134
  miscarriage, 151–2
  morning sickness, 134
  and para-umbilical hernia, 124–5
  pain during, and fibroids, 96
  piles in, 169
  and painful intercourse, 193
  raised blood pressure in 34, 175–6
    see also blood pressure, high
  sickness in, 176–8
    see also hernia, hiatus
  and stretch marks, 213–14
  and thrush, 228
  unwanted, 178–80
    operation, 179–80

and vaginal discharge, 246
and varicose veins, 247
and vitamin deficiency, 252
and vomiting, 253
and wrist pain and tingling fingers, 257
Pregnancy Advisory Service, 180
premature babies
　low vitamin stores and rickets in, 37
　and undescended testicles, 225
　and vitamin deficiency, 252
premature ejaculation, 194–5
premenstrual tension (PMT), 180–1
　see also periods
pre-senile dementia (Alzheimer's disease), 72–4
prolapsed disc (slipped disc), 24, 26
prostate problems, 181–4
　cancer, 47, 181–2
　enlargement, 182–4
　and impotence, 192
　and incontinence, 133
　inflammation, 184
　and NSU, 159
　and painful intercourse, 193
psoriasis, 184–6
　and itching, 140
　and rash, 186
　and unsightly nails, 155
　see also arthritis
psychiatric problems and alcoholism, 6
pubertal mastitis (tender breasts in adolescence), 41
puberty
　and abnormal cervical smear, 50
　and breast development, 41–2
pubic lice (crabs), 65–6
pulse rate
　increased, and asthma, 20
　and heatstroke, 122
　see also heart beat
puncture marks/wounds
　accidental, 68–9
　from drug abuse, 79
pyelonephritis, 242

R

rabies, 32
rages
　and hypomania, 144
　and tantrums, 217
rashes, see skin, rashes
Raynaud's disease, see cold hands and feet
rectal bleeding, 168–9
red cell production, difficulties in, and anaemia, 9–10
redness, see skin, redness on
Reiter's disease and NSU, 159
repeated gestures (tics), 230–1
restlessness
　and hyperactivity, 128–9
　and hypomania, 144
　too much thyroid, 230
rheumatoid arthritis (an inflammatory joint disease), 18–19

and anaemia, 9
ribs, broken, 43
rickets, 37
　and knock knees, 142
　and vitamin D deficiency, 252
ringing in the ear, see tinnitus
ringworm and itching, 139
ring stuck on finger, 187
rubella, see German measles
running fast, difficulty with and flat feet, 97
runny nose, see nose, runny

S

sadness and depression, 74
saliva
　blood in, and cancer, 47
　glandular fever transmitted through, 108
salivation and epilepsy, 89
salmonella food poisoning, 103–4
salmon patch (birthmark, stork mark), 31
salt shortage and heatstroke, 122
Samaritans, 75
sarcomas (tissue cancers), Kaposi's, and AIDS, 3
scabbing
　and bites and stings, 32
　and scabies, 187
scabies, 187–8
　and itching, 139
scalding, 46
　see also burns
scaling, see skin, scaling
scalp
　and cradle cap, 66
　irritation from headlice, 119
　itching, 140
　and psoriasis, 185
　scaly, and fungal infection, 112
　and soft spot, 66
　tension and headache, 116
scarlet fever, 188
　and infection of middle ear, 85
　and rash, 186
　see also convulsions, febrile
scarring, see skin, scarring
schizophrenia, 74, 188–90
Schizophrenia Association of Ireland, 190
school
　learning problems and hyperactivity, 129
　poor attendance/performance in
　　and drug abuse, 79
　　and glue sniffing, 109
　refusal, 190–1
　　and anxiety, 14
　starting and bedwetting, 28
sciatica (nerve pain aka neuralgia), 24, 26
SCODA (Standing Conference on Drug Abuse), 5, 80
Scottish AIDS Monitor, 5
screening
　for breast cancer, 48
　for cervical cancer (smear test), 48, 49–51
　　abnormal, 49–51

seasickness, 237
seborrhoeic eczema, 66
— and itching, 140
secondary hypertension, 34
secretiveness, increased, and drug sniffing, 109
self-examination for breast lumps, 39
self-neglect and drug abuse, 79–80
senile dementia, 72–3
sensitisation to household products and itching, 139
separation from a parent and bedwetting, 28
sexual intercourse
  and AIDS, 4
  anal and NSU, 159
  bleeding after
    and abnormal cervical smear, 49
    and cervical erosion, 52
  and cervical smear tests, 50
  and crabs, 65
  and cystitis, 70–1
  at early age, and cervical cancer, 51
  foreskin pulled back, para-phimosis, 100
  foreskin drawn forward, phimosis, 101
  and genital herpes, 106
  and gonorrhoea, 110
  painful, see under sexual problems
  and PID, 163
  vigorous, causing bruising, and swelling vagina, 245
sexual problems, 191–5
  absence of orgasm, 191
  and alcoholism, 5
  and anorexia nervosa, 12
  and infertility, 135–6
  loss of interest
    and baby blues/post-natal depression, 23
    and depression, 74
  painful intercourse, 193
    and dry vagina, 244
    and fibroids, 96
    and PID, 163
    and thrush, 228
    and vaginal irritation, 246
    see also episiotomy; foreskin problems; genital herpes; NSU; pelvic infection; periods, painful; piles; prostate problems; thrush; vaginal problems
  premature ejaculation, 194–5
  see also impotence
Sexually Transmitted Disease Clinics, 5
sexually transmitted diseases
  acquired immune deficiency syndrome see AIDS
  and cervical cancer, 51
  crabs, 65–6
  gonorrhoea, see gonorrhoea
  jaundice, see jaundice
  non-specific urethritis see NSU
  syphilis, see syphilis
shaking
  and alcoholism, 6
  and anxiety, 14
  and too much thyroid, 230
  and tranquilliser addiction, 236

and tremor, **238–9**
shingles, **195–6**
  and chicken pox, 52, 53
  and depression, 74
  and ear ache, 81
  and vertigo, 249
  and viral illness, 250
shiny tongue, 233
shivery feeling, and flu, 97
shock, **196–7**
  anaphylactic, and allergy 8, 115
  from bites and stings, 32
  reactions
    and anti-allergy injections, 8, 115
    and bereavement, 28
  see also allergy; burns; heart attack
shoes, ill-fitting
  and bunions, 45–6
  and flat fleet, 97
  and in-growing toenails, 138
  and limp, 143
  and nail problems, 155
shoulder pain, **197–8**
  and bursitis, 89
  dislocated, 78–9
  and gallstones, 102
  frozen shoulder, **198–9**
  and neck, stiff and painful, 156–8
  and swollen elbow, 89
  tendonitis, 88, 199
  see also arthritis; dislocation; elbow, pain; gout
sickle cell anaemia, 9
  and gallstones, 102
  and jaundice, 141
silent heart attack, 120
simple (brown) mole (birthmark), 30
sinusitis, **199–200**
  and colds, 54, 55
  and ear ache, 81
  and general swelling of eyelids, 93
  and headache, 116
skin problems and symptoms
  acne, 1–2
  see also hair problems
  and AIDS, 3, 4
  allergies, 8
    and dermatitis, 8
    and eczema, 8
  bites on 32–3
  blemishes, 30–2
  see also birthmarks
  blisters, see blisters
  blue from holding breath, and tantrums, 217
  boils, 35–6
  brown patches
    café au lait spot (birthmark), 30
    simple (brown) mole (birthmark), 30
  bruising
    from broken bones, 42
    from falls, and alcoholism, 6
    and meningitis, 147
    Mongolian blue spots mistaken for, 30
    temporary, and forceps delivery, 30
  burns, 46–7

282

carbuncles, 35
changes in colour and hyperactivity, 129
cold and wet, and shock, 196
cracking, and eczema, 86–7
crusty, and eczema, 86–7
discharge and itching, 139
discoloration
   and dislocation, 78
   and varicose veins, 247
eczema, 86–7
flaking
   and eczema, 86–7
   and itching, 139
flushed
   and raised temperature
   hot, and menopause, 148
grafting, and birthmarks, 31
hives, 127–8
impetigo, 132
infections and diabetes, 76
and in-growing toenails, 137–8
itchy, *see* itching
Kaposi's sarcoma, and AIDS, 3
lipomas, 143–4
loss of elasticity
   and dehydration in infants, 105
   and stretch marks, 213–14
moles, *see* moles
numb, *see* numbness
outside eye, 95
pallor of
   and anaemia, 9
   in pregnancy, 174
   and anorexia nervosa, 12
   and hyperactivity, 129
   and shock, 196
peeling, and sunstroke, 216
pins and needles, **169–70**
psoriasis, **184–6**
purple rash, 186
rashes, **186**
   and allergy, 8
   and chicken pox, 52–3
   and German measles, 107–8
   and glandular fever, 108
   and itching, 139
   and measles, 145–6
   nappy, 155–6
   and scabies, 187
   and scarlet fever, 188
   and viral illness, 251
   see also allergy; hives; itching; scarlet fever
redness on
   bites and stings, 32
   blisters, 33
   boils, 35
   and breast infection, 37, 39
   burns, 46
   chilblains, 53
   cold sores, 56
   eczema, 86–7
   fungal infection, 112
   German measles, 107
   hives, 127–8

impetigo, 132
   and itching, 139
   and measles, 145
   and mouth ulcers, 153
   port wine stain (birthmark), 31
   and psoriasis, 184–5
   and rash, 186
   and scabies, 187
   and scarlet fever, 188
   strawberry naevus (birthmark: *carernous haemangioma*), 31–2
   and stretch marks, 214
   and sunburn, 216
   and thrush, 228
scabs, *see* scabs
scaling
   and athlete's foot, 22
   and cradle cap, 66
   and eczema, 86–7
   and fungal infection, 112
   and psoriasis, 185
scarring
   and acne, 1
   and birthmarks, 30
   and bites and stings, 32
shingles, *see* shingles
sore(s), *see* eczema, 86–7
splinters, **207–8**
stings on, 32–3
stretch marks, **213–14**
sunburn, **216–17**
tingling, *see* tingling
tumours, *see* tumours
warts, *see* warts
weals and rashes, 186
yellow from jaundice, 140–1
skull fracture, **117–18**
   and meningitis, 147
   and soft spot, 206
   see also head injuries
sleep problems, **200–6**
   and baby-blues/post-natal depression, 22
   and bereavement, 29
   early morning waking and hypomania, 144
   insomnia and sleep problems in adults, **200–2**
      and anxiety, 14, 15
      and depression, 74
      and headache, 116
      and tension, 221–2
      and tiredness, and too much thyroid, 230
      see also anxiety; depression
   and menopause, 149
   nightmares, **202–3**
      and anxiety, 14
   night terrors in children, **202**
   oversleeping and drug abuse, 79
   sleepwalking in children, **203–4**
   and tension, 221
   and tranquilliser addiction
   wakefulness in children, **204–6**
      and hyperactivity, 128–9
   see also dreams; nightmares
slipped disc (prolapsed disc), 24, **26**

283

smear test, cervical, 49–51
  abnormal, **49–51**
smell(s)
  difficulty with, and hayfever, 114
  peculiar, and migraine, 150
smoking
  and angina, 11
  and bad breath, 27
  and bronchitis, 44–5
  and cancer
    and blood in saliva, 47
    of lungs, 64
  and cough, 64
  and cramp, 67
  and duodenal ulcer, 240
  and gastritis, 103
  and heart attack, 121
  and hiatus hernia, 125
  and high blood pressure, 34
  and hoarseness, 128
  and indigestion, 134–5
  and irritable colon, 138
  and menopause, 148
  and palpitations, 162
  and pneumonia, 172
  and Raynaud's disease, 56
  and stomach ulcers, 240
  and stroke, 215
sneezing
  and allergy, 8
  and colds, 54
  exacerbating pain, and backache, 24
  and hayfever, 114
  and hernia, 123
  and incontinence 132
  and para-umbilical hernia, 124
  and pneumonia, 172
snoring and adenoids, 2
social problems
  and alcoholism, 5, 6–7
  and hyperactivity, 129
soft spot, **206**
  and cradle cap, 66
  sunken, and dehydration in infants, 105
  tense and bulging, and meningitis, 147
  see also cradle cap
solvent abuse *see* glue-sniffing
sores
  cold, *see* cold sores
  and crabs, 65
  and eczema, 86–7
  and impetigo, 132
  infected, and drug abuse, 80
  and scabies, 187
sore throat, *see* throat, sore
speech
  difficulty, 206–7
    broken, and asthma, 20
    and deafness, 71
    and head injury, 118
    nasal, and adenoids, 2–3
    slurred, and glue sniffing, 109
  loss of, and stroke, 214
  rapid, and mania, 144–5

  vague, and schizophrenia, 188
sperm count low, and infertility, 135
spine
  and backache, 24–6
  broken, 43
  injuries, and incontinence, 133
  and prolapsed disc (slipped disc), 24, 26
  and sciatica, 24, 26
  see also arthritis; neck, stiff and painful
spinning sensation (vertigo), **249–50**
  see also dizziness
spleen, enlarged, and glandular fever, 108
splinter, **207–8**
spots
  from acne, 1–2
  from bites and stings, 32
  café au lait (birthmark), 30
  on chest, tummy and head, and chicken pox, 53
  Mongolian blue (birthmark), 30
  see also birthmarks
sprains, **208–9**
  and swelling, 88
squint, **209–10**
stammer, **206–7**
staphylococcus
  and food poisoning, 104
  and impetigo, 132
  see also boils
sterilisation
  female, **210**
  male (vasectomy), **210–11**
  male or female, **211**
sticky eyes in infants, 93–4
stiffness
  and rheumatoid arthritis, 18
  neck, **156–8**
stings
  and bites, 32–3
  nettle and hives, 127
stitches and cuts, 68
stomach
  -ache
    and chicken pox, 53
    and constipation, 61
    and cough, 64
    and cystitis, 69
    and tension, 221
  cancer of, and indigestion, 134
  cramps
    and gastritis, 103
    and gastroenteritis, 104
    and irritable colon, 138
    and painful periods, 167
  disorders
    and alcoholism, 6
    and anxiety, 14
    appendicitis, 16–17
    and beta blocking drugs, 16
    grumbling appendix, 17
    peritonitis, 16
    and raised temperature, 220
    and sickness in pregnancy, 177–8
  fibroids as painless lumps in, 96

284

pain
  and gallstones, 102
  and gastroitis, 103
  and gastroenteritis, 104
  and indigestion, 134
  and migraine, and young children, 149–50
  and mumps, 154
  and painful periods, 167
  and PID, 163
  and tonsillitis, 234
  and urine infection, 243
pot belly and alcoholism, 6
spots on, and chicken pox, 53
swelling inside, and glandular fever, 108
ulcers, 240–1
  and anaemia, 9, 10
  and gastritis, 103
stork mark (birthmark salmon patch), 31
strawberry naevus (birthmark: *cavernous haemangioma*), 31–2
streptococcus
  and impetigo, 132
  and scarlet fever, 188
stress, 212–13
  and alcoholism, 6
  and amenorrhoea, 166
  and angina, 11
  and anxiety, 15
  and backache, 24
  and cold sores, 56
  and diarrhoea, 77
  and headache, 116
  and hyperventilation, 130
  and impotence, 191–2
  and incontinence, 122
  and indigestion, 134
  and irregular, unexpected periods, 165–6
  and irritable colon, 138
  and manic depression, 45
  and migraine, 150
  and palpitations, 162
  and school refusal, 190
  and tension, 221–2
  and tics, 231
  and tremor, 238
  and wakefulness in children, 204–5
stretching
  and backache, 24
  for cramp, 67
stretch marks, 213–14
stroke, 214–16
  and confusion, 60
  and fainting, 96
  and fits, 90
  and high blood pressure, 34, 90
  and incontinence, 133
  and obesity, 160
  and thrombosis, 226
  see also depression
Stroke Association, 216
student's elbow (inflamed swollen elbow), 89
styes (swellings amongst eyelashes), **94–5**
subarachnoid harmorrhage (internal bleeding)
  and headache, 116

suicide
  and depression, 74–5
  and manic depression, 144–5
sunburn, **216–17**
  see also heatstroke
sunstroke, 122
  see also heatstroke
surgery and impotence, 192
swallowing, difficulty, in
  and anxiety, 14
  and mumps, 154
  and tension, 221
  and tonsillitis, 233–4
sweating
  and AIDS, 3
  and anxiety, 14
  and asthma, 20
  and diabetes, 76
  and flu, 97
  and heart attack, 120
  and heatstroke, 122
  and hyperventilation, 130
  and menopause, 148
  and obesity, 160
  and palpitations, 162
  and pneumonia, 172
  and raised temperature, 220
  and shock, 196
  and too much thyroid, 230
  and urine infection, 243
sweat rash under armpits and itching, 140
swelling
  of ankles, *see* ankles, swelling
  and arthritis, 88
  from bites and stings, 32
  blisters, 33
  and breast infection, 37
    and breast lumps, 39
  and broken bones, 42, 88
  and burns, 47
  from chilblains, 53
  and dislocation, 78–9, 88
  of elbow (olecranon bursa), **88–9**
  amongst eyelashes (styes), **94–5**
  inside eyelid, **95**
  of eyelids, **93**
  of eyes and hayfever, 114, 115
  of face and hives, 127
  of fingers, **187**
  and frozen shoulder, 198
  ganglions, 101
  glandular
    and glandular fever, 108
    and mumps, 153–4
  and itching, 139
  of joints, and rheumatoid arthritis, 18
  and sprain, 88
  of testicles, **22–4**
  of vagina, at entrance, 245
  in wrist pain and tingling fingers, **237–8**
  see also fluid retention
symptoms, lack of immediate, and AIDS, 3

285

syphilis
   and AIDS, 3
   and dementia, 73
systolic blood pressure, 33

T

tampons
   and cystitis, 70
   and vaginal discharge, 246
tantrums, 217–219
taste, difficulty with, and hayfever, 114
tattooing
   and AIDS, 4
   and birthmarks, 31
   and jaundice, 141
TB (tuberculosis)
   and cough, 64
   and meningitis, 147
   and pleurisy, 171
   and pneumonia, 172
   and swollen testicles, 222–3
tearfulness and baby blues/post-natal depression, 22, 23
teeth, problems with
   and comforters, 59
   damaged by stomach acid, and bulimia nervosa, 14
   decay, 27
   extraction and gout, 111
   and headache, 116
   and sinusitis, 200
   see also toothache
teething, 219–20
temperature, high/raised 220–1
   and bronchiolitis, 44
   and colds, 55
   and febrile convulsions, 62, 63
   and flu, 97
   and measles, 145
   taking the temperature, 221
   upset and heatstroke, 122
   and whooping cough, 256
   see also convulsions, febrile
tenderness
   of area around broken bones, 42
   of breasts in adolescence (pubertal mastitis), 41
   of sprain, 208
   and thrombophlebitis, 227
tendonitis, 87–8
tennis elbow, 87–8
tension, 221–2
   and alcoholism, 6
   and anxiety, 14
   and baby blues/post-natal depression, 22
   and backache, 24
   premenstrual (PMT), 180–1
   and tranquilliser addiction, 236
   see also anxiety; headache; indigestion; insomnia; neck problems; piles; stress; tranquilliser addiction
Terence Higgins Trust, 5

termination of pregnancy, 178–80
testes problems, 222–5
   and infertility, 135
   mild pain and mumps, 154
   and NSU, 159
   swollen testicles, 222–4
      and gonorrhoea, 110
      see also mumps
   twisted testicles, 224
   undescended testicles, 224–5
thalassaemia
   and anaemia, 9
   and gallstones, 102
   and jaundice, 141
thigh, dislocated, 78
thirst, excessive, and diabetes, 76
threadworms, 225–6
throat
   and adenoids, 2, 84
   cancer of, and alcoholism, 6
   catarrh and allergy, 8
   dry, and hayfever, 114
   and flu, 97
   operation and glue ear, 84
   sore/infected 233–4
   and acute bronchitis, 44–5
   and allergy, 8
   and chicken pox, 53
   and colds, 54
   and glandular fever, 108–9
   and gonorrhoea, 110
   and infection of middle ear, 85
   and measles, 145
   and mumps, 154
   and psoriasis, 185
   and scarlet fever, 188
   and tonsillitis, 233–4
thrombophlebitis, 227–8
   and varicose veins, 247
thrombosis, 226–7
   and ankle-swelling, 12
   deep-vein thrombosis, 226–7
   and heart attack, 119–21
   and heart failure, 122
thrush, 228–9
   from cracked nipples, 41
   and cystitis, 70
   and infected nails, 154
   and itching, 139
   in mouth, and AIDS, 3, 4
   and nappy rash, 156
   and painful intercourse, 193–4
   and vaginal discharge, 246
   see also nappy rash
thumb(s)
   broken, 43
   sucking, and comforters, 58–9
thyroid problems, 229–31
   and amenorrhoea, 238
   and anxiety, 15
   and confusion, 60
   and dementia, 73
   and irregular periods, 165
   and palpitations, 162

and thinning hair, 113
too little thyroid hormone (hypothyroidism, myxoedema), 229–30
and hoarseness, 128
too much thyroid hormone (Grave's disease, hyperthyroidism, thyrotoxicosis, toxic goitre), 230–1
and tremor, 238
thyrotoxicosis, 230
tics, 231–2
tinea pedis (ringworm causing athlete's foot), 22
tingling
backache, 24, 25
bites and stings, 32–3
in fingers, and too little thyroid, 230
genital herpes, 106
hands, and anaemia, 9
and hyperventilation, 130
and migraine, 150
and neck, stiff and painful, 156
and pins and needles, 170
and stroke, 214
tinnitus, 232–3
and vertigo, 249
tiredness
and anaemia, 9
in pregnancy
and angina, 11
and baby blues/post-natal depression, 23
and cancer, 47
and cold sores, 56
and constipation, 61
and diabetes, 76
and glandular fever, 108
and heart failure, 121
and hysterectomy, 131
and impotence, 192
and menopause, 148
and PMT, 181
and sleeping difficulty, and too much thyroid, 230
and stress, 212
toe(s)
and athlete's foot, 22
big toe joint and gout, 111
and bunions, 45–6
chilblains on, 53–4
cold, 55–6
and beta-blocking drugs, 16
-nails
ingrowing, 137
problems *see* nail problems
pigeon, and bowlegs, 36
see also feet
tongue problems, 233
and epilepsy, 91
'strawberry', and scarlet fever, 188
swelling and hives, 121
ulcers on, *see* mouth ulcers
uncomfortable, 9
tonsillitis, 233–4
and adenoids, 3
and bad breath, 27

and ear ache, 81
and glue air, 84
and infection of middle ear, 85
and scarlet fever, 188
see also adenoids; flu; glandular fever; glue ear
toothache, 234–5
and bad breath, 27
and ear ache, 81
see also teeth, problems with
torticollis (wry neck), 158
toxic goitre, *see* thyroid problems, too much thyroid traction
for backache, 26
for broken legs, 43
tranquilliser addiction, 235–7
see also anxiety; drug(s), addiction; sleep problems
trapped nerve in neck
and cervical spondylosis, 157
and headache, 116
travel sickness, 237
and diarrhoea, 77
and vomiting, 253
trembling and too much thyroid, 230
tremor, 238–9
and anxiety, 16
trichomonal vaginitis, 246
tuberculosis, *see* TB
tumours, 47
brain, *see* brain tumours
and hoarseness, 128
removal of, 48
and swollen testicles, 222–3
see also cancer(s)

U

ulceration
and chilblains, 54
and varicose veins, 247
ulcers, 239–41
and alcoholism, 6
bleeding, and anaemia, 9, 10
duodenal, 239–40
and anaemia, 9, 10
from genital herpes, 106
and indigestion, 134
mouth, *see* mouth ulcers
stomach, *see* stomach ulcers
and vomiting, 253
ultrasound examination/treatment
for backache, 26
for breast lumps, 39
umbilical
hernia 124–5
problems in the newborn, 241–2
unwanted pregnancy, 178–80
urine
alteration of regular pattern, and cancer, 47
dark, and jaundice, 140
infection, 242–4
and confusion, 60

urine *Contd.*
    and cystitis, 71
    and incontinence, 133
    and vomiting, 253
    see also cystitis; foreskin problems; NSU and nappy rash, 155–6
  pass(ing)
    desire to
      and enlargement of prostate, 183
      and migraine, 150
    interference with, and fibroids, 96
    pain, on
      and balanitis, 99
      and genital herpes, 106
      and gonorrhoea, 110
      and NSU, 159
      and phimosis, 100–1
      and swollen testicles, 222
      and threadworms, 225–6
      and urine infection, 243
  passage
    infection of (non-specific urethritis, NSU), 158
    unexplained bleeding from, and cancer, 47
  problems
    cystitis, **69–71**
    and diabetes, 76
    and enlargement of prostate, **182–4**
    and incontinence, **132–3**
    and inflammation of prostate, 184
  tests
    for boils, 36
    for cystitis, 70
    for high blood pressure, 35
  see also bedwetting; bladder problems; incontinence
urticaria (hives, nettlerash) **127–8**
  and itching, 139
  and weals from rash, 186

V

vaccination for flu, **98**
vaginal problems, **244–7**
  discharge, **245–6**
    and fibroids, 96
    and gonorrhoea, 110
    and PID, 163
    and thrush, 228
    see also cervical problems; miscarriage; pelvic infection; periods; thrush
  dry, **244**
    and painful intercourse, 194
    see also sexual problems
  and genital herpes, 106
  irritation, **246–7**
    see also warts, genital
  pain at entrance to vagina, 193
  and painful intercourse, 193
  secretions and cervical erosion, 52
  swelling at entrance, 245
  and threadworm, 226
  and thrush, **228–9**
  see also cervical problems
vaginismus and painful intercourse, 193
varicella zoster (chicken pox virus), 53
varicose eczema, 247
varicose veins, **247–8**
  and anaemia in pregnancy, 174
  and ankle-swelling, 12
  and swollen testicles, 222, 224
  and thrombophlebitis, 226–7
vasectomy (male sterilisation) 210–11
venereal disease, *see* sexually transmitted disease
vertigo **249–50**
  and tinnitus, 232
  see also dizziness
veruccas, **248–9**
  see also corns; warts
viral illness, **250–1**
  post–viral syndrome, 251
  see also AIDS; colds; convulsions, febrile; flu; gastroenteritis; genital herpes; rashes; shingles
vision, temporary loss of, and stroke, 214–15
visual disturbances, **92–6**
  from cataracts, **48–9**
  and diabetes, 76
  and fainting, 96
  and hyperventilation, 130
  and pre-eclampsia, 176
  and stroke, 214
  see also eye problems
vitamin deficiency, **251–3**
  and alcoholism, 6
  of B12, and anaemia, 9
  and confusion, 60
  and dementia, 73
  and flu, 98
  see also anaemia; bowlegs; pregnancy problems; rickets
voice
  deepens, too little thyroid, 230
  hoarse
    and colds, 54
    and croup, 67–8
  husky, and alcoholism, 6
  and speech difficulty, 206–7
vomit(ing), **253–4**
  and appendicitis, 16
  and drug abuse, 80
  and gastritis, 103
  and gastroenteritis, 103–4
    in infants, 104–5
  and headache, 116–17
  and head injury, 118
  and hernia, 123
  and indigestion, 134
  induced
    and anorexia nervosa, 13
    and overeating (bulimia nervosa), 14
  inhalation of
    and drug abuse, 80

and febrile convulsions, 63
and measles, 145
and meningitis, 147
and migraine, 150
and painful period, 167
and pneumonia (of babies), 172
and pre-eclampsia, 176
and scarlet fever, 188
and sickness in pregnancy, 176–7
and stomach ulcers, 240
and tinnitus, 232
and tonsillitis, 234
and travel sickness, 237
and urine infection, 243
and whooping cough, 256
repeated, and alcoholism, 6
and vertigo, 249
see also alcoholism; appendicitis; colds; diarrhoea; drug abuse; gallstones; glue-sniffing; ear problems; gastritis; gastroenteritis; jaundice; head injury; migraine; pelvic infection; pregnancy problems; travel sickness; ulcers; urine infection

vulva
cancer of, 247
itching of, 139
and vaginal irritation, **246–7**

W

warts, 64, **254–5**
genital, **255–6**
and abnormal cervical smear, 50
and cervical cancer, 51
and vaginal irritation, 246
veruccas, **248–9**
wasp stings, 32
weakness
and anaemia, 9
in pregnancy, 174
and backache, 24, 25
and gastroenteritis, 104
and head injury, 118
and heart attack, 120
and heatstroke, 122
and stroke, 214–15
and vertigo, 249
see also tiredness
weight
control and prevention
of arthritis, 18
of backache, 25
of diabetes, 76
of heart attack, 121
of hiatus hernia, 125
of high blood pressure, 35
of obesity, 161–2
of stroke, 215
of varicose veins, 247–8
gain
excessive *see* obesity
and stretch marks, 214
and too little thyroid, 230
loss
and AIDS, 3
and anaemia, 9
in anorexia nervosa, **12–14**
see also bulimia nervosa
and baby blues/post-natal depression, 23
and cancer, 47
and diabetes, 76
and drug abuse, 79
and glue sniffing, 109
and mania, 144
and rheumatoid arthritis, 18
Weight Watchers Enquiries, 162
Wertheim's hysterectomy, 131
wet cough, 64
wheezing
and asthma, 19, 21, 44
and bronchiolitis, 44
and bronchitis, 45
cough, 64
and hayfever, 114
whooping cough, **256–7**
and bronchitis, 45
and cough, 65
and pneumonia, 172
winter depression, 75
womb
abnormal shape, and infertility, 136
fibroids (benign growths), **96–7**
inflamed neck of (cervix), and gonorrhoea, 110
and miscarriage, 151–2
and PID, 163
prolapse of, 130
removal of, *see* hysterectomy
Woman's Health Concern, 149, 181
Women's Health, 51
Women's Nationwide Cancer Control Campaign 51
wounds and cuts, **68–9**
wrist(s)
broken, 43
ganglions on, 101
pain and tingling fingers, **257–8**
and pins and needles, 170
see also shoulder pain
sprain, 208–9
wry neck (torticollis), **158**

Also available from Cedar

Dr. CHARLES SHEPHERD

Living with M.E.

It is estimated that there are over 100,000 people suffering from M.E. in Britain today. M.E. is short for *myalgic encephalomyelitis*, a term which relates to the parts of the body affected: *myalgic*, the muscles; *encephalo*, the brain; and *myelitis*, the nerves. The principal symtoms are intense muscle fatigue and brain malfunction following a flu-like infection.

Until recently, many people suffering from M.E. had great difficulty in finding a diagnosis and a way of dealing effectively with the disease. This guide provides much-needed basic information about M.E. The symptoms are described in detail and there is also information on the viruses thought to be responsible for M.E., what triggers it and who can get it. Additional problems, such as disordered sleep, depression, pain in the joints and difficulties with the eyes, ears and balance are also discussed.

'A well-researched, up-to-date guide written from an orthodox medical viewpoint . . . the one to buy for any sufferer who wants information based on science, not speculation.'
  M.E. Action Campaign Newsletter

Editor: Dr. JAMES BEVAN

Sex and Your Health

The recent spread of AIDS has brought the relationship between sex and health to the forefront of the public debate. It has also given rise to a maze of misinformation about sex and sexual problems.

In this book – the first encyclopedic survey of the subject – nine experts disentangle the medical facts from the myths and explain, simply and authoritatively, the physiology and psychology of sex-related health problems.

- The anatomy and physiology of sex
- Main methods of contraception
- Causes of male and female infertility
- Physical problems that affect sexuality
- Ageing and sexuality
- Sexually transmissible diseases
- The psychology of sex
- Deviation from the sexual norm
- Sexuality in the social context

DALE ALEXANDER

The New Arthritis and Common Sense

Dale Alexander has spent over thirty years studying the science of nutrition as a means of avoiding sickness and disease. During the course of his research he has found convincing evidence that the onset and severity of arthritis can often be directly related to a person's eating habits.

Here he explains his findings on food assimilation, and gives a clearly-presented drug-free method (complete with suggested menus) to reduce the suffering caused by arthritis.

Following the huge success of the first edition of *Arthritis and Common Sense* this new, revised edition expands on Dale Alexander's unique theories on sickness and health.

Over one million copies of *Arthritis and Common Sense* sold worldwide

JANE R. HIRSCHMANN and
CAROL H. MUNTER

Overcoming Overeating

Conquer your obsession with food

- Lose weight naturally
- Enjoy the food you most desire
- Forget your preoccupation with eating and weight
- Discover the freedom of no restraints
- Give up dieting forever

Overcoming Overeating makes this all possible, for the authors have returned eating to its natural place in life, so that food becomes something to be enjoyed rather than feared.

Concentrating on the normal physiological hunger that we all experience, Jane R. Hirschmann and Carol H. Munter help you to break out of the lonely cycle of diet, binge, recrimination and self-loathing. Both practical and reassuring, they offer radical, realistic guidance on how to conquer an obsession and restore the compulsive eater's self-esteem.

'*Overcoming Overeating* will stand out from the crowd of diet books for its caring response to the compulsive eater.'

Susie Orbach, author of *Fat is a Feminist Issue*

GEOFF WATTS

Irritable Bowel Syndrome

Until recently, little was known about IBS, a condition identified by a collection of symptoms which include stomach pain and discomfort, constipation and/or diarrhoea. For some people it is no more than a minor inconvenience – for others it can be painful, and utterly debilitating. Its cause remains largely mysterious, and no one as yet has come up with a comprehensive cure. Now this up-to-date, authoritative and practical handbook covers all aspects of the problem, and discusses at length its symptoms and treatments. The author assesses both orthodox and alternative treatments, and gives invaluable advice about what to do if you are a sufferer.

Dr. ROGER MORGAN

Help for the Bedwetting Child

Bedwetting is one of the commonest problems of childhood – and one which few parents, and even fewer children talk to other people about. It is also a problem for many teenagers and young people. This is an invaluable handbook for both parents and professionals, and is suitable for the older child to read himself. It explains how bedwetting occurs, and why an understanding of it is essential for the success of its management and treatment. It stresses how bladder control problems *can* be overcome by a carefully planned learning technique, adjusted according to a consistent record of progress. The author, Dr Roger Morgan, gained his doctorate in 1973 for work on the treatment of bedwetting. He runs bedwetting treatment clinics, and has written and taught widely on the subject.

A Selected List of Cedar Books

While every effort is made to keep prices low, it is sometimes necessary to increase prices at short notice. Mandarin Paperbacks reserves the right to show new retail prices on covers which may differ from those previously advertised in the text or elsewhere.

The prices shown below were correct at the time of going to press.

☐	7493 0791 9	**New Arthritis and Common Sense: A Complete Guide to Effective Relief**	Dale Alexander £4.99
☐	7493 0046 9	**Sex and Your Health**	James Bevan £4.99
☐	7493 0938 5	**The Courage to Heal**	Ellen Bass and Laura Davis £7.99
☐	7493 0098 1	**Divorced Parenting**	Dr Sol Goldstein £4.50
☐	7493 1033 2	**Carbohydrate Addict's Diet**	Dr Rachael Heller and Dr Richard Heller £4.99
☐	7493 0246 1	**Overcoming Overeating**	Jane Hirschmann & Carol Munter £3.99
☐	7493 0322 0	**Women, Sex and Addiction**	Charlotte Davis Kasl £4.99
☐	7493 1079 0	**Help For the Bed-Wetting Child**	Dr Roger Morgan £4.99
☐	7493 0933 4	**The Amazing Results of Positive Thinking**	Norman Vincent Peale £4.99
☐	7493 0821 4	**The Power of Positive Living**	Norman Vincent Peale £4.99
☐	7493 0715 3	**The Power of Positive Thinking**	Norman Vincent Peale £4.99
☐	7493 1023 5	**The Power of the Plus Factor**	Norman Vincent Peale £4.99
☐	7493 1041 3	**How to Survive in Spite of Your Parents**	Dr Margaret Reinhold £5.99
☐	7493 1018 9	**When Am I Going to be Happy**	Dr Penelope Russianoff £5.99
☐	7493 0733 1	**When You and Your Mother Can't be Friends**	Victoria Secunda £5.99
☐	7493 0724 2	**Living with ME: A Self Help Guide**	Dr Charles Shepherd £4.99

All these books are available at your bookshop or newsagent, or can be ordered direct from the publisher. Just tick the titles you want and fill in the form below.

Mandarin Paperbacks, Cash Sales Department, PO Box 11, Falmouth, Cornwall TR10 9EN.

Please send cheque or postal order, no currency, for purchase price quoted and allow the following for postage and packing:

UK including BFPO   £1.00 for the first book, 50p for the second and 30p for each additional book ordered to a maximum charge of £3.00.

Overseas including Eire   £2 for the first book, £1.00 for the second and 50p for each additional book thereafter.

NAME (Block letters) ....

ADDRESS..

....

☐ I enclose my remittance for ....

☐ I wish to pay by Access/Visa Card Number

Expiry Date